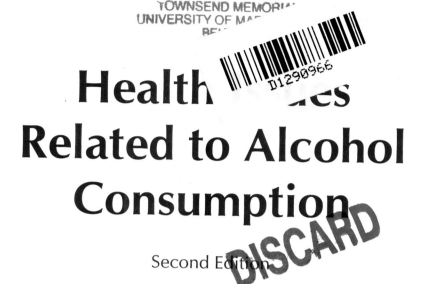

Health Issues Related to Alcohol Consumption

Second Edition

DISCARD

Ian Macdonald

Editor

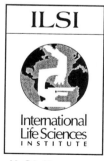

ILSI

International Life Sciences INSTITUTE

ILSI Europe

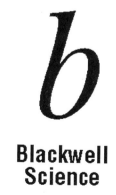

Blackwell Science

Copyright © 1999 International Life Sciences Institute

ILSI
1126 Sixteenth Street, N.W.
Washington, D.C. 20036, USA
Telephone: +1 202 659 0074
Telefax: +1 202 659 8654
E-mail: ilsi@ilsi.org
Home Page: http://www.ilsi.org

ILSI Europe
83 Avenue E. Mounier, Box 6
B-1200, Brussels, Belgium
Telephone: +32 2 771 00 14
Telefax: +32 2 762 00 44
E-mail: publications@ilsieurope.be

First edition published in 1993
Second edition published by Blackwell Science Ltd in 1999

Blackwell Science Ltd
Editorial Offices:
Osney Mead, Oxford OX2 0EL
25 John Street, London WC1N 2BL
23 Ainslie Place, Edinburgh EH3 6AJ
350 Main Street, Malden MA 02148 5018, USA
54 University Street, Carlton, Victoria 3053, Australia
10 Rue Casimir Delavigne, 75006 Paris, France

Printed and bound in Great Britain by
MPG Books Limited, Bodmin, Cornwall

ISBN 1-57881-064-7 (printed paper case)
ISBN 1-57881-062-0 (paperback)

Contents

Authors

Prof. E. Abel
C.S. Mott Center
Growth and Development
275 East Hancock Avenue
Detroit, Michigan 48201, USA

Prof. H. Begleiter
State University of New York
Health Science Center at Brooklyn
Department of Psychiatry
450 Clarkson Avenue, Box 1203
Brooklyn, New York 11203, USA

Prof. F. Cavallo
University of Torino
Department of Public Health and
Microbiology
Via Santena, 5 bis
I-10126 Torino, Italy

Dr. P. Charles
Aarhus Amtssygehus
Department of Endocrinology and
Metabolism
Tage Hansenesgade 2
DK-8000 Aarhus C, Denmark

Prof. P. Couzigou
Hôpital Haut-Lévêque
Hepato Gastro Enterology Department
Avenue de Magellan
F-33604 Pessac, France

Dr. J. de Vries
Wageningen Agricultural University
Department of Human Nutrition and
Epidemiology
P.O.Box 8129
NL-6700 EV Wageningen,
The Netherlands

Sir R. Doll
University of Oxford
Clinical Trial Service & ICRF
Cancer Studies Unit
Radcliffe Infirmary
Oxford OX2 6HE, United Kingdom

Dr. D. Forman
University of Oxford
ICRF Cancer Epidemiology Unit
Gibson Laboratory
Radcliffe Infirmary
Oxford OX2 6UE, United Kingdom

Dr. K. Grant
Wake Forest University
Bowman Gray School of Medicine
Dept. of Physiology and Pharmacology
Medical Center Boulevard
Winston-Salem, North Carolina
27157-1083, USA

Prof. D. Grobbee
University of Utrecht
Julius Center of Patient Oriented Research
P.O. Box 85500
NL-3508 GA Utrecht, The Netherlands

Dr. C. Guerri
Instituto de Investigaciones Citologicas
Fundacion Valenciana de Investigaciones
Biomedicas
Amadeo de Saboya, 4
E-46010 Valencia, Spain

Dr. P. Hoffman
Univeristy of Colorado - School of
Medicine
Department of Pharmacology
Health Sciences Center
4200 East Ninth Avenue
Box C236
Denver, Colorado 80262, USA

Prof. E. Jéquier
Université de Lausanne
Faculté de Médecine
Institut de Physiologie
7, Rue du Bugnon
CH-1005 Lausanne, Switzerland

Dr. H. Kalant
University of Toronto
Department of Pharmacology
MSB 4326
Toronto, Ontario M5S 1A8, Canada

Dr. A. Kardinaal
TNO - Nutrition and Food Research
Institute
Utrechtseweg 48
P.O. Box 360
NL-3700 AJ Zeist, The Netherlands

Prof. U. Keil
University of Münster
Institute of Epidemiology & Social
Medicine
Domagkstrasse 3
D-48129 Münster, Germany

Dr. K. Kiianmaa
National Public Health Institute
Alcohol Research Center
P.O. Box 719
SF-00101 Helsinki, Finland

Prof. F. Kok
Wageningen Agricultural University
Division of Human Nutrition &
Epidemiology
Biotechnion
Bomenweg, 2
NL-6703 HD Wageningen,
The Netherlands

Dr. K. Laitinen
Näkinkaari 8 D 8
SF-02320 Espoo, Finland

Dr. C. La Vecchia
Istituto di Ricerche Farmacologiche
"Mario Negri"
Via Eritrea, 62
I-20157 Milan, Italy

Dr. P. Lemmens
Maastricht University
Department of Medical Sociology
Peter Debeyeplein 1
NL-6229 HA Maastricht, The Netherlands

Prof. H. Little
Durham University
Department of Psychology
South Road
Durham DH1 3LE, United Kingdom

Prof. I. Macdonald
University of London
Hillside
Fountain Drive
London SE19 1UP, United Kingdom

Prof. K. McPherson
University of London
School of Hygiene and Tropical Medicine
Department of Public Health & Policy
Health Promotion Sciences Unit
Keppel Street
London WC1E 7HT, United Kingdom

Dr. P. Pietinen
National Public Health Institute
Department of Nutrition
Mannerheiminitie, 166
SF-00 300 Helsinki, Finland

Dr. M. Plant
Alcohol and Health Research Group
City Hospital
Greenbank Road
Edinburgh EH 10 5SB, United Kingdom

Dr. K. Poikolainen
Järvenpää Addiction Hospital
SF-04480 Haarajoki, Finland

Dr. A. Prentice
MRC International Nutrition Group
Public Health Nutrition Unit
London School of Hygiene and Tropical
Medicine
49-51 Bedford Square
London WC1B 3DP, United Kindgom

Prof. S. Renaud
INSERM - Unité 330
Université de Bordeaux II
F- 33076 Bordeaux cedex, France

Dr. E. Rimm
Harvard School of Public Health
Department of Epidemiology and
Nutrition
665 Huntington Avenue
Boston, Massachusetts 22115, USA

Prof. J. Rodés
Hospital Clinico i Provincial de Barcelona
Servicio de Hepatologia
Villarroel 170
E-08036 Barcelona, Spain

Dr. E. Rubin
Jefferson Medical College
Department of Pathology, Anatomy and
Cell Biology
111 South 11th Street
Philadelphia, Pennsylvania 19107, USA

Prof. M. Salaspuro
University of Helsinki
Research Unit of Alcohol Diseases
Tukholmankatu 8F
SF-00290 Helsinki, Finland

Prof. T. Sorensen
Copenhagen Health Services
Institute of Preventive Medicine
Kommunehosptalet
DK-1399 Copenhagen, Denmark

Dr. B. Tabakoff
University of Colorado
Department of Pharmacology
Health Sciences Center
4200 East Ninth Avenue
Campus Box C236
Denver, Colorado 80262, USA

Prof. K. Westerterp
Maastricht University
Department of Human Biology
P.O. Box 616
NL-6200 MD Maastricht, The Netherlands

Dr. R. Woutersen
TNO - Toxicology & Nutrition Institute
Department of Biological Toxicology
Utrechtseweg 48
P.O. Box 360
NL-3700 AJ Zeist, The Netherlands

Foreword

This publication results from a project organised by ILSI Europe which is a branch of the International Life Sciences Institute (ILSI). ILSI is a non-profit, world-wide foundation established in 1978 to advance the understanding of scientific issues relating to nutrition, food safety, toxicology and environmental safety. ILSI's standards, the quality of the research it supports and the world-wide as well as regional meetings and symposia it sponsors are recognised by the scientific community throughout the world. Additionally, ILSI is affiliated with the World Health Organisation as a non-governmental organisation of international significance and has specialised consultative status with the Food and Agriculture Organisation of the United Nations. ILSI Europe receives its funding from member company dues, governmental projects and publication sales.

Although alcohol has been one of the most studied and researched substances consumed by man, there are few sources one can consult for an objective review of the current state of scientific knowledge in this very broad area.

In 1993, the first edition of "Health Issues Related to Alcohol Consumption" was published which resulted from an international scientific project conducted by the International Life Sciences Institute-ILSI Europe, Brussels. The present book is an updated and extended edition appearing under the same title.

Most of the chapters from the first book have been revised by the medical expert panels in the light of the most recent scientific publications. The reviews on cancer of the intestinal tract and on liver disease were judged by the respective panels not to require modification. For the sake of completeness these are reprinted here in their original version. The former reviews on the subject of hypertension, stroke and coronary heart disease have been drawn together into one, covering the cardiovascular system.

Two additional alcohol-related health issues have been reviewed. The complex field of alcohol and the central nervous system was studied by an international expert panel. The possible effects of alcohol intake on bone metabolism is the subject of a second new chapter.

In the course of the project most panels discussed the question of the reliable measurement of alcohol intake in epidemiological studies. A special expert panel has addressed the issue in this book. Finally, the question regarding what should be understood by "moderate" alcohol consumption is elaborated separately.

ILSI Europe gratefully acknowledges the invaluable contributions made by all medical experts within a tight time schedule. All reports have been peer reviewed by scientific experts. ILSI Europe is confident that this second edition will find a broad readership among those who are interested in a balanced review of the relationship between the consumption of alcoholic beverages and human health.

Peter de Vogel
Former Chairman of the ILSI Europe Alcohol Task Force

Executive Summary

Overview of the Health Issues Related to Alcohol Consumption

I. Macdonald
University of London, United Kingdom

Introduction

The role of beverages containing alcohol has been a prominent feature of life in many societies. For as long as alcohol has been consumed, and that is millennia, the relationships between drinking and various aspects of health have been explored.

Under the auspices of the International Life Sciences Institute-ILSI Europe, leading scientists were invited in 1992 to review critically and objectively the state of information available on the relationship between alcohol consumption and nine important health issues: hypertension, stroke, coronary heart disease, digestive tract cancers, liver disease, breast cancer, pregnancy, overweight, and genetics. This group of scientists included epidemiologists, clinicians, toxicologists, and other biomedical researchers. The task assigned was to appraise what we know and, equally important, what we do not know about alcohol and especially moderate consumption, as it pertains to a wide range of biomedical considerations. The result was the publication of the book "Health issues related to alcohol consumption" ILSI Press 1993.

Recently it was determined to update the project with this new edition, which includes additional new topics and combines some of the topics from the original book. Again, nine panels were formed, each with its own chairman. Each panel was asked to address the relationship between alcohol consumption and one of the following areas: moderate drinking, assessment of intake, genetics, body weight, the cardiovascular system, pregnancy, breast cancer, bone, and the central nervous system. All panels were asked the following:

(1) To list possible associations between specific biomedical conditions and the consumption of alcohol.

(2) For each possible association or hypothesis, to assess the progress reached in achieving a scientific consensus, including whether a consensus exists, the specific content of the consensus, and the body of research that allows the consensus to form. The panels were also asked to address whether the consensus reached far enough to cover a relationship between biomedical consequences and a particular dose or range of dosage, and whether the intakes are consistent across the population.

(3) To identify issues where a scientific consensus does not exist and, in such cases, to identify the gaps in knowledge or contradictory

results that preclude such a consensus, and to specify research tasks necessary for shifting each possibility to a thorough consensus, confirmation, or dismissal.

(4) To determine whether there are cases:
 - where a hypothesis is supported by epidemiological findings that demonstrate a relationship between alcohol consumption and a biomedical effect, but where a causal relationship cannot be confirmed because of the absence of clinical, laboratory or animal research defining a mechanism;
 - where the findings are too dependent on a particular piece of research to permit consensus; or
 - where it is recommended that increased attention be paid to contrary evidence.

Also included as appendices to this book are two chapters from the first edition, Alcohol and Liver Diseases and Cancers of the Digestive Tract and Larynx. The panel chairmen considered that so few new findings have been reported since the 1993 edition that an update on these subjects was not necessary.

This overview is intended to summarise the reports of the nine panels plus the appendices; readers interested in the details can refer to the full chapter.

The reader will note that different panels have used differing measurements of the amounts of alcohol consumed by subjects in medical research. This reflects differences in the measurements employed in the studies themselves. A number of the panel reports measure consumption in grams of pure ethanol consumed. In most countries, a standard serving of beer, wine, or spirits varies between 8 to 12 g of ethanol.

Moreover, several of the panels have noted serious methodological problems in the consumption measurements employed in the currently available studies reviewed by the panels, especially those of the non-experimental observational studies. Measurement of alcohol intake in the studies is usually based on self-reporting by the subjects of the study, and this can result in recall errors. Specifically, people in general, and heavy drinkers in particular, often underreport their intake. In other words, subjects may not recall (or wish to admit) precisely how many grams or millilitres they drank per day or what proportion of a mixed drink consumed consisted of alcohol. Because of this underreporting, the threshold amounts of alcohol consumption associated with certain health risks may in fact be higher than those indicated in the existing studies. Alternatively, persons reporting as teetotallers may have been former heavy drinkers, and indeed self-styled abstainers have been found to have alcohol in their urine. Here again, such misclassification may cast doubt on the precise consumption figures shown in the research literature.

Additional methodological problems include a number of "confounding factors", such as age, sex, body mass index, diet, physical activity, smoking, coffee consumption, educational attainment, Type A/B behaviour, socioeconomic status and medical history, that may be factors in particular health problems in persons who have been the subjects of the reported studies. For example, a generally poor nutritional condition could possibly play a significant role in various health problems associated with heavy drinking. In most of the investigations, adjustments could be made for many of these confounding factors, but for some this was not possible because the relevant information was not available or assessment was too difficult.

It is worth noting that the ILSI Europe panels did not address every aspect of alcohol and health or every system of the human body. The panels were charged with considering or updating nine specific issues, with an emphasis on the health effects of moderate consumption. Some topics involving the neuropathological consequences of alcohol use, such as the psychiatric effects of alcohol abuse and injuries from drinking and driving, have not been addressed by the panels.

Moderate Drinking: Concepts, Definitions and Public Health Significance

The term "moderate", when referring to the amount of alcohol ingested, can be used in at least five senses. The oldest sense is "non-intoxicating" but it is also used as "statistically normal", "non-injurious", "problem-free" and "optimal". However, regardless of definition it is difficult to specify moderate intake quantitatively because intakes are still frequently expressed in "units" or "drinks" and there is no uniform international definition of a standard drink.

The idea of "optimal" level of alcohol intake is based on the demonstration that overall mortality in a population, or mortality or morbidity due to certain specific causes, is lower among those who drink lightly than those who drink more heavily or who do not drink at all. For those diseases which do not show such a "J-shaped" or "U-shaped" relation between degree of risk and level of alcohol intake, it is not possible to talk of an optimal level.

In a review of 28 scientific papers the lower limit of moderate intake ranged from 4.5 to 50 g/day and the upper limit range was 24–80 g/day. Contributing to this wide scatter is the variability arising from the relatively low level of accuracy in estimating alcohol intake.

It is not possible to give any exact advice on moderate drinking. Estimates based on epidemiological studies (because they are under-evaluations, a notable safety margin is included) suggest that for an average adult man the optimal level is about 10–19 g/day and the non-injurious level is about 30–40 g/day. For an average woman the respective levels are <10 g/day and about 10–20 g/day. These estimates of the optimal and non-injurious levels of alcohol intake are valid only for the average adult. Variation in body size and composition has a marked influence on the blood alcohol concentrations produced by the same amount of alcohol and must be taken into account. Differences in individual drinking patterns also introduce additional variation in the degree of health risk associated with any given daily intake of alcohol.

The wise drinker will bear in mind the words of Aristotle "The temperate man keeps a middle course in these matters … such pleasures as conduce to health and fitness he will try to obtain in a moderate and right degree; as also other pleasures so far as they are not detrimental to health and fitness, and not ignoble, nor beyond his means."

Assessment of Alcohol Consumption

It is well known that assessment of dietary intake is prone to errors. However, assessment of alcohol intake poses a larger problem because, for example, alcohol is not considered as a normal food substance, it has a highly symbolic value and drinking is influenced by cultural differences and social norms.

Methods used to assess alcohol consumption may be divided into those that use official data such as sales statistics, and those in which the individual is aware of the investigation, such as self-reporting. An important disadvantage of sales statistics is that they do not provide information about the manner and amount of alcohol consumption of specific groups or individuals.

Self-reporting includes face-to-face interviews, telephone interviews and self-administered questionnaires. The major types of self-reporting ask for a summary of drinking, for example, the quantity-frequency method and lifetime drinking history, or for current drinking, for example, diaries and recalls. In general, data collected from self-reports are sufficiently reliable for ranking subjects according to intake and can be used for associations in epidemiological studies but are unreliable for assessing actual individual intakes. Common errors in assessing alcohol intake in surveys include selection bias, non-response, under- or overestimation of portion size and recall bias.

Biological markers can be an important for assessing objective intake but currently their sensitivity and specificity are relatively low.

It is not easy to state which method is the closest to real intake because a gold standard is lacking, but the quantity/frequency method and the prospective diary are probably the closest to real intake, provided they cover the different types of alcoholic beverage and deal with the problem of standard units.

Alcohol and Genetics

It has long been observed that alcoholism runs in families and more recently epidemiological and experimental studies have provided substantial evidence for the role of heredity in alcoholism and also in disease in organs resulting from alcohol. It is now widely accepted that the genetic predisposition to develop alcoholism is, unlike, for example, cystic fibrosis, dependent on the interaction of these genetic factors with environmentally determined precipitating factors. Alcoholism is thus a complex disorder.

Studies on ethanol intake in animals and the development of animal models are made possible by the fact that a variety of animals voluntarily consume ethanol. Breeding experiments with animals differing in their preference to consume alcohol voluntarily and new statistical methods (including a technique called Quantitative Trait Loci) has greatly extended the understanding and identification of the genes involved. The development of genetic engineering techniques has also allowed progress to be made in identifying specific genes in alcoholism. At present the risk and the protective genes influencing ethanol-related traits in animals have not been specifically extrapolated to humans.

In man, a very large collaborative study (Collaborative Study on the Genetics of Alcoholism) has been implemented whose purpose is to identify genes which predispose to the development of alcoholism.

Candidates considered for genetic involvement in alcoholism that have been studied include the dopamine receptor in the brain, monoamine oxidase activity in blood platelets, lymphocyte and platelet adenylate cyclase activity, serotonin transporter and receptor mechanisms, as well as alcohol and acetaldehyde metabolism.

Turning to end organ effects of alcoholism, the fact that only 20-30% of chronic alcoholics develop liver cirrhosis, has led to a search for the genotypes of this and other alcohol-related organ injuries. So far studies have produced no convincing results.

The ability to genetically predict a person's reaction to alcohol and the use of molecular biology in therapy are important goals yet to be achieved.

Alcohol and Body Weight

Nation-wide studies indicate that 10–30 g of alcohol daily is the average per capita consumption which is 3–9% of daily energy intake in the Western diet. However, there is no consensus on the relationship between moderate drinking and body weight and epidemiological studies are almost equally divided between those which show a positive correlation, those which show a negative correlation and those which show no correlation.

In recent years there have been several studies that have looked at the possible reasons for this discrepancy in epidemiological findings on the relationship between alcohol and body weight. One possibility is that alcohol has influence on the amount of food eaten and, despite the errors arising from dietary studies in free-living people, in 11 out of 12 studies alcohol use was associated with a raised total energy intake in both men and women. For social drinkers the mean increment in energy intake would be close to 10% but for heavy drinkers it can reach over 30%. In most of these studies the non-alcohol food energy remained constant irrespective of drinking level.

Studies carried out in the laboratory on the "aperitif" effect of alcohol, which is supposed to increase appetite, have been few and inconclusive with either showing an increase in food intake or changes in the subjective feelings of hunger or fullness or, in one study, showing no effects. In free-living people drinkers tend to consume more energy than non-drinkers and among the drinkers energy intake is higher on days when alcohol is drunk. This, however, may be due to the fact that alcohol consumption often occurs at special meals and in company.

Does alcohol affect the body's expenditure of energy? The gross energy of alcohol is 7.1 kcal/g or 29.7 kJ/g and after consumption very little is lost in breath, urine or sweat, it cannot be stored and it is principally metabolised in the liver. This metabolic handling of alcohol has a cost in terms of energy and several studies have reported figures of around 17% for the energy of the ingested alcohol used in its metabolism to carbon dioxide and water. So a large increase in heat dissipation after ethanol intake is not an explanation for the apparent lack of weight gain when excess energy as alcohol is consumed. The general conclusion is that no mysterious loss of energy results from moderate alcohol intake in healthy subjects.

Laboratory studies on energy and nutrient balances show that ethanol is a nutrient that the body utilises with an efficiency close to that of carbohydrates and that alcohol calories do count. Thus, all these studies do not explain the epidemiological evidence of no clear correlation between alcohol use and body weight. Controlled metabolic experiments show that habitual alcohol use in excess of energy needs favours lipid storage. Thus, ethanol acts as a preferred fuel.

Possible explanations for this discrepancy include the possibility that alcohol could be associated with or induce a higher level of physical activity. Also there are suggestions that the increase in heat production after alcohol ingestion could be higher in thin individuals than in fat subjects because thin persons lose heat easier. Furthermore, subjects who are overweight systematically underscore energy intake more than lean subjects. Thus, the expected positive relation between alcohol intake and body weight could be due to under-reporting in subjects who are overweight. Also, a negative correlation between alcohol use and body weight, as often observed in women, could be due to a high degree of under-reporting in this sex.

The mechanism(s) behind the relation between alcohol consumption and the maintenance of energy balance is for future research.

Alcohol and the Cardiovascular System

There is abundant epidemiological and clinical evidence to show that light to moderate drinking is associated with a reduced risk of coronary heart disease, total and ischaemic stroke and total mortality in middle-age and elderly men and women. There is little basis to expect one particular beverage to be more effective in reducing risk than another and the effect appears to be due to alcohol itself, though the discussion continues.

The evidence suggests that there is a U-shaped relation between alcohol and coronary heart disease and the threshold at which the right side of the U begins to increase could be as few as 2 or as many as 6 drinks/day. Though vascular disease takes a long time to develop it is not known how long alcohol needs to be consumed, in light to moderate quantities, in order to have an effect on reducing the manifestations of vascular disease.

There is considerable evidence to support the suggestion that moderate drinking reduces the risk for coronary heart disease both by inhibiting the formation of atheroma and decreasing the rate of blood coagulation.

Observational and interventional studies provide strong support for the view that alcohol use is an important lifestyle factor in raising the blood pressure and that a causal association exists between the use of 30–60g/day and blood pressure elevation in men and women.

The two subtypes of stroke are (1) where there is a blockage (ischaemia) of a cerebral artery (75–85% of all strokes) and (2) cerebral haemorrhage. Light and moderate habitual drinkers have a slightly lower risk of ischaemic stroke, whereas heavy drinking, both regular and short-term, is an independent risk factor for haemorrhagic stroke. Binge drinking is associated with an increased risk of both ischaemic and haemorrhagic stroke.

Alcohol use in moderation appears to promote cardiovascular health and guidelines adopted in the USA and UK suggest that individuals may achieve some benefit if daily consumption is limited to 2–3 drinks.

Alcohol and Pregnancy

Considerable advances in the understanding of the foetal alcohol syndrome (FAS) and related abnormalities resulting from prenatal alcohol exposure have been made since 1993. As it is over 35 years since the first scientific reports were published, it is possible to study potential prenatal alcohol-related harm in older children and adults. In 1996, a new diagnostic paradigm was developed in which maternal alcohol exposure was more clearly stated to be part of the diagnosis (although certain features of FAS can occur without a history of maternal alcohol use).

Changes have also been made in the diagnosis of foetal alcohol effects (FAE). As there is no single anomaly of the foetus specific to, or consistently associated with, lower levels of maternal alcohol use during pregnancy, there may be a tendency to over-diagnose FAE.

The level and, in particular, the pattern of maternal drinking has received further attention but no consistent picture of alcohol-related foetal harm has emerged in relation to lower levels of maternal drinking. However, there are critical periods during gestation, for example early pregnancy, when heavy maternal drinking is particularly risky.

There is no consistent evidence for a clear-cut relationship between the adverse effects in pregnancy on the foetus or on the child and lower levels of maternal alcohol use. Information is insufficient to state where exactly this threshold lies but it may be around 30–40 g/day, a level well above that defined as moderate drinking for non-pregnant women. On the other hand, no level of maternal drinking can be established that is absolutely safe for the foetus.

FAS is related to a variety of adverse influences other than heavy maternal drinking. These include the mother's socioeconomic status, her nutritional status, the extent of prenatal care, lifestyle, age, smoking and drug use, as well as her genetic make-up. The general health of alcohol-dependent women is often poor with immune deficiency and liver damage increasing the risk of poor outcome to the pregnancy.

Follow-up studies of children born to mothers drinking "light to moderate" amounts during pregnancy tend to show no lasting impairment. Some studies have found behavioural or school problems in these groups. Even so, it is difficult to show that this is necessarily attributable to maternal drinking during pregnancy rather than to environmental or other factors.

Experimental data have shown that ethanol can interfere with all stages of brain development and that the effects are dose-dependent. The effects are also dependent on the time in pregnancy the drinking occurs; for example, exposure to high levels during the early formation of the embryo produces significant changes. Binge drinking and heavier drinking during the foetal "brain growth spurt" in the last three months of pregnancy may induce functional deficits in specific areas of the brain.

Animal models have provided evidence that foetal alcohol effects are dose-dependent and have clearly demonstrated that the peak maternal blood alcohol concentration and the pattern of drinking (e.g. bingeing) are the most important determinants of the magnitude of alcohol-related birth defects. Different aspects of development may be sensitive to different levels of alcohol.

The search for the underlying mechanisms of foetal alcohol damage goes on. Possible factors include acetaldehyde toxicity, placenta dysfunction, impaired foetal nutrition, foetal hypoxia, abnormal prostaglandin metabolism and free radical formation.

Alcohol and Breast Cancer

Some 70 studies for a causative association between alcohol and the risk of breast cancer are reviewed and the accumulated evidence suggests the possibility of a weak association between alcohol use and breast cancer. The most likely causative relationship exists for large amounts of consumption. Since the evidence for an association between alcohol intake and breast cancer is all non-experimental and since the cause of this tumour remains largely unexplained, the interpretation of the evidence is necessarily problematic.

Considering first the epidemiological evidence, the findings are of limited value because of the many possible confounding variables that cannot be or were not adequately measured. These include the exact measurement and timing of the alcohol intake, the accuracy of the recall of the intake of alcohol some 20–30 years ago, the type of drink (wine, beer, spirits), psychological stress, the use of oral contraceptives, socioeconomic status, tobacco use and body mass as well as many important dietary factors.

The combination of several individual epidemiological studies (meta-analysis) shows a considerable variation between some of them, in the estimated relative risks of alcohol consumption and breast cancer. Most of these estimates are not significant and are not consistent at any drinking level.

Some investigators have reported that the risk of breast cancer is associated with a specific type of drink, such as wine or beer, whereas others did not find such a specific association.

Concerning the quantity of alcohol consumed, it is probably not possible for anyone to provide exact quantitative data and in addition there is much under-reporting, so it is not possible to demonstrate a strong and consistent relationship, based on epidemiological evidence, between the risk of breast cancer and a particular dose of alcohol.

In spite of intensive investigation, evidence for a casual relationship between moderate or "social" drinking among women and breast cancer is lacking. Even a causal link at higher levels of consumption is most likely to be seriously compromised by unknown confounders. Any recommendations that women should limit their alcohol use to reduce the risk of breast cancer can only be supported in terms of reduction from excessive drinking.

Alcohol and Bone

The incidence of osteoporosis, leading to hip fracture, has increased in most industrial countries in recent years. It is a disease with a significant morbidity, mortality and economic impact. Many factors connected with lifestyle and nutrition have been held responsible, among them alcohol.

The effects of alcohol on bone differ depending on the dose and duration of its use. Different effects are observed as a result of moderate consumption, of acute heavy drinking and of alcohol abuse.

Acute alcohol intoxication enhances urinary excretion of calcium with a drop in the blood calcium level. Both blood magnesium and its urinary excretion are increased after alcohol ingestion, and these alcohol-induced changes in mineral metabolism are dose-dependent. Bone formation is depressed.

With the exception of a few studies, the overall conclusion is that moderate drinking is not likely to have adverse effects on bone density. In some studies a positive association has been observed between moderate alcohol use and risk of hip and forearm fracture, and there is some indication that age may play a role, particularly in women. Moderate drinking does not change serum calcium, magnesium, phosphate or their urinary excretion. The levels of vitamin D and the absorption of calcium remain unchanged.

Although the evidence suggests that chronic alcohol abuse adversely affects bone mineral density, it may well be that clinical effects only become apparent after a long period of abuse. Nevertheless, chronic alcohol abuse seems to be associated with an increased risk of fractures. Chronic alcohol abuse brings about profound changes in mineral metabolism such as low serum calcium and phosphate levels and magnesium deficiency. These lead to deranged bone quality and may adversely affect bone quality. There is evidence that the physiological response of the parathyroid glands to produce parathyroid hormone is impaired by alcohol.

In summary, acute alcohol intoxication has a short-term effect on bone metabolism, moderate drinking does not derange mineral metabolism and abuse easily leads to fracture.

Alcohol and the Central Nervous System

The effects of alcohol on the central nervous system include a reduction in anxiety, feelings of pleasure, sedation, muscular incoordination, aggression, alterations in cognition as well as changes in social interaction. Beverage alcohol has a relatively simple structure, and in order to see physiological and behavioural effects, considerably higher blood alcohol concentrations (BACs) are required as compared to other psychoactive drugs. These comparative differences in chemical structure and dose indicate that alcohol's mode of action in the brain is inherently different from that of psychoactive compounds. Specific receptors in the brain are utilised by psychoactive drugs to initiate actions but no such receptors have been identified for alcohol. The mode of action of alcohol seems to be that of a modulator of certain neurotransmitter systems in the brain.

Individuals differ extensively in their responses to alcohol and these differences in response are affected by genetic factors, the environment and by previous experience. The character, intensity and duration of alcohol's actions are also affected by its rate of absorption, its distribution in the body and the rate of its metabolism so that, for example, the question "what dose of alcohol impairs motor performance?" will not be a single number but a range of values and will, furthermore, also be determined by the complexity of the task.

Alcohol increases social interaction and conversation whereas the same dose decreases performance of a non-verbal task. The reinforcing effects of alcohol, such as an increase in speech, are restricted to the rising limb of the BAC curve. Certain individuals find even low doses of alcohol aversive and a significant proportion of the population choose not to drink even when alcohol is freely available. The aversive and rewarding properties of alcohol are probably mediated by different neural mechanisms, and it is the balance between these two properties that affects alcohol intake.

Turning to the biochemical and electrophysiological effects in the brain of alcohol, at the cellular level, signalling by the major excitatory and inhibitory systems of the brain seem to be the target of alcohol's action, and within these systems there is differential sensitivity. Alcohol also alters the release of transmitter substances in particular areas of the brain. These transmitter substances may have a direct effect on the excitability of neurons (ionotrophic effect) or may stimulate the production of molecules known as "second messengers", which then trigger a cascade of reactions within neurones (metabotropic effect). Some of these neural systems affected by alcohol, adapt during periods of chronic alcohol ingestion and this may generate tolerance, physical dependence and craving.

There is clearly much to be learned about the effects of alcohol on the central nervous system, both in the context of "social" drinking and in the generation of physical dependence.

Alcoholic Beverages and Cancers of the Digestive Tract and Larynx

Ethanol is not a carcinogen by standard laboratory tests. Animal experiments suggest, however, that, given by mouth, it may act as a co-carcinogen in the production of cancers in the oesophagus and possibly also in the non-glandular (fore)stomach, but not in the glandular stomach or pancreas. The evidence relating to the production of colorectal cancer is conflicting, and no conclusion can be drawn from it.

Epidemiological evidence shows that the consumption of alcoholic beverages increases the risk of developing cancers of the mouth (other than the salivary glands), pharynx (other than the nasopharynx), and larynx; that the risks are principally due to the presence of ethanol and increase with the amount consumed; that the risks are increased by increased smoking, each agent approximately multiplying the effect of the other; and that, in the absence of smoking, the risks in developed countries are small unless consumption is exceptionally heavy. The risks may be diminished by a diet rich in fruit and green vegetables, but the evidence is inconclusive. Whether the co-carcinogenic effects of different alcoholic beverages depend solely on the presence of ethanol and are unaffected by its concentration or by the presence of congeners (other constituents in alcoholic beverages) is uncertain.

The epidemiological evidence also suggests that there may be some direct relationship between the consumption of alcohol and colorectal cancer. The apparent relationship is quantitatively moderate, and even with heavy consumption a doubling of the relative risk can be excluded. No apparent difference exists between the susceptibility of men and women or of the two sites (colon and rectum), or between the effect of different types of alcoholic beverage. The nature of the observed relationship remains in doubt: it may be causal, it may be due to confounding between the consumption of alcoholic beverages and some other dietary factor that increases the risk of the disease, and it may be due, at least in part, to the selective publication of positive results. Research aimed at discovering whether the association can be explained by confounding with dietary habits should be encouraged.

The balance of the evidence suggests that alcoholic beverages do not cause cancers of the stomach or pancreas, but it does not rule out the possibility altogether. Alcohol may contribute specifically to the production of cancer of the gastric cardia and, indirectly through the production of chronic (calcifying) pancreatitis, to cancer of the pancreas; but the evidence is insufficient for any conclusion to be reached.

Alcohol and Liver Disease

There is strong evidence for a direct relationship between the toxicity of alcohol and liver damage. The liver plays a major role in the metabolism of alcohol. By the action of alcohol dehydrogenase, alcohol is transformed to acetaldehyde, which in turn is rapidly oxidized in the liver to acetate by aldehyde dehydrogenase. Acetaldehyde is a very potent and reactive compound, and it has been suggested that it is one of the major factors in the pathogenesis of alcoholic liver disease.

There is a firm consensus about the association between chronic excessive drinking and the development of fatty liver, perivenular fibrosis, acute alcoholic hepatitis and liver cirrhosis. The potential for developing these conditions is higher in individuals who, for a period of time, have had a daily excessive intake of alcohol. Whereas the consensus about the qualitative association between excessive drinking and the development of the above-mentioned hepatic lesions is well established, there is much uncertainty about the dose-effect relationship.

The key mechanism in the genesis of fatty liver is due to the alcohol-induced change in the redox state of the liver. Excessive alcohol intake may produce liver damage by other mechanisms, such as promotion of lipid peroxidation and toxicity associated with an activation of the microsomal alcohol-oxidizing system. Although there is some evidence that both mechanisms may play a role in the development of alcohol-induced injury to the liver, further studies are required to reach a definite consensus. Nutritional studies have also been implicated, but data are insufficient to establish a critical role.

It is considered that chronic alcoholism constitutes a significant public health problem. Four prospective studies have assessed the relationship between daily alcohol use reported at the start of the study and subsequent cirrhosis mortality during long-term follow-up. In one study it was found that, among subjects reporting drinking at least 50 g/day, the number of those who develop cirrhosis after 10–15 years was about 2% per year. Many studies have demonstrated a very close correlation between total alcohol use in populations and mortality from cirrhosis. Although the incidence of heavy drinkers is higher among men, women are more sensitive to the development of liver injury. Individuals drinking intermittently had a lower incidence of liver damage. Abstinence will reverse, improve or delay progression of alcoholic liver disease depending on the stage of the lesion, which also indicates that alcohol is responsible for the liver damage.

The fact that only a minor proportion of alcohol abusers develop the most severe forms of liver damage, cirrhosis in particular, indicates that other causal factors may be involved. Despite years of research, no consensus has been reached on any one such factor. Current research focuses on genetic factors, viral infections and specific nutritional disturbances.

Chapter 1

Moderate Drinking: Concepts, Definitions and Public Health Significance

H. Kalant
University of Toronto and Centre for Addiction and
Mental Health, Toronto, Ont., Canada

K. Poikolainen
Järvenpää Addiction Hospital, Haarajoki, and
National Public Health Institute, Helsinki, Finland

Abstract

Despite widespread interest in the health effects of moderate drinking, there is no universally accepted definition of "moderate". The term is used in at least five different senses, with different implications.

1. The oldest sense is *non-intoxicating*, and its focus is on the immediate adverse events, such as accidental trauma and interpersonal violence, for which the risk is clearly increased by intoxication. It is difficult to define quantitatively, because genetic factors and acquired tolerance result in large individual differences in the amounts that can be drunk without producing intoxication.

2. Moderate has also been defined as *statistically normal*, i.e. corresponding to the average or modal amount that is typical of drinkers in a given population. This can be measured reasonably accurately, but differs substantially from one population or culture to another, and bears no clear relationship to the risk of chronic health or social problems.

3. The definition of moderate as *non-injurious* reflects primarily a medical preoccupation with alcohol-related disease.

4. A similar but broader definition of moderate as *problem-free* is concerned not only with health but also with social problems in such areas as interpersonal relations, work performance and legal and economic difficulties. Both of these definitions are difficult to translate into quantitative terms, because of individual and environmental influences that affect the risk of harm at a given level of intake.

5. The definition of moderate as *optimal*, in terms of the lowest overall morbidity or mortality in a population, reflects the growing body of epidemiological literature relating habitual levels of alcohol intake to the degree of risk for various types of health outcome in that population. This approach permits objective quantitative definition, but only for those outcomes which show a U- or J-shaped relation between intake and level of risk.

Regardless of the type of definition, problems of several types make it difficult to specify "moderate" intake quantitatively. One is the fact that intakes are still frequently expressed in "drinks" or "units" that vary with beverage type, culture and era. It is extremely important to adopt a uniform international definition of a "standard drink" or, better still, to adopt the practice of expressing individual intakes in amounts (grams) of absolute alcohol per kg body weight per day. Another problem is the inherent variability in accuracy of recall by the drinker. Still another is the influence of drinking pattern (e.g. binge drinking versus regular daily drinking) on the risk of problems at any given long-term average level of intake.

Because of these difficulties, it is not yet possible to specify a "moderate" level of intake that will be useful in giving advice to the individual drinker. On a population basis, the optimal level is probably in the range of 10–19 g alcohol a day for the average adult man and less than 10 g for a woman. But the physician, in giving advice, should take into account individual differences in body size, age, and special situations that can increase the degree of risk, such as pregnancy, inherently hazardous activities such as driving, and the presence of various diseases and medications.

Concepts of Moderation

The concept of moderation in relation to eating, drinking and other behaviours is a very old one in human history, as exemplified by the ancient Greek Golden Rule of "moderation in all things". It has usually been considered a moral issue rather than primarily a health concern. In recent years, however, the topic of moderate drinking of alcoholic beverages has received a great deal of scientific and clinical attention, because of evidence relating individual levels of consumption to the level of risk of various types of disease. Despite this interest, there is no universally accepted definition of moderation in current use. Even the previous edition of this book (Verschuren 1993) contains very few references to moderation, and no definition of it.

In the absence of such an agreed definition, it is not surprising that the literature contains widely different applications of the term "moderate". A comparison of average daily amounts defined as light, moderate and heavy in a sampling of recent publications from various countries (Table 1) shows that the lower limit of "moderate" alcohol intakes ranges from 4.5 to 50 g a day, and the upper limit from about 24 to 80 g a day. These examples are not necessarily a representative sample of the whole literature, and are meant only to illustrate the range of variation.

The problem is compounded when one examines what the drinking public understands by "light", "moderate" and "heavy" drinking (Abel et al. 1995). A questionnaire survey conducted in several American cities revealed that the threshold quantities of consumption by which the respondents defined these levels of intake varied as a function of age,

Table 1
Examples of variation in definition of moderate drinking
(g/day absolute alcohol)

Reference	Country	Original units[1]	Drinking category		
			light	moderate	heavy
Abel et al. 1995	USA	drinks/day	19-33	34-49	>50
Beilin et al. 1996	Australia	drinks/day		10-40	
Camargo 1996	USA	drinks/day		<27 M, <12 W	
Carmelli et al. 1995	USA	drinks/day[2]	0.5-7	7.5-29.5	30+
Carpenter et al. 1998	USA	drinks/day	<13.5	13.5-27	>40
Colditz et al. 1985	USA	g/day	0.1-8.9	9-34	>34
de Labry et al. 1992	USA	drinks/yr[3]	...	1-42	43+
Glaser 1994	USA	drinks/mon		4.5-26.7	
Goldberg et al. 1994	USA	g/day	1-12	12-31	32+
Harper et al. 1988	Australia	g/day		30-80	>80
Herbert et al. 1993	USA	oz/day		12-24	>24
Jenkins et al. 1992	UK	units/wk[4]		<23.7	
Karkkainen et al. 1990	Finland	g/day		60	
La Grange et al. 1995	USA	g/yr	<2.0	2.7-38	
Lazarus et al. 1991	USA	drinks/mo	M 0.4-20 W 0.4-13.5	M 20.7+ W 14+	
Mello et al. 1987	USA	drinks/day	16.6±2.9	52.4±2.6	106±9
Mills et al. 1987	USA	drinks/day	<13.5	13.5-27	
Orgogozo et al. 1997	France	drinks/day	1-24	36-48	60+
Pajarinen et al. 1996	Finland	g/day		<40	>80
Palomaki et al. 1993	Finland	g/week	<21.4	21.4-42.8	>42.8
Paunio et al. 1994	Finland	drinks/day[3]	14	28-70	84+
Rostand et al. 1990	France	glasses/wk[5]	0-8.6	10-28.6	>30
Sanchez-Craig et al. 1984	Canada	drinks/wk		<39	>39
Scragg et al. 1987	New Zealand	g/day	1-9	10-34	35+
Shaper et al. 1988	UK	units/wk[6]	1-19	20-54	55+
van 't Veer et al. 1989	Netherlands	g/day	1-4		30+
Wannamethee et al. 1996	UK	drinks/day[6]	9-18	27-54	>54
Wannamethee et al. 1997	UK	units/wk[6]	1-19	20-54	55+

[1] Where the originals have expressed the amounts as drinks or units per day, week, month or year, they have been converted into g/day, on the basis of the alcohol content of a standard drink in the respective country (Table 4), except when the authors have specified an alcohol content per drink or unit, as indicated below.
[2] drink = 15 g ethanol.
[3] drink = 14 g ethanol.
[4] unit = 7.9 g ethanol.
[5] glass = 10 g ethanol.
[6] drink or unit = 8-10 g of ethanol; 9 g used for calculations above.

education, income, sex and personal drinking habits and tolerance of the respondents. They also varied according to the drinking situation in question, being different for weekdays, weekends and social events.

The lack of an accepted definition may be due in part to the fact that concepts of moderation held by clinicians and researchers have changed. For many decades, moderate drinking was seen simply as the antithesis of heavy drinking, but as a result of epidemiological studies of various types in the past decades, moderate drinking has also come to be seen as part of a continuum ranging from total abstinence through light and moderate to heavy drinking. This change in concept will be discussed in some detail here. As a necessary preliminary to that discussion, it is useful at this point to review briefly the various meanings that different authors have given to the term "moderate drinking".

Moderate as Non-Intoxicating

The English word "moderation", and its equivalents in French, Italian, Spanish and various other European languages, is derived from the Latin *moderare*, meaning to control or restrain. When it is used in relation to alcohol use, it carries the clear implication that alcohol tends to give rise to impulsive and excessive consumption, which must be controlled or restrained in order to avoid some undesired consequence. This concept is implied or clearly stated in various definitions of moderate drinking in earlier literature. In his classic study on alcohol and mortality, Pearl (1926) defined moderate drinking as non-intoxicating intake, not exceeding about two pints of beer a day. Haggard et al. (1942) defined the moderate drinker as one who

> *does not seek intoxication and does not expose himself to it. He uses alcoholic beverages as a condiment and for their milder sedative effects. Alcohol constitutes neither a necessity nor a considerable item in his budget.*

This definition is geared specifically to the absence of acute intoxication and its attendant risks. The wide public support for present-day campaigns against drinking-driving, and the legal issues concerning the role of alcohol in family and other violence (de Vente et al. 1998), attest to the importance most societies attach to the avoidance of intoxication. Such a definition is thus primarily socially motivated, and its medical aspects relate mainly to emergency medicine, and to the human and economic costs of the continuing care of those with permanent injuries caused by alcohol-related accidents.

Moderate as Statistically "Normal"

An alternative approach to the definition of moderate intake could be based on the levels of consumption typical of the majority in a population. Cahalan et al. (1969) proposed that drinking levels should be defined in terms of both frequency of drinking and amounts drunk per occasion, including the "typical" amount and the highest amount per occasion. They gathered such data and categorized drinking as none, occasional, light, moderate and heavy, in operational terms that are clear but for which a theoretical rationale is not apparent.

In order to take into account the important variable of the drinker's body size, Vogel-Sprott (1974) studied a group of regular drinkers and obtained data on age, weight, type of beverage drunk, number of drinks per drinking occasion, and frequency of drinking occasions, from which she was able to calculate the consumption in grams of absolute alcohol per kg per occasion, or per week. She suggested that "normal" should be defined as at or near the mean value for the respective age group, and "heavy" should mean at least one standard deviation above the respective group mean. In these terms, a moderate intake would presumably mean normal (as so defined) or less.

Another approach to define "normal" would be to study the lifetime drinking habits among drinkers who do not meet the diagnostic criteria for alcoholism. Retrospective interviews of a US random-digit dialling sample of social drinkers in New York State found that in this group alcohol use remained rather constant at an average of about 5–10 drinking days per month and about 3–4 drinks (42–56 g of ethanol) per drinking occasion (York 1995).

A problem that comes to mind at once is that the norm differs considerably from one culture to another, and even with sex and educational level within a culture (Abel et al. 1995). Another problem is that a "moderate" intake, as defined statistically or culturally, is not necessarily a harmless intake. For example, a definition of moderate drinking in 19th century France, cited by Haggard et al. (1942) and by Babor et al. (1987), was "not more than one litre of wine a day, for an active man". In modern terms, this is equal to a daily intake of about 7 standard North American drinks, 8 standard French drinks, or nearly 12 standard British units. In contrast, most of the entries in Table 1 give 1–3 drinks a day as a moderate intake. In Chile, Marconi (1959) defined a moderate drinker as one whose alcohol intake provides less than 20% of the total energy of the diet. At a typical dietary energy intake of 10 MJ/day (2400 kcal/day), this would mean an alcohol intake providing less than 2 MJ (480 kcal) a day and, if alcohol yields 29 kJ/g (7 kcal/g), this would mean just under 70 g alcohol or about 5–6 standard drinks a day. Such intakes, if sustained on a long-term basis, are enough to put the "moderate drinker" into the range in which the risk of liver cirrhosis or of mortality from several causes of death is significantly increased (Péquignot 1958, Rankin et al. 1975, English et al. 1995, Poikolainen 1995).

Moderate as Non-Injurious

Other definitions of moderate drinking, however, have been primarily medically motivated, and refer to the avoidance of harm that may result from the cumulative effects of *chronic* ingestion of excessive (i.e. "immoderate") amounts of alcohol. This is reflected in a recent comment (Werner 1996) that "the very designation "moderate" implies that such drinking is presumed to be generally uninjurious". If this definition of moderate were generally adopted, it would necessarily follow that there could be no adverse health consequences of moderate drinking, and the upper limit of moderate intake would be just below the minimum daily consumption shown to give rise to organic malfunction of some type.

The quest for such a limit has a long history. Anstie, a nineteenth-century British physician and one of the founders of the modern discipline of public health, concluded from his clinical observations that a healthy adult man could drink, on a daily basis, beverages containing a total of 43 ml absolute alcohol (equivalent to about 100–115 ml of 80-proof spirits containing 32% alcohol (w/v), i.e. about four British or three US or Canadian drinks) without risk of deterioration of health (Baldwin 1977, Babor et al. 1987). Anstie's limit, as this quantity is named, did not include any reference to drinking pattern, as opposed to average amount, and one can only suppose that the typical British drinking pattern was one of daily intake of a more or less constant amount.

Moderate as Problem-Free

Drinking-related harms include not only problems with physical health, but also social and mental problems. One broad definition of moderate drinking could be problem-free drinking. In the past two decades, there have been a number of studies of brief interventions aimed

Table 2

Recommended upper limit of alcohol intake for controlled or problem-free drinking, in brief interventions to reduce excessive alcohol intake

Authors and year	Sex of drinker	Recommendation "no more than"	Equivalent amount of alcohol, g/day
Heather et al. 1986	M	50 units/wk	57
	F	35 units/week	40
Heather et al. 1987	M	139 units/month	37
	F	79 units/month	21
Wallace et al. 1988	M	18 units/wk	21
	F	9 units/week	10
Scott et al. 1990	F	14 units/wk	20
Anderson et al. 1992	M	210 g/wk	30
Babor et al. 1992	M	4 drinks/occasion, 5 days/wk	34
	F	3 drinks/occasion, 5 days/wk	26
Richmond et al. 1995[*]	M	35 drinks/week	50
	F	21 drinks/week	30
Fleming et al. 1997[*]	M	14 drinks/week	24
	F	11 drinks/week	19

[*] Screening cut-off point for problem drinkers.
M, men; F, women.

at reducing excessive drinking rather than stopping drinking altogether (e.g. Fleming et al. 1997, Heather et al. 1986, 1987, Sanchez-Craig et al. 1995). The excessive drinkers in these studies are advised, on the basis of their individual characteristics, either to abstain or to drink in a controlled and problem-free way. In these studies, the recommended upper limit of daily alcohol intake has varied from 21 to 57 g alcohol for men and from 10 to 40 g for women (Table 2).

A problem-free level of alcohol intake has been defined empirically in one brief-intervention study, by comparing intakes in drinkers with and without problems at one-year follow-up, who had initially the same level of problems at baseline (Sanchez-Craig et al. 1995). Problems were assessed in the areas of health, interpersonal relationships, aggression, work performance, finances and the law. Based on the upper limit of the

95% confidence interval, this analysis found that problem-free drinking did not exceed a weekly intake of 218 g for men and 163 g for women (averaging 31 g/day for men and 23 g/day for women). The maximum problem-free amounts consumed on any drinking day were 54 g for men and 41 g for women. The amount consumed on any single day was an important predictor of the presence or absence of problems, but the frequency of drinking appeared to have little influence. Governments and learned bodies in various countries have also put forward analogous recommendations for *sensible*, *safe* or *acceptable* drinking levels (Table 3). The recommended upper limit has varied from 24 to 60 g alcohol a day for men and from 12 to 36 g for women. These recommendations do not differ much from the advice given to the target populations of the brief interventions for reducing excessive drinking.

Moderate as Optimal

In the past twenty years or so, numerous studies have found that moderate drinkers have lower total mortality, and less coronary heart disease, cholelithiasis, diabetes and dementia than either abstainers or heavy drinkers (English et al. 1995, Facchini et al. 1994, Rimm et al. 1995, Orgogozo et al. 1997, Thun et al. 1997, Attili et al. 1998). The dose-response curve relating mean daily alcohol intake to morbidity or mortality is therefore U-shaped or J-shaped (de Labry et al. 1992, Poikolainen 1995, Werner 1996). This relationship appears to be independent of beverage type (Rimm et al. 1996) since it has been found in populations consisting predominantly of wine drinkers (e.g. Renaud et al. 1998) and in others made up chiefly of beer drinkers (e.g. Keil et al. 1997). Such findings suggest that, instead of searching for the highest harmless level of alcohol intake, it might be better to attempt to identify the optimal level. In this sense the optimal level would be that which corresponds to the nadir, the lowest point on the J- or U-shaped curve. Some recent research of this type agrees remarkably well with Anstie. For example, Klatsky (1996) defines moderate drinking as "the area [under the curve] below the level at which overall net harmful effects are seen in population surveys, about three drinks a day. Thus, I call less than three drinks per day "moderate" or "lighter" drinking, and define heavy drinking as three or more drinks per day".

Table 3
Upper limit of alcohol intake for problem-free or sensible drinking, as recommended by governmental or learned bodies

Country and agency	Recommended limit	Alcohol equivalent, g/day
Australia		
National Health and Medical	M 28 units/week	36
Research Council[1]	F 14 units/week	18
Canada		
Ministry of Health of Ontario[1]	M 14 drinks/week	27
	F 14 drinks/week	27
Finland		
State Alcohol Monopoly[2]	M 24 drinks/week	41
	F 16 drinks/week	27
France		
Academy of Medicine[3]	M 3-5 glasses of wine/day	60
	F 1.5-3 glasses of wine/day	36
UK		
Department of Health[4]	M 4 units/day	32
	F 3 units/day	24
British Medical Association[5]	M 21 units/week	24
	F 14 units/week	16
USA		
Department of Health[1]	M 2 drinks/day	24
	F 1 drink/day	12
American Heart Association[6]	2 drinks/day	24
NIAAA[7]	M 2 drinks/day	24
	F 1 drink/day	12
	Over 65: 1 drink/day	12

M, men; F, women.
[1] Sanchez-Craig et al. 1995. [2] Sillanaukee et al. 1992. [3] David 1992.
[4]Department of Health 1995. [5] British Medical Association 1995.
[6] Pearson 1996. [7] O'Connor et al. 1998.

Implications of Different Concepts of Moderation

1. The concept of "moderate" as non-intoxicating has essentially a short-term reference. Damage that might be attributable to acute intoxication would be confined largely to trauma of various kinds, and to the dramatic and obvious functional disturbances of the central nervous system, such as alcohol poisoning, alcohol-drug interactions and lowering of the seizure threshold during hangover or withdrawal (Mucha et al. 1979). These acute effects are essentially reversible, and even fatal poisoning is due mainly to functional depression of the respiratory centre, which can recover fully if the individual is kept alive by mechanical ventilation. However, in experimental studies in which artificial ventilation had been applied, death due to circulatory arrest occurred at even higher blood alcohol concentrations (Wallgren et al. 1970). The older concept that alcohol is a "protoplasmic poison" that causes death of a certain number of neurons on each exposure (Edmondson et al. 1956) is not supported by empirical evidence at alcohol concentrations that would be achievable by voluntary consumption.

Moreover, this concept of "moderate" suffers from an important shortcoming in that it fails to take account of the effect of differences in both "innate" or initial tolerance and acquired tolerance. Modern genetic studies have made it clear, for example, that the offspring of alcoholic biological parents are significantly more resistant to the acute intoxicating effects of alcohol than the offspring of non-alcoholic parents, even when the two groups of offspring have had similarly small experience with alcohol (Schuckit 1992, Pollock 1992). In addition to this initial difference, the regular drinker acquires a greater level of tolerance, so that a greater amount of alcohol can be consumed daily without producing subjective or objective signs of intoxication (Kalant et al. 1971, Kalant 1996b, Deitrich et al. 1996). Moreover, a large consumption may still not constitute a considerable item in the budget if the drinker is reasonably affluent and the cost of alcohol is relatively low. Such a definition may therefore be expected to lead to very wide variations in the range of actual daily intake that would be considered moderate (in the sense of non-intoxicating), and consequently a very wide range of risk of later-stage organic and functional disturbances of various organ systems.

2. The concept of moderate as statistically normal has the clear advantage that it permits an empirically defined reference standard, but

carries no implications with respect to damage. In a heavy-drinking society, the norm of consumption may well be high enough to carry a significantly elevated risk of organic damage of all kinds, as has been the experience in various countries. This definition of moderate also creates difficulties for popular education campaigns, because the argument that even moderate drinking is potentially harmful seems self-contradictory and can be mistaken for a prohibitionist or temperance message.

3.   As noted earlier, the concept of moderate as non-injurious implies that moderate drinking carries *no* risk of damage to any organ system. The problem remains, however, of how to discover the non-injurious level. As is shown in Table 1, there is a wide range of intakes considered moderate by different observers. It seems possible that drinkers at the heavier end of this range may indeed suffer long-term health consequences. If this is so, the observer is then forced to conclude either that moderate drinking is harmful, or that the level initially accepted as moderate is, after all, not moderate. Another problem is that this concept of moderate drinking is commonly thought to refer only to damage due to chronic organic disease.

4.   The concept of moderate drinking as problem-free drinking has the advantage that it is defined in terms of the avoidance of all possible social, mental, physical health and intoxication-related harms. However, because cultural and situational factors may strongly influence social harms, this concept of moderation is less universally valid than those based primarily on physical health.

5.   The concept of moderate drinking as the optimal level corresponding to the lowest overall rate of morbidity or mortality has much to commend it. Like the statistical definitions of moderate drinking, it is also empirically defined, but in addition it can have a predictive value with respect to the risk of damage in an individual drinker. It implies maximal health benefits and minimal risk, and is likely to be more universally valid in different societies than the concepts based on statistical norms or freedom from problems. This definition of moderate is applicable only if there is a U-shaped or J-shaped curve that permits the identification of a level of drinking at which harm is minimal. Such a shape has been found for cardiovascular and some other diseases, but for some other groups of diseases the shape of the curve has not yet been clarified (e.g. Kearney et al. 1995, Rimm et al. 1995).

In the case of the nervous system (see Chapter 9) the relationship has not yet been explored as thoroughly as for the cardiovascular system (see Chapter 5). Early studies (Parker et al. 1974) suggested that there is a linear relation between the amount habitually consumed per drinking occasion and the decrease in cognitive function; the implication was that *any* amount of drinking, even at what is usually regarded as a social level, causes some cumulative loss of neurons or neuronal function. The later difficulties in confirming or rebutting this view have been reviewed in detail recently (Eckardt et al. 1998, Parsons et al. 1998). On the other hand, under certain circumstances acute administration of alcohol may actually improve memory, possibly by preventing conflicting information from retroactively preventing the conversion of the immediate short-term memory into a long-term or permanent one (Hewitt et al. 1996, Tyson et al. 1994). This is not clearly related to a specific position on a dose-effect curve.

Similarly, heavy chronic drinking can cause a loss of neurons in various brain structures, and associated cognitive impairment, but light drinking may possibly have a protective effect (Eckardt et al. 1998). Light drinkers have been reported to show less age-related loss of logical memory than non-drinkers (Farmer et al. 1987) and a small but statistically significant advantage over non-drinkers on various cognitive tests (Hendrie et al. 1996), especially in women (Dufouil et al. 1997, Forette et al. 1998), but there was a deleterious effect for heavier drinkers (Hendrie et al. 1996). Even more direct evidence was obtained in prospective studies of cognitive function in ageing populations: a smaller loss of memory over a three-year period (Herbert et al. 1993) and a lower incidence of Alzheimer's disease (Orgogozo et al. 1997) was seen in light drinkers than in non-drinkers.

If the risk of a particular type of health problem increases linearly or exponentially with increasing alcohol intake, showing no threshold level and no minimum, so that all levels of alcohol use carry a higher risk than non-drinking, then it is impossible to talk of moderate drinking (as so defined) with respect to that problem. Examples of this type of relation include liver cirrhosis, large bowel cancer (Longenecker et al. 1996) and traffic accidents.

It is clear that the shape of the dose-response curve linking alcohol intake and health outcome varies with the specific outcome measure under study. Numerous authors have pointed out that the J-shaped curve relating total mortality rate to alcohol intake is the result of the blending of the alcohol effects on the separate mortality rates for all separate diseases. For example, increasing alcohol intakes appear to produce a progressive lowering of the death rate from coronary heart disease, at least up to a certain level of heavy intake. At a certain intake, however, for example above three drinks a day in some studies, this beneficial effect is offset by rapidly rising mortality rates from hypertensive heart disease, stroke, upper digestive tract cancers and various other causes. Thus, if we wish to define moderate consumption in terms of an optimal level, we need an overall indicator of health, rather than a specific type of disease, as the outcome measure. Depending on our interest, such an indicator can be total mortality, incidence of any functional incapacity, incidence of disease of any type, or a subjective report of health status (e.g. good, average or bad). The difficult problem common to all concepts of moderate drinking is how to estimate these levels.

Difficulties in Estimating Moderate Levels

The emphasis on long-term cumulative effects on health makes the working definition of moderate drinking subject to much variation. The onset of some such effects offers a less sharp end-point than acute intoxication and its attendant social and physical consequences. The latency of chronic adverse effects on health may be long and it is more difficult to prove the causal role of alcohol in relation to these effects than to those due to acute intoxication. In the interim, the socially accepted level of drinking may be more likely to be defined in terms of variable and culture-dependent criteria (Cahalan et al. 1969), including traditional patterns of use and social acceptance of different levels of use and intoxication (Vogel-Sprott 1974).

There are several problems in the estimation of the moderate levels. First, estimates of use based on questionnaire data can give different results, depending on the questions asked. For example, general questions about overall drinking yield different amounts than specific questions that inquire about each beverage type (beer, wine, spirits), and questions about the amount drunk in the past one or two weeks yield different results than those that inquire about the past month or year (Dawson 1998). Another problem is the common practice of expressing alcohol use in traditional units such as drinks, glasses or bottles. Transformation to a common unit is needed. Universal comparability can be achieved by expressing alcohol intake in grams of absolute ethanol. In the transformations, average alcohol contents of beer, wine, spirits or other beverage types are commonly used. This is one source of error. The consumption of beverages is typically ascertained as self-reported numbers of drinks, and a drink is usually defined as the typical serving volume of a beverage in a bar or other drinking establishment in the particular region under study. These "standard drinks" are useful in collecting the data on alcohol intake. A problem, however, is comparability. Various authors have called attention to the lack of uniformity of the "standard drinks", which vary not only from country to country, but also from one beverage type to another (Lemmens 1994, Miller et al. 1991, Stockwell et al. 1994, Turner 1990). A recent publication (ICAP 1998) has addressed the problem of the lack of a universal "standard drink", and lists official government definitions of standard drinks in seventeen countries, which range from 6 g alcohol in Austria to 19.75 g in Japan (Table 4). However, even the official definitions may vary. For example, both 12 g and 14 g have been presented as the official figure in the USA (ICAP 1998, O'Connor et al. 1998). For each study cited here, we have used the same figure for alcohol content of "a drink" that was used by the original authors.

Although there are practical reasons for the variation in the alcohol content of the "standard drinks", the comparison of data between countries and regions would be greatly facilitated by the uniform expression of alcohol intakes in grams of absolute alcohol and by the adoption of a uniform international definition of a "standard drink".

The relatively low level of accuracy of present methods in estimating alcohol intake (see Chapter 2) makes it difficult to ascertain the actual moderate levels of consumption. Recall of alcohol intake by the drinker is subject to some random error, although this is not as great as might be expected. The test-retest reliability has been found to be reasonably good, the reliability coefficients varying from 0.80 to 0.90 (O'Malley et al. 1983). A serious problem, however, is that most subjects underestimate their alcohol intake. In population surveys, the average extent of underestimation reported varied between 29% and 83% of the actual intake (Pernanen 1974, Polich 1981, Simpura 1987). If the degree of underestimation is not linked to the actual level of intake (i.e. if the absolute amount of underestimation is the same at all levels of intake), it will not affect the conclusions about the shape of the dose-effect curve and will not alter in general terms the relation between the degree of health risk and the rank order of alcohol intake. The quantitative definition of moderate or optimal level of alcohol use, however, will be unrealistically low.

Table 4
Alcohol content of a "standard drink" (in g absolute ethanol) as defined in various countries

Country	Size of standard drink (g alcohol)
Australia	10
Austria	6
Canada	13.5
Denmark	12
Finland	11
France	12
Hungary	17
Iceland	9.5
Ireland	8
Italy	10
Japan	19.75
Netherlands	9.9
New Zealand	10
Portugal	14
Spain	10
UK	8
USA	14

Data from International Center for Alcohol Policies, ICAP Report 5 (1998).

On the other hand, if the degree of underestimation is directly proportional to the actual alcohol use (i.e. if the absolute amount of underestimation is progressively larger at progressively higher levels of intake), conclusions about dose-response relationships will be unreliable. There is some evidence that heavy drinkers underestimate their alcohol intake more than light drinkers do (Uchalik 1979, Poikolainen 1985). This is likely to exaggerate the increase of health risks related to high levels of alcohol intake.

The best way to obtain more accurate information on the optimal level of alcohol intake would be to do large-scale randomized trials of healthy abstainers, assigned to groups either to continue abstaining or to begin use of "moderate" amounts of ethanol. The end-points of such trials could include levels of various risk factors for major diseases, the incidence of disease and injury, and mortality. For the present, however, such trials may not be feasible for various reasons (Renaud et al. 1993).

Significance of Drinking Pattern in the Definition of Moderate Drinking

Most studies relevant to the foregoing discussion have focused on the individual's average level of alcohol use over a period of time. The effects on health and on social problems of various types, however, are related not only to the average level, but also to the pattern of drinking (Midanik et al. 1996). For example, an Australian study (McElduff et al. 1997) found the lowest risk of coronary heart disease at the level of one to two drinks (each containing 10 g of ethanol) per day on five or six days a week, in both men and women. In these groups, men had 64% less coronary heart disease (CHD) than abstinent men, and women had a 61% lower risk than their abstinent counterparts. However, there was a significant increase in CHD risk among men who drank nine or more drinks a day on one or two days a week, as well as among those who drank this amount daily. Compared with lifelong abstainers, these two groups had odds ratios for CHD of 2.62 and 2.40 respectively. This and other evidence reviewed recently (Poikolainen 1998) suggests that light and frequent drinking is beneficial, while large amounts drunk infrequently are harmful with respect to CHD, even though long-term average daily use might be the same.

There is a large body of literature demonstrating that for any given amount of alcohol drunk, the maximum blood alcohol concentration (BAC) and the area under the concentration-time curve are less when the alcohol is drunk with a meal than when it is taken in the absence of food (Kalant 1996a). Thus, those who regularly drink alcohol only with meals would be expected to have a lower risk of health effects directly related to the peak BAC than drinkers who usually take alcohol in the absence of food. However, the risk of effects related to alcohol metabolism rather than the peak BAC, such as the production of fatty liver (Lieber 1997), would not be expected to differ between the two types of drinker unless the presence of food diminishes the total amount of alcohol absorbed from the gastrointestinal tract.

Advice on Moderate Drinking

It is impossible to give any exact advice on moderate drinking. However, the results from epidemiological studies, taken at their face value, may provide conservative estimates of moderate drinking. Because these are underestimates, a notable safety margin is included. As to total mortality, these estimates suggest that for the average adult man, the optimal level is ca. 10–19 g alcohol a day and the non-injurious level is ca. 30–40 g a day. For the average adult woman, the respective levels are <10 g and ca. 10–20 g a day (English et al. 1995, Poikolainen 1995). As to morbidity data such as hospitalizations, absenteeism and self-reported subjective health status, these intake levels are of the same magnitude (Poikolainen 1996).

The estimates of non-injurious and optimal levels of alcohol use derived from epidemiological studies are valid for the "average" adult. Such average data for a population overlook individual differences. For example, variation in body size and composition has a marked influence on the BAC produced by the same amount of ethanol in different individuals (Kalant 1996a). Thus, what is moderate for a large young man may be heavy for a small elderly woman. Estimates would be better if the important variables of the drinker's body size and composition were taken into consideration.

Advice to the general public should consider individual differences and situational factors. It should include the following.

- It is best to avoid intoxication.
- Abstaining is the only safe choice in situations with increased risk of accidents, for example in sports activities, or in the operation of motor vehicles or other machinery.
- Abstinence is probably the safest choice in pregnancy, because the minimum level of alcohol use associated with foetal damage is not known with certainty (see Chapter 6). Occasional light drinking (e.g. one or two drinks a week) may have no adverse effects, but it is not yet possible to be certain that this is true, especially with respect to the most subtle types of functional alteration (Larroque et al. 1998).
- Abstinence is the only safe choice if one has a disease that is aggravated even by small amounts of alcohol (e.g. alcohol dependence, depression, hypertension, liver cirrhosis or peptic ulcer) or is using drugs that have significant adverse interactions with alcohol.
- Abstainers who contemplate starting moderate drinking for health reasons should bear in mind that (1) protection from coronary heart disease by alcohol has been clearly demonstrated only in the middle-aged and elderly, and in those with relatives having a history of coronary heart disease, and (2) moderate drinking exposes the user to the potential risk of alcohol dependence, especially if the abstainer's parents are or have been alcohol-dependent.

What is known by science at present, and what will be known in the future, can only be the best current approximation to reality. There will always remain individual differences, and some of them may call for modification of the general advice. The wise drinker will bear in mind the general principles enunciated by Aristotle:

> *"The temperate man keeps a middle course in these matters. He takes no pleasure at all in the things that the profligate enjoys most, on the contrary, he positively dislikes them; nor in general does he find pleasure in wrong things, nor excessive pleasure in anything of this source; nor does he feel pain or desire when they are lacking, or only in a moderate degree, not more than is right, nor at the wrong time et cetera. But such pleasures as conduce to health and fitness he will try to obtain in a moderate and right degree; as also other pleasures so far as they are not detrimental to health and fitness, and not ignoble, nor beyond his means."*

Conclusions

Various definitions of moderate drinking have been put forward, with quite different conceptual bases and different implications for the risk of physiological malfunction and organic damage. Probably the most uniformly valuable definitions are those based on epidemiological studies of the relationship between alcohol intake and the relative risk of different types of disturbance. Such studies are fairly numerous and extensive with respect to the liver, cardiovascular system, cancer, and total morbidity and mortality rates. For clinically useful predictive ability, as well as for possible clues concerning pathogenetic mechanisms and potential inter-ventions, much more evidence of this type is required with respect to other organ systems and disease processes, using operationally defined criteria for "light", "moderate" and "heavy" drinking, and sufficiently detailed measurement data taking into consideration variability due to body size, beverage characteristics, and drinking pattern. Assessment and comparison of data from many countries would be greatly facilitated by the uniform expression of alcohol intakes in grams of absolute alcohol and by the adoption of a uniform international definition of a "standard drink".

References

Abel EL, Kruger ML (1995) Hon v. Stroh Brewery Company: what do we mean by "moderate" and "heavy" drinking? Alcohol Clin Exp Res 19: 1024–31.

Anderson P, Scott E (1992) The effect of general practitioners' advice to heavy drinking men. Br J Addict 87: 891–900.

Aristotle (1926) The Nicomachean ethics, chapter III, xi, 8. Heineman, London.

Attili AF, Scafato E, Marchioli R, et al. (1998) Diet and gallstones in Italy: the cross-sectional MICOL results. Hepatology 27: 1492–98.

Babor TF, Grant M, eds. (1992) Project on identification and management of alcohol-related problems. Report on Phase II. A randomized clinical trial of brief interventions in primary health care. World Health Organization, Geneva.

Babor TF, Kranzler HR, Lauerman RJ (1987) Social drinking as a health and psychosocial risk factor. Anstie's limit revisited. Rec Dev Alcohol 5: 373–402.

Baldwin AD (1977) Anstie's alcohol limit. Am J Publ Health 67: 679–81.

Beilin LJ, Puddey IB, Burke V (1996) Alcohol and hypertension: kill or cure? J Hum Hypertension 10 (Suppl 2): S1–S5.

British Medical Association (1995) Guidelines on sensible drinking. BMA, London.

Cahalan D, Cisin IH, Crossley HM (1969) American drinking practices: a national study of drinking behavior and attitudes. Monograph 6, Rutgers Center of Alcohol Studies, New Brunswick, NJ.

Camargo CA Jr (1996) Case-control and cohort studies of moderate alcohol consumption and stroke. Clin Chim Acta 246: 107–19.

Carmelli D, Swan GE, Page WF, et al. (1995) World War II-veteran male twins who are discordant for alcohol consumption: 24-year mortality. Am J Public Health 85: 99–101.

Carpenter CL, Morgenstern H, London SJ (1998) Alcoholic beverage consumption and lung cancer risk among residents of Los Angeles County. J Nutr 128: 694–700.

Colditz GA, Branch LG, Lipnick RJ, et al. (1985) Moderate alcohol and decreased cardiovascular mortality in an elderly cohort. Am Heart J 109: 886–89.

David J-P (1992) Vin et alimentation: la place du vin dans l'hygiène alimentaire. Bull O.I.V. 65: 739–40.

Dawson DA (1998) Volume of ethanol consumption: effects of different approaches to measurement. J Stud Alcohol 59: 191–97.

Deitrich RA, Radcliffe R, Erwin VG (1996) Pharmacological effects in the development of physiological tolerance and physical dependence. In: Begleiter H, Kissin B (eds.), The pharmacology of alcohol and alcohol dependence. Oxford University Press, New York, pp. 431–76.

de Labry LO, Glynn RJ, Levenson MR (1992) Alcohol consumption and mortality in an American male population: recovering the U-shaped curve. J Stud Alcohol 53: 25–32.

Department of Health, UK (1995) Sensible drinking: report of an inter-departmental working group, December 1995. Department of Health, Wetherby, UK, 105 pp.

de Vente W, Wiers RW, van den Brink W, et al. (1998) Alcohol use and domestic aggression. University of Amsterdam.

Dufouil C, Ducimetière P, Alpérovitch A (1997) Sex differences in the association between alcohol consumption and cognitive performance. Am J Epidemiol 146: 405–12.

Eckardt MJ, File SE, Gessa GL, et al. (1998) Effects of moderate alcohol consumption on the central nervous system. Alcohol Clin Exp Res 22: 998–1040.

Edmondson HA, Hall EM, Myers RO (1956) Pathology of alcoholism. In: Thompson GN (ed.), Alcoholism. C.C Thomas, Springfield, IL, pp. 233–90.

English DR, Holman CDJ, Milne E, et al. (1995) The quantification of drug caused morbidity and mortality in Australia, 1995 edition. Commonwealth Department of Human Services and Health, Canberra.

Facchini F, Ida Y-D, Reaven GM (1994) Light-to-moderate alcohol intake is associated with enhanced insulin sensitivity. Diabetes Care 17: 115–19.

Farmer ME, White LR, Abbott RD, et al. (1987) Blood pressure and cognitive performance: the Framingham Study. Am J Epidemiol 126: 1103–14.

Fleming MF, Barry KL, Manwell LB, et al. (1997) Brief physician advice for problem alcohol drinkers: a randomized controlled trial in community-based primary care practices. J Am Med Ass 277: 1039–45.

Forette F, Seux M-L, Thijs L, et al. (1998) Detection of cerebral aging, an absolute need: predictive value of cognitive status. Eur Neurol 39 (Suppl. 1): 2-6.

Glaser FB (1994) In: Kishline A, Moderate Drinking: The New Option for Problem Drinkers. See Sharp Press, Tuczon, AZ, p. vi.

Goldberg RJ, Burchfiel CM, Reed DM, et al. (1994) A prospective study of the health effects of alcohol consumption in middle-aged and elderly men: the Honolulu program. Circulation 89: 651–59.

Haggard HW, Jellinek EM (1942) Alcohol Explored. Doubleday, Garden City, NY, p. 12.

Harper C, Kril J, Daly J (1988) Does a "moderate" alcohol intake damage the brain? J Neurol Neurosurg Psychiatry 51: 909–13.

Heather N, Campion PD, Neville RG, et al. (1987) Evaluation of a controlled drinking minimal intervention for problem drinkers in general practice (the DRAMS scheme). J Roy Coll Gen Pract 37: 358–63.

Heather N, Whitton B, Robertson I (1986) Evaluation of a self-help manual for media-recruited problem drinkers: six-month follow-up results. Br J Clin Psychol 25: 19–34.

Hendrie HC, Gao S, Hall KS, et al (1996) The relationship between alcohol consumption, cognitive performance, and daily functioning in an urban sample of older black Americans. J Am Geriat Soc 44: 1158–65.

Herbert LE, Scherr PA, Beckett LA, et al. (1993) Relation of smoking and low-to-moderate alcohol consumption to change in cognitive function: a longitudinal study in a defined community of older persons. Am J Epidemiol 137: 881–91.

Hewitt GP, Holder M, Laird J (1996) Retrograde enhancement of human kinesthetic memory by alcohol: consolidation or protection against interference? Neurobiol Learning Memory 65: 269–77.

ICAP [International Center for Alcohol Policies] (1998) What is a "standard drink"? ICAP Reports No. 5. ICAP, Washington, DC.

Jenkins R, Harvey S, Butler T, et al. (1992) A six year longitudinal study of the occupational consequences of drinking over "safe limits" of alcohol. Br J Ind Med 49: 369–74.

Kalant H (1996a) Pharmacokinetics of ethanol: absorption, distribution, and elimination. In: Begleiter H, Kissin B (eds.), The pharmacology of alcohol and alcohol dependence. Oxford University Press, New York, pp. 15–58.

Kalant H (1996b) Current state of knowledge about the mechanisms of alcohol tolerance. Addiction Biol 1: 133–41.

Kalant H, LeBlanc EA, Gibbins RJ (1971) Tolerance to, and dependence on, some non-opiate psychotropic drugs. Pharmacol Rev 23: 135–91.

Karkkainen P, Jokelainen K, Roine R, et al. (1990) The effects of moderate drinking and abstinence on serum and urinary beta-hexosaminidase levels. Drug Alcohol Depend 25: 35–38.

Kearney J, Giovannucci E, Rimm EB, et al. (1995) Diet, alcohol, and smoking and the occurrence of hyperplastic polyps of the colon and rectum (United States). Cancer Causes Control 6: 45–56.

Keil U, Chambless LE, Doring A, et al. (1997) The relation of alcohol intake to coronary heart disease and all-cause mortality in a beer-drinking population. Epidemiology 8: 150–56.

Klatsky AL (1996) Alcohol and hypertension. Clin Chim Acta 246: 91–105.

La Grange L, Anton RF, Garcia S, et al. (1995) Carbohydrate-deficient transferrin levels in a female population. Alcohol Clin Exp Res 19: 100–103.

Larroque B, Kaminski M (1998) Prenatal alcohol exposure and development at preschool age: main results of a French study. Alcohol Clin Exp Res 22: 998–1040

Lazarus NB, Kaplan GA, Cohen RD, et al. (1991) Change in alcohol consumption and risk of death from all causes and from ischaemic heart disease. Br Med J 303: 553–56.

Lemmens PH (1994) Alcohol content of self-report and "standard" drinks. Addiction 89: 593–601.

Lieber CS (1997) Ethanol metabolism, cirrhosis and alcoholism. Clin Chim Acta 257: 59–84.

Longenecker MP, Enger SM (1996) Epidemiologic data on alcoholic beverage consumption and risk of cancer. Clin Chim Acta 246: 121–41.

Marconi J (1959) The concept of alcoholism. Q J Stud Alcohol 20: 216–35.

McElduff P, Dobson A (1997) How much alcohol and how often? Population based case-control study of alcohol consumption and risk of a major coronary event. Br Med J 314: 1159–64.

Mello NK, Mendelson JH, Palmieri SL (1987) Cigarette smoking by women: interactions with alcohol use. Psychopharmacology 93: 8–15.

Midanik LT, Tam TW, Greenfield TK, et al. (1996) Risk functions for alcohol-related problems in a 1988 US national sample. Addiction 91: 1427–37.

Miller WR, Heather N, Hall W (1991) Calculating standard drink units: international comparisons. Br J Addict 86: 43–48.

Mills JL, Graubard BI (1987) Is moderate drinking during pregnancy associated with an increased risk for malformations? Pediatrics 80: 309–14.

Mucha RF, Pinel JPJ (1979) Increased susceptibility to kindled seizures in rats following a single injection of alcohol. J Stud Alcohol 40: 258–71.

O'Connor PG, Schottenfeld RS (1998) Patients with alcohol problems. New Engl J Med 338: 592–602.

O'Malley PM, Bachman JG, Johnston LD (1983) Reliability and consistency in self-reports of drug use. Int J Addict 18: 805–24.

Orgogozo J-M, Dartigues J-F, Lafont S, et al. (1997) Wine consumption and dementia in the elderly: a prospective community study in the Bordeaux area. Rev Neurol (Paris) 153: 185–92.

Pajarinen J, Savolainen V, Perola M et al. (1996) Glutathione S-transferase-M1 "null" genotype and alcohol-induced disorders of human spermatogenesis. Int J Androl 19: 155–63.

Palomaki H, Kaste M (1993) Regular light-to-moderate intake of alcohol and the risk of ischemic stroke. Is there a beneficial effect? Stroke 24: 1828–32.

Parker ES, Alkana RL, Birnbaum IM, et al. (1974) Alcohol and the disruption of cognitive processes. Arch Gen Psychiatry 31: 824–28.

Parsons OA, Nixon SJ (1998) Cognitive functioning in sober social drinkers: a review of the research since 1986. J Stud Alcohol 59: 180–90.

Paunio M, Heinonen OP, Virtamo J, et al. (1994) HDL cholesterol and mortality in Finnish men with special reference to alcohol intake. Circulation 90: 2909–18.

Pearl R (1926) Alcohol and longevity. Alfred A. Knopf, New York.

Pearson TA (1996) Alcohol and heart disease. Circulation 94: 3023–25.

Péquignot G (1958) Enquête par interrogatoire sur les circonstances diététiques de la cirrhose alcoolique en France. Bull Inst Nat Hygiène 13: 719–49.

Pernanen K (1974) Validity of survey data on alcohol use. In: Gibbins RJ, Israel Y, Kalant H, et al. (eds.), Research advances in alcohol and drug problems, Vol. 1. Wiley, New York, pp. 355–74.

Poikolainen K (1985) Underestimation of recalled alcohol intake in relation to actual consumption. Br J Addict 80: 215–16.

Poikolainen K (1995) Alcohol and mortality: a review. J Clin Epidemiol 48: 455–65.

Poikolainen K (1996) Alcohol and overall health outcomes: a review. Ann Med 28: 381–84.

Poikolainen K (1998) It can be bad for the heart, too: drinking patterns and coronary heart disease. Addiction 93: 1757–59.

Polich JM (1981) Epidemiology of alcohol abuse in military and civilian populations. Am J Public Health 71: 1125–32.

Pollock VE (1992) Meta-analysis of subjective sensitivity to alcohol in sons of alcoholics. Am J Psychiatry 149: 1534–38.

Rankin JG, Schmidt W, Popham RE, et al. (1975) Epidemiology of alcoholic liver disease: insights and problems. In: Khanna JM, Israel Y, Kalant H (eds.), Alcoholic liver pathology. Addiction Research Foundation, Toronto, pp. 31–41.

Renaud S, Criqui MH, Farchi G, et al. (1993) Alcohol drinking and coronary heart disease. In: Verschuren PM (ed.), Health issues related to alcohol consumption. ILSI Europe, Brussels, pp. 81–123.

Renaud SC, Gueguen R, Schenker J, et al. (1998) Alcohol and mortality in middle-aged men from eastern France. Epidemiology 9: 184–88.

Richmond R, Heather N, Wodak A, et al. (1995) Controlled evaluation of a general practice-based brief intervention for excessive drinking. Addiction 90: 119–32.

Rimm EB, Chan J, Stampfer MJ, et al. (1995) Prospective study of cigarette smoking, alcohol use, and the risk of diabetes in men. Br Med J 310: 555–59.

Rimm EB, Klatsky A, Grobbee D, et al. (1996) Review of moderate alcohol consumption and reduced risk of coronary heart disease: is the effect due to beer, wine, or spirits? Br Med J 312: 731–36.

Rostand A, Kaminski M, Lelong N, et al. (1990) Alcohol use in pregnancy, craniofacial features, and fetal growth. J Epidemiol Commun Health 44: 302–06.

Sanchez-Craig M, Annis HM, Bornet AR, et al. (1984) Random assignment to abstinence and controlled drinking: evaluation of a cognitive-behavioral program for problem drinkers. J Consult Clin Psychol 52: 390–403.

Sanchez-Craig M, Wilkinson A, Davila R (1995) Empirically based guidelines for moderate drinking: 1-year results from three studies with problem drinkers. Am J Public Health 85: 823–28.

Schuckit MA (1992) Advances in understanding the vulnerability to alcoholism. In: O'Brien CP, Jaffe JH (eds.), Addictive states. Raven Press, New York, pp. 93–108.

Scott E, Anderson P (1990) Randomized controlled trial of general practitioner intervention in women with excessive alcohol consumption. Drug Alcohol Rev 10: 313–21.

Scragg R, Stewart A, Jackson R, et al. (1987) Alcohol and exercise in myocardial infarction and sudden coronary death in men and women. Am J Epidemiol 126: 77–85.

Shaper AG, Wannamethee G, Walker M (1988) Alcohol and mortality in British men: explaining the U-shaped curve. Lancet ii: 1267–73.

Sillanaukee P, Kiianmaa K, Roine R, et al. (1992) Alkoholin suurkulutuksen kriteerit. Suom Lääkäril 47: 2919–21.

Simpura J, ed. (1987) Finnish drinking habits: results from interview surveys held in 1968, 1976 and 1984. Finnish Foundation for Alcohol Studies, Helsinki.

Stockwell T, Lemmens PH (1994) Would standard drink labelling result in more accurate self-reports of alcohol consumption? Addiction 89: 1703–06.

Thun MJ, Peto R, Lopez AD, et al. (1997) Alcohol consumption and mortality among middle-aged and elderly U.S. adults. N Engl J Med 337: 1705–14.

Turner C (1990) How much alcohol is in a "standard drink"? An analysis of 125 studies. Br J Addict 85: 1171–75.

Tyson PD, Schirmuly M (1994) Memory enhancement after drinking ethanol: consolidation, interference, or response bias? Physiol Behav 56: 933–37.

Uchalik D (1979) A comparison of questionnaire and self-monitored reports of alcohol intake in a nonalcoholic population. Addict Behav 4: 409–13.

van 't Veer P, Kok FJ, Hermus RJ, et al. (1989) Alcohol dose, frequency and age at first exposure in relation to the risk of breast cancer. Int J Epidemiol 18: 511–17.

Verschuren PM (ed) (1993) Health Issues Related to Alcohol Consumption. ILSI Europe, Brussels.

Vogel-Sprott M (1974) Defining "light" and "heavy" social drinking; research implications and hypotheses. Q J Stud Alcohol 35: 1388–92.

Wallace P, Cutler S, Haines A (1988) Randomised trial of general practitioner intervention in patients with excessive alcohol consumption. Br Med J 297: 663–68.

Wallgren H, Barry H III (1970) Actions of alcohol, vol. 1. Elsevier, Amsterdam, pp. 189–90.

Wannamethee SG, Shaper AG (1996) Patterns of alcohol intake and risk of stroke in middle-aged British men. Stroke 27: 1033–39.

Wannamethee SG, Shaper AG (1997) Lifelong teetotallers, ex-drinkers and drinkers: mortality and the incidence of major coronary heart disease events in middle-aged British men. Int J Epidemiol 26: 523–31.

Werner M (1996) Assessing moderate alcohol consumption as a personal risk factor. Clin Chim Acta 246: 5–20.

York JL (1995) Progression of alcohol consumption across the drinking career in alcoholics and social drinkers. J Stud Alcohol 56: 328–36.

Chapter **2**

Assessment of Alcohol Consumption

J.H.M. de Vries
Wageningen Agricultural University, The Netherlands

P.H.H.M. Lemmens
Maastricht University, The Netherlands

P. Pietinen
National Public Health Institute, Helsinki, Finland

F.J. Kok
Wageningen Agricultural University, The Netherlands

Abstract

One of the major problems in health studies on alcohol is to assess alcohol intake accurately. Several methods are available but they all have their specific errors such as underreporting, overreporting or mis-estimation of portion sizes. When selecting a method it is important to define in detail the type of information required to answer the question in order to choose the best approach for assessing alcohol intake.

It is more difficult to assess the intake of alcohol than of nutrients, because alcohol is not considered a normal food constituent. It has a highly symbolic value and its consumption is influenced by cultural differences and social norms.

Methods to assess alcohol use can be divided into intrusive estimates based on self-reports and biological markers, and less intrusive estimates including collateral reports and sales figures. Self-reports may be conducted by several methods such as face-to-face interviews, telephone interviews or self-administered questionnaires. The main types of self-reports are methods asking for a summary of drinking, for example the quantity-frequency method and the lifetime drinking history, or for actual drinking, for example, diaries and recalls. Most of them can be applied easily and are relatively cheap, but they suffer from socially desirable answering. In general, self-reports are sufficiently reliable for ranking subjects according to alcohol intake and can thus be used for identifying associations between alcohol use and the outcome of disease in epidemiological studies. However, they are not accurate enough for assessing actual individual intakes needed to set sensible limits for acceptable alcohol use.

Although indirect methods are less intimidating than self-reports, it is not clear whether they are more valid. Moreover, they are not useful for assessing alcohol intake for every study purpose.

Several types of error commonly occur in the assessment of alcohol use by self-reports and collateral reports. Major examples, important to take into consideration in surveys, are selection bias, non-response, incomplete time sampling, mis-estimation of portion size and recall bias.

Biological markers of alcohol use include ethanol and methanol concentrations, liver enzymes, 5-hydroxytryptophol, HDL-cholesterol, fatty acid ethyl esters and carbohydrate-deficient transferrin. An important advantage of markers is that they are an objective measurement of intake. Biological markers differ in their suitability for assessing recent or chronic alcohol use. Because their sensitivity and specificity are relatively low, they cannot be used for assessing moderate or actual use but are, at best, suitable for the ranking of individuals according to intake.

It is clear that methods for assessing alcohol use have serious limitations, and that their errors may seriously influence the outcome of health surveys. The accuracy of self-reports appears to be very similar. Therefore, the most important task is to choose the most appropriate method for the aim of the study. Up to now, biological markers were not suitable for use in large-scale surveys. For future studies, it will be important to improve existing techniques, and to develop new and more accurate ones.

Glossary

Bias: error in the measurement

Biological marker or biological measurement: component in the body reflecting the effect of an exposure

Case-control study: a study in which subjects are selected according to their disease status and further classified according to their exposure status

Categorical analysis: statistical approach of data in which the variables of interest are classified into categories

Distributional analysis: statistical approach of data in which the distribution of the exposure in the population is determined

Epidemiological study: study in which the association between exposure and the occurrence of disease is investigated

Food frequency questionnaire: technique including a set of questions about how many times portions of specific foods are used. This technique is often applied in large-scale nutritional surveys

Non-differential reporting: non-random measurement in reports, by which subjects may be erroneously classified according to intake

Precision: lack of random error

Random measurement error: sources of variation in a measurement that cannot be predicted. The average value of many repeated measurements is the true value

Recall bias: errors in reporting by the respondents

Reliability: capacity of a technique to give the same result on repeated application

Reproducibility: reproducibility is reliability

Response effect: measurement error caused, for example, by interviewer effects, memory failure or motivation of the respondents, resulting in false reports

Selection bias: error caused by the fact that the relation between exposure and disease is different for those who participate and those who should be theoretically eligible for study, including those who do not participate

Sensitivity of the technique: the probability that someone who is truly exposed will be classified as exposed by the technique

Specificity of the technique: the probability that someone who is truly unexposed will be classified as unexposed

Systematic measurement error: non-random sources of variation. The mean of repeated measures does not approach the true value

Validity: lack of systematic error

Introduction

One of the crucial problems in clarifying the relationship between alcohol use and health outcomes is the difficulty in assessing alcohol intake accurately. It is well known that assessment of dietary intake in general is prone to errors (Willett 1998), but assessment of alcohol intake is an even larger problem because of its social stigma (Caetano 1998). Several methods have been developed for the determination of alcohol intake (Alanko 1984, Room 1998, Rehm 1998, Litten et al. 1992), but they all have their specific problems.

All methods suffer from measurement error, both systematic and random error, but the scope for error differs from method to method. Sources of error include underreporting or overreporting of intake and incorrectly estimating portion sizes. When selecting a method, it is of utmost importance to define in detail the type of information required (Beaton 1994, Cameron et al. 1988). Based on this information, and bearing in mind the study population, the available time, finances and equipment, the best method can then be selected.

In order to assess what type of information is required, Beaton (1994) suggested the following four approaches to data analyses:

(1) estimation of mean intakes of a group or comparison of mean intakes across categories of individuals

(2) distributional analyses, for example to determine the proportion of

individuals with inadequate or excessive intakes
(3) correlation and regression analyses to assess relations between intake levels and outcome measurements
(4) categorical analyses to classify individuals by intake, and by occurrence of disease, as is common in epidemiological studies.

The second approach, distributional analyses, needs the most detailed data because information is required about actual individual intake. There is a general rule that the more detailed a measure, the less reliable the assessment will be (Bingham et al. 1988). Thus, achieving accurate information using the second approach will be the most difficult. On the other hand, for the third approach, correlation and regression analyses, subjects have only to be ranked according to drinking level, which requires less accurate methods. Thus, systematic errors are acceptable in some epidemiological studies because they occur in a linear fashion over the whole range of intake, but are not suitable in distributional analyses (Willett 1998).

Furthermore, it is important to select a method appropriate for the population or subgroup to be studied because they may differ in drinking behaviour (Caetano 1998, Fitzgerald et al. 1987). This means that for patients different approaches have to be selected than for healthy subjects, and for adults versus adolescents. Also, a method appropriate for assessing habitual alcohol use in population studies may not be suitable to identify heavy drinkers in clinical studies (Levine 1990).

A method has to be chosen for the right reference period. For example, if one wants to know whether moderate alcohol use protects against coronary heart disease, it is important which reference period one has in mind when asking this question. Is it current alcohol use or intake over a longer period of time (Lemmens et al. 1995)?

Thus, in selecting a method it is important to define in detail the type of information required to answer the question in order to choose the best approach for assessing alcohol intake, bearing in mind the type of information required. Therefore, an overview is provided of specific problems in the assessment of alcohol intake, the most frequently used methods, their suitability for different purposes, and their pros and cons. This overview is limited to healthy subjects and does not include patients or subjects who suffer from alcohol abuse.

Problems of Assessing Alcohol Use in Surveys

There are several reasons why it is more difficult to assess alcohol intake accurately than, for example, energy intake. An important reason is that alcohol intake may vary extensively (Fitzgerald et al. 1987, Göransson et al. 1994) among cultures and also between and within subjects. Social norms and their relationship to drinking play an important role in these differences (Caetano 1998). An example given by Ahlström (Caetano 1998) illustrates this point. In many countries alcohol is generally drunk between meals. People in these countries may, for example, enjoy a glass of wine in the afternoon. However, for many other cultures drinking between meals is indicative of alcohol dependence.

Cultural differences are also expressed in the variety of settings in which alcohol is consumed. In some populations alcohol is only drunk during meals, whereas in other populations it is associated with certain events, for example, as an aside to watching TV, sporting events or other social activities (Caetano 1998). In addition, the number of different types of alcoholic beverages consumed varies from country to country. In some countries, such as Hungary and Italy, most subjects drink just one type, namely wine, whereas in other countries, such as Belgium and Denmark, a broader range of beverages is consumed.

Large differences in drinking patterns exist not only between but also within populations. Individual drinking behaviour is strongly determined by social context and norms. Alcohol is often drunk in the company of other people and can be seen as a highly symbolic activity. Some drink small amounts frequently whereas others drink large amounts infrequently (Chenet et al. 1997). Also, moderate drinking can alternate with binge drinking and heavy drinking may change to non-drinking.

Drinking patterns also differ between men and women and among age categories (Caetano 1998). Women drink substantially less than men (Lemmens 1991) and probably show larger variations in their drinking pattern over the year (Lemmens et al. 1993, Lemmens 1998). Also, young people have drinking patterns that differ from those of adults. For example, the proportion of abstainers is much lower among young people than among the elderly (Caetano 1998).

Subjects also vary in motives to drink. It is important to know why they drink in order to correctly interpret study results because some reasons, for example reduction of stress, may interfere with the outcome of disease and cause bias (Lemmens et al. 1995).

Although it is not always possible to take into account all of the problems mentioned, it is important to be aware of the fact that alcohol is often not seen as a food constituent but has a highly symbolic value. Whenever possible, methods to assess alcohol intake should be selected or adjusted such that measurement errors due to these problems are avoided.

Methods Used to Assess Alcohol Use

The methods or techniques available to assess alcohol use include intrusive estimates based on self-reports and biological markers and less obtrusive ones such as collateral reports and sales figures (Litten et al. 1992, Midanik 1982, 1988, Fenekes et al. 1999, Rehm 1998).

Self-Reports

Methods based on self-reports include interviews, self-administered questionnaires, and diaries (Table 1). The quality of the data collected by these methods is not only determined by the order and the structure of the questions asked, but also by the mode of the report and characteristics of the respondent, such as their age and culture (Caetano 1998).

Modes of Self-Reports (Willett 1990, Rehm 1998)

An important feature of a method is the mode in which it is administered. Modes of self-reporting include face-to-face interviews, telephone interviews, diaries and records administered by computer or by tape. Not every mode is suitable for every study: the best mode of self-reporting depends on the research question and on the study population or sub-group (Cameron et al. 1988). For instance, if only a limited number of respondents in a population is literate, a diary is not a good choice, and in remote areas a face-to-face interview will not be a real option. Thus, every mode has its pros and cons.

An advantage of *a face-to-face interview* is that the interviewer may help the respondent by reminding him or her of the occasions of intake, or may ask additional questions to clarify an answer. The use of key questions and memory aids may be crucial to obtain accurate information about the type and quantity of the beverages consumed.

Table 1
Overview of methods to assess alcohol use

Self-reports
  Modes
    face-to-face interview
    telephone interview
    self-administered questionnaire
    diary
    taped question
    computer interview
  Types
  summary of drinking
    quantity-frequency method
    extended quantity-frequency method
    graduated frequency method
    periodic-specific normal week
    lifetime drinking history
  actual drinking
    prospective and retrospective diaries
    recall method

Non-intrusive measurements
  Types
    collateral report
    official record
    other: randomized response, bogus-pipeline
    direct observation, refuse analysis

On the other hand, the results of this type of interview may be affected by interviewer bias, i.e. error due to the influence of the interviewer, for example, by behavioural factors, and social desirability (Willett 1998). Social desirability is a response effect caused by a perceived threat. Thus, when the perceived threat is high, a larger response effect is to be expected. There are large individual and cultural differences in the perception of threats. An example is that heavy drinkers may feel threatened when their drinking is discussed but moderate drinkers may even think they are doing the right thing and feel no threat. This will lead to differences in response between both groups of drinkers.

An *interview by telephone* (Cohen et al. 1995) has the same advantages as the personal interview but is probably less threatening and may hence suffer less from the tendency to give socially desirable answers. On the other hand, respondents may feel less involved in the study because they do not have visual contact with the interviewer. This probably explains the lower response rates for this method. Other disadvantages of this method are that no visual aids can be used, less time is available and the environment of the interview may be less controlled by the interviewer.

Self-administered questionnaires may be handed out or sent by mail. Important advantages of *questionnaires* are that they are cheaper and less confronting than interviews. However, they cannot always be applied because the respondents have to be more or less literate, depending on the complexity of the questionnaire. Also, they have lower response rates than interviews (Rehm 1998). Other disadvantages of this mode are that respondents, intentionally or unintentionally, miss questions or provide unclear answers. Also, control over the situation is less for self-administered questionnaires than for personal interviews, and therefore the setting in which the questions are administered could be a matter of concern. For example, questionnaires administered to adolescents in their classroom may be less threatening than those completed at home, and may therefore yield more reliable results (Caetano 1998).

Self-reports by *diaries* also require respondents to be literate. Another problem of this method is that respondents become aware of their behaviour during the period of recording and tend to change their behaviour towards more acceptable norms (Schoeller 1990).

For a group of respondents who are not literate and who would prefer to hear the questions rather than read them, the questions could be administered by the use of *taped questions* on a "walkman" (Caetano 1998). In general, new automated techniques (Midanik 1998) could make certain methods cheaper and more accessible. One example of such a technique is the touch-tone phone (Searles et al. 1995) used to record intake on the previous day over a longer period. The use of *computerized interviews* might also lead to less socially desirable answering, resulting in higher values of reported alcohol intake (Midanik 1988).

Finally, data on alcohol use may be collected as part of a complete nutritional assessment. This may be an advantage because in that context respondents are less aware of answering sensitive questions about their alcohol use and this might give more reliable answers (King 1998).

TYPE OF METHOD

Techniques to assess alcohol use can be roughly classified into methods that ask for a summary of drinking, such as quantity-frequency methods and lifetime drinking histories, and methods that ask for actual current intake, such as prospective and retrospective diaries and recall methods (Rehm 1998, Feunekes et al. 1999, Litten et al. 1992). Techniques can differ in the way they are conducted, the assessment mode and the reference period they are supposed to cover. Some methods ask for alcohol in general, whereas others may ask for specific beverages. Data may also be collected as part of a complete nutritional assessment or as part of a life-style questionnaire.

METHODS THAT ASK FOR A SUMMARY OF DRINKING

The hypothesis of quantity-frequency methods is that people report their modal frequency and modal quantity, such that their habitual alcohol use can be calculated by multiplying reported frequency and quantity. Thus, respondents are asked to summarize their alcohol intake and to report their typical consumption over a certain period of time, usually between one month and one year (Lemmens et al. 1992).

For most studies, it is important to assess both frequency and quantity, for example when the relationship of alcohol use with coronary heart disease is being investigated. If the questionnaires are limited to questions about the frequency of drinking, no information is provided about level and variability of consumption (Levine 1990).

The quantity-frequency method (Feunekes et al. 1999)

The simplest technique in this category is the quantity-frequency method, in which respondents are asked to report their usual daily use of any alcoholic beverage. It consists in one question to assess the average frequency (how often do you drink?) combined with one question about the average quantity drunk (how many drinks per occasion?).

The extended quantity-frequency method (Feunekes et al. 1999)

In order to take the variability of drinking behaviour into account and to avoid bias related to unstable drinking patterns, the quantity-frequency method is sometimes extended to include questions on variability of drinking habits. This extended method is called the extended quantity-frequency method or the quantity-frequency-variability method (Lemmens et al. 1992). Questions added to the questionnaire concern the respondent's alcohol use during specific periods such as during the weekend and periods of heavy drinking, and where the alcohol is consumed, for example, at home or in a bar.

The graduated frequency method (Feunekes et al. 1999)
The graduated frequency method also accounts for variability in drinking patterns. Frequency of alcohol use is estimated over the full range of quantities consumed. Thus, alcohol use is estimated first for the largest quantity drunk and consecutively for all smaller amounts.

Period-specific normal week (Rehm 1998, Romelsjö et al. 1995)
Another method dealing with variability in intake is the period-specific normal week (PSNW) technique. Respondents answer questions about alcohol use during a typical week. Because intake is reported for a whole week, this technique accounts for differences in consumption between workdays and weekend days.

Lifetime drinking history (Lemmens 1998b, Russell et al. 1997)
Researchers may want to cover drinking over a more extended period of time (Lemmens 1998b, Swanson et al. 1997) to investigate, for example, relations between chronic, long-term alcohol use and the occurrence of disease in epidemiological studies. With a history of lifetime drinking the respondent is asked to summarize drinking behaviour over a long period of time, sometimes over their lifetime. The lifetime history method may be obtained either by a face-to-face interview or by a self-administered questionnaire.

METHODS THAT ASK FOR ACTUAL DRINKING

The principle underlying these methods is that respondents recall or record what they actually have drunk in the recent past, sometimes immediately after consumption.

Prospective and retrospective diaries (Feunekes et al. 1999)
For self-reports based on a diary respondents record their alcohol intake for specific days in a booklet or diary. The respondents may report their consumption either prospectively or retrospectively. The greater the number of days included in the survey, the more the variability of intake is taken into account. However, an instant and steady decline in the number of reported drinks has been observed in some monitoring studies (W. Dijkstra, personal communication).

Recall methods (Feunekes et al. 1999)

These methods consist of a series of (random) recalls of use over a period short enough for the respondent to remember the actual intake of alcohol. It may be helpful to ask time-reference questions, for example about employment or residence. One 24-hour recall or only a few will not be sufficient to assess habitual alcohol use because the number is too limited to account for variability in intake.

The Time-Line Follow-Back method is an example of a so-called aided or assisted recall method. By this method respondents recall their intake day-by-day with the help of a calendar or other memory cues. A specific and popular example is the weekly recall method. As the name of the method indicates, respondents recall retrospectively their drinking 7 days before the day of the interview (Lemmens et al. 1992). Recalls should not cover a period longer than 1 or 2 weeks because accurate reporting declines considerably when the reference period is extended (Mäkelä 1971).

ADVANTAGES AND DISADVANTAGES OF SELF-REPORTS

Advantages and disadvantages of self-reports in general

Self-reports are suitable for use in small studies and in large-scale surveys for epidemiological research. They can be easily applied and most of them are relatively cheap, depending on the effort needed to gather the data. Self-reports are non-invasive, unlike many biological markers, and they can easily be adjusted to the needs of the survey. In addition, they can provide beverage-specific information.

The most important disadvantage of these methods is that questions about drinking are threatening and may easily yield socially desirable answers. However, in an anonymous questionnaire this problem is partly removed. Another general problem of self-reports is that the memory capacity of respondents is limited.

Advantages and disadvantages of modes of self-reports

Not each mode of administration is suitable for each study group. For example, in many parts of the world, reaching respondents by phone or mail or interviewing them face-to-face could be difficult or not acceptable (Caetano 1998). For mailed questionnaires and diaries, people have to be literate and motivated. Response rates to telephone interviews appear to be lower than to personal interviews. However, it was shown recently that response rates are increasing, which will improve the quality of results (de Leeuw 1992). It is important to evaluate the costs of the methods, the skills of the staff, the purpose of the study and the characteristics of the respondents to make the best choice of mode.

Advantages and disadvantages of methods that ask about a summary of drinking

An important advantage of these methods is that they may cover a longer period of time. A shortcoming is that respondents report their modal drinking, whereas the researcher is mostly interested in average drinking (Duffy et al. 1992). Moreover, these methods do not account for variability in alcohol use. Although one may correct for episodes of atypical drinking, there is neither a standard procedure nor knowledge of the way respondents estimate their alcohol use. It is thought to be a cognitively difficult task to summarize drinking behaviour (Midanik et al. 1991).

Although more complex frequency methods deal better with the problem of variability and averaging intake, they may have higher non-response rates (Rehm 1998), especially when the questions are administered in the form of questionnaires. Also lifetime drinking histories suffer from response and memory error, but if one is interested in chronic long-term alcohol use it is the only possible method.

Frequency methods may be administered by personal interviews or by mailed questionnaires. They both require experienced research groups. Face-to-face interviews require trained interviewers and questionnaire experts able to devise questionnaires with high quality on the wording of the questions, routing, lay-out and pre-testing. Obviously, it is less troublesome if questionnaires validated for the population of interest can be used.

Advantages and disadvantages of methods that ask about actual drinking

An important advantage of methods that ask about actual drinking is that respondents do not have to evaluate their drinking pattern but can directly recall or report what they actually consume. Furthermore, diaries and recall methods often provide information about specific beverages.

A problem of these methods is that they are sensitive to temporal variation in individual drinking behaviour. They provide data about actual drinking over a certain period of time and are, therefore, capable of demonstrating variability between drinking occasions. However, the shorter the recall period and the larger the time variation, the more likely it is that these methods do not cover typical periods (Lemmens et al. 1992) and are not representative of usual intake (Romelsjö et al. 1995).

On the other hand, the accuracy of recalls decreases rapidly with a longer reference period. That is why the diary method is thought to be better than the weekly recall: there is a shorter interval between consumption and reporting.

A specific disadvantage of a diary is that people become aware of their behaviour and, therefore, tend to change their drinking pattern. In addition, diaries may be impractical to use in epidemiological studies and probably suffer from selection bias: the proportion of abstainers will often be higher than with other methods (Rehm 1998).

Although aided recalls yield higher estimates of alcohol use, it is questionable whether they are always the best choice. Aided recalls take a lot of time in interviews, they are costly and it is not yet clear if they improve accuracy.

Finally, depending on the mode of administration, some methods may have to deal with interviewer effects.

ACCURACY OF METHODS BASED ON SELF-REPORTED INTAKES

Under- and over-reporting

It is difficult to determine whether self-reports underestimate or overestimate actual intake because gold standards against which assessment techniques can be validated are lacking. Sometimes, sales figures are used as a reference (Midanik 1982, 1988) but, as will be discussed, these have their own problems. As a consequence, only so-called convergent validity can be determined by comparing one method with another. A high correlation between two methods does not necessarily mean that a method is valid because errors of methods are often interrelated, for example when they both suffer from underreporting (Willett 1998).

An assumption often made in the literature is that higher estimates of alcohol intake are more valid because they cover a larger part of sales figures. This may be true for the average consumption of a population but higher individual intakes may also be biased because of overreporting. Also, the extent of underreporting is not necessarily the same for all subjects. For example, heavy drinkers might be more likely to underreport their alcohol use than light drinkers. In addition, heavy drinkers are thought to be less likely to participate in surveys than other groups. Therefore, it is not a real option to correct estimated alcohol use for a specific factor as is sometimes done.

Conclusions of reviews comparing different methods of self-reporting are not consistent. Feunekes et al. (1999) have reviewed 33 methodological papers published between 1984 and 1995 in which alcohol intake was assessed by different types of self-reports. They showed that the mean level of intake estimated by retrospective diaries was 20% lower than that estimated by quantity-frequency methods or prospective diaries. This finding is not in line with reviews that report higher estimates for diaries than for quantity-frequency methods (Rehm 1998, Lemmens et al. 1992, Midanik 1988).

The inconsistent results of these reviews could be caused by differences in the way the methods are administered. For example, the context or the time frames in which questionnaires were applied probably differed among studies (Feunekes et al. 1999, Rehm 1998). It has been shown that studies in which questions about alcohol intake are embedded in a food frequency questionnaire show better agreement with diaries (Flegal 1990, Giovanucci et al. 1998).

Some studies corroborate the notion that the more supportive the information that is given the better is the recall (Romelsjö et al. 1995). A large number and a large range of answering categories may indeed increase reported intakes (Hughes et al. 1988). An example is the graduated frequency method, which consistently results in higher estimates of intake than the quantity-frequency method (Rehm 1998). Also, a period-specific normal week (PSNW) method yields higher estimates than an unspecific quantity-frequency method, especially in societies where weekend drinking is common (Rehm 1998). Another example is a 30-day recall differentiating for beverage and depending on memory, which appeared to be more efficacious and valid than other methods (Embree et al. 1998). On the other hand, if a questionnaire becomes too complex, it may increase non-response. In addition, for some purposes a simple question could be as valid as an extended questionnaire (Parker et al. 1996, Feunekes et al. 1999), and then it is probably better to select the least complicated method.

In line with the idea that the more is asked, the higher the estimates of alcohol use will be, beverage-specific questions yield higher estimates than questions asking only for total alcohol use (Rehm 1998). When the type of beverage, such as beer, wine or spirits, was asked, estimates were about 20% higher (Feunekes et al. 1999). Thus, if the assumption is true that higher estimates are more valid, beverage-specific questions improve the validity of the method. On the other hand, too many questions may result in overreporting. Also, bias may be introduced when reporting errors differ among the various beverage types. The difference in mortality pattern found in some studies (Rimm et al. 1996) between subject groups differing in intake of wine, beer or spirits might be explained by this type of reporting error. Thus, light wine drinkers would have to overreport while heavy drinkers of spirits would have to underreport their intake. Other studies (Ferraroni et al. 1996, Grönbæk et al. 1996), however, demonstrate that reporting errors are similar for wine, beer and spirits and that they cannot explain the different mortality patterns seen between groups with different drinking patterns (Farraoni et al. 1996, Grönbæk et al. 1996).

Additional questions about drinking patterns and the context of drinking also provided higher estimates of alcohol use (Göransson et al. 1994, Single et al. 1994). However, overlap between different contexts might also result in overreporting (Rehm 1998).

In some cultures underreporting could be greater than in others (Romelsjö et al. 1995, Moreiras et al. 1996). This could be due to differences in drinking patterns among countries. It is assumed that regular patterns are easier to recall than patterns with a wide variability (Lemmens et al. 1992). Under-coverage could be caused, for example, by underreporting of heavy drinking. The average level of intake is probably less important because populations with a light alcohol use of about 4 drinks per week report in a similar way as those with a higher level of about 10 drinks per week (Feunekes et al. 1999). Also, reporting could be more reliable in countries where drinking is a socially acceptable habit. In the Seneca study, a better relative validity of reported alcohol intake was seen for the southern than for the northern centres (van Staveren et al. 1996, Moreiras et al. 1996).

Not only differences between types of technique but also between specific features within similar techniques are thought to cause either underreporting or overreporting. For instance, questionnaires only asking about frequencies are more prone to underreporting than questionnaires asking about both frequency and quantity (Lemmens et al. 1992, Alanko 1984). In addition, it has been suggested that the duration of the reference method or the mode of administration could play a role. However, this could not be confirmed by Feunekes et al (1999).

Reproducibility and validity of self-reports

In general, self-reports are reliable in a clinical or research setting, where subjects do not drink alcohol and questionnaires are processed anonymously and confidentially. Test-retest correlations appear to be reasonably good for self-reported intakes. Feunekes et al. (1999) calculated weighted averages from 11 studies (Pietinen et al. 1988, Giovanucci et al. 1998, Munger et al. 1992, Ocké et al. 1996, Midanik et al. 1989, 1994, Williams et al. 1985, 1994, Lemmens et al. 1992, Longnecker et al. 1992, Webb et al. 1991) of 0.84–0.88, ranging from 0.75 to 0.99 in the separate studies (Table 2). Of course, these high correlations might be explained by consistent under- or overreporting by the same method.

Assessment of alcohol intake embedded in food frequency questionnaires show high reproducibility, especially if compared with other food items (King 1994). These questionnaires are probably less threatening than alcohol-specific questionnaires, which show lower test-retest associations (Rehm 1998, Feunekes et al. 1999, Embree et al. 1991). Nevertheless, serious misclassification of alcohol intake by food frequency questionnaires is seen between non-drinkers and moderate drinkers (Ferraroni et al. 1996). Thus, a food frequency questionnaire is probably only a valid method to collect data on alcohol intake in regular drinkers.

There are only small differences in reproducibility between the various techniques, as reviewed by Feunekes et al (Table 2). Also, the reliability of lifetime drinking estimates (Lemmens 1998b) is, in general, quite acceptable. Reproducibility correlation coefficients for these methods range between 0.67 and 0.90.

In addition, the association between different methods, the relative validity, appears to be quite acceptable. Feunekes et al. (1999) calculated weighted averages from 12 studies between 0.63 and 0.73 (Table 2), ranging from 0.32 to 0.90 in separate studies.

Table 2
Ranking of individuals according to alcohol use: weighted averages of test-retest and validity correlations[a] of currently available methods[b]

Method	QF	Extended QF	RD	PD	24-h recall
QF	0.88 (0.75–0.99) $n = 1211$	–	–	–	–
Ext. QF	0.63 (0.59–0.90) $n = 24045$	0.88 (0.83–0.98) $n = 317$	–	–	–
RD	0.67 (0.66–0.74) $n = 5855$	0.66 (0.66)	n.a.	–	–
PD	0.71 (0.61–0.90) $n = 1722$	0.73 (0.57–0.89) $n = 2002$	0.65 (0.51–0.65) $n = 948$	0.84 (0.84) $n = 399$	–
24-h recall (series)	0.68 (0.32–0.90) $n = 165$	n.a.	n.a.	n.a.	n.a.

[a] Test-retest correlations are on the diagonal axis; all others are correlations between methods. In parenthesis: range (minimum and maximum value). n = total number of subjects included.

[b] QF, quantity-frequency method; Ext. QF, extended quantity-frequency method; RD, retrospective diary; PD, prospective diary. n.a., no data available.

After: Feunekes et al. (1999)

For the validity of a method it is also important to know whether there is a linear or a non-linear relationship between true and reported consumption (Figure 1) or, in other words, whether there is differential or non-differential misclassification. If underreporting is linearly related to the level of intake, serious bias in estimates of health risks can occur, but it will still be possible to rank subjects according to their alcohol intake. Therefore, correlation or regression analysis, the third approach suggested by Beaton (1994), may perform well. However, if underreporting is non-linearly related to the level of intake, it will not be possible to rank subjects properly. Feunekes et al. (1999) found an indication of systematic or non-differential reporting errors, as the differences in underreporting between the methods were larger at high than at low intakes. In addition, several studies show that incidental, unusually high alcohol intake is underreported (Romelsjö et al. 1995). However, other studies report that errors are, in general, linearly related to intake (Lemmens 1991), and also Feunekes et al. (1999) conclude that individuals can be classified reasonably well according to their drinking level.

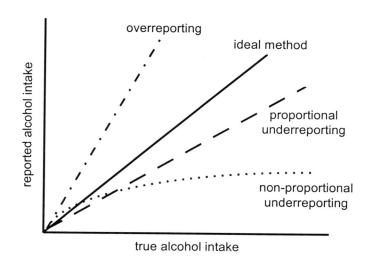

Figure 1
**Alcohol intake reporting: hypothetical curves of reported
alcohol use versus true intake. After: Feunekes et al. (1999)**

Thus, associations between alcohol intake and disease or health can be validated by self-reporting in epidemiological studies. However, because it is not possible to determine the actual level of alcohol consumption by self-reports, it is difficult to set sensible limits for acceptable intake.

Non-intrusive Estimates (Table 1)

Some estimates of alcohol intake are more indirect than self-reports because respondents are not aware of them. An advantage could be that they are less threatening and more objective. However, these assessments have their own disadvantages.

TYPES OF NON-INTRUSIVE ESTIMATES

Collateral reports (Midanik 1982)

Collateral reports are provided by a significant "other" person, for example, a spouse or a friend. These reports are often used to test the validity of self-reports (Midanik 1988). Studies using collateral reporting as a reference method are not consistent in their conclusions about the validity of self-reports: they range from not being accurate at all to being extremely accurate (Caetano 1998, Lemmens 1991, Midanik

1988). Some important factors affecting the accuracy of these reports are the perceived threat of the interview situation, the subject's daily routine making behaviour more or less predictable, and the frequency of contact between the subject and the collateral (Midanik 1982, Lemmens 1991).

Official records

Per capita sales figures are often used to determine alcohol use in a population. The accuracy of estimates of consumption depends on the accuracy of sales statistics and on the validity of the assumption that alcoholic beverages sold in a particular period are equivalent to consumption in that period (Lemmens et al. 1992). A major drawback of sales figures is that they do not provide information about alcohol consumption in certain groups or individuals. For example, for some age categories they will overestimate intake, while for others they will underestimate intake. This could be one of the reasons why sales figures are often not comparable to self-reports (Midanik 1988). Other reasons are that sales reports do not include untaxed alcohol, such as alcohol sold in duty-free shops, and home-brewn alcohol (Midanik 1982).

Other techniques

There are other possibilities for assessing alcohol consumption indirectly. These include the randomized response technique (the respondent may choose between a sensitive and a non-sensitive question), the bogus-pipeline (the respondent is told that the questionnaire is cross-checked with a physiological test), direct observation and refuse analysis.

ADVANTAGES AND DISADVANTAGES OF INDIRECT ESTIMATES

Indirect methods are less threatening than self-reports (Lemmens 1991), and therefore socially desirable answers are less likely. However, because a gold standard is lacking it is very hard to say whether self-reports or indirect methods, such as collateral reports, provide the most valid individual intake data.

Several studies (Midanik 1982, Höyer et al. 1999, Single et al. 1994) have shown that self-reported alcohol use in population surveys covers only 40–60% of alcohol sales. Nevertheless, sales figures may underestimate consumption because they do not include all alcoholic beverages available and do not provide information for specific population groups. Therefore, sales figures are more suitable for ecological studies to assess differences in intake of the population over time than to estimate individual consumption.

Sources and Assessment of Errors (Lemmens et al. 1991)

There are several types of error that commonly occur in the assessment of alcohol use (Table 3). These cannot be completely avoided but, if the type and sources of error are known, it is at least possible to account for them when interpreting the results. Therefore, it is important to assess any possible errors in a survey.

NON-COVERAGE OF THE SOURCE POPULATION

This type of error is introduced if the source population is not covered by the study population. An example is found in sales figures which could provide overestimation for a specific age category. When sales figures are used as a reference for self-reports, the false conclusion could be drawn that self-reported intakes are under-estimated. This type of error can be demonstrated by determination of alcohol use in sub-samples not covered by the sampling frame.

SELECTION BIAS

A common error in epidemiological studies is selection bias in the reference group (Rehm 1998, Ruchlin 1997). For example, a reference group of non-drinkers may consist of both former drinkers and lifetime abstainers. Both groups are very different because a large number of former drinkers have stopped drinking for health reasons, which may not be true for lifetime abstainers. In addition, young abstainers differ markedly from older ones. To assess and avoid this type of selection bias, it is necessary to distinguish between the various subgroups by asking additional questions about the drinking history of the respondents (Rehm 1998).

Non-Response (Embree et al. 1991)

Rates of non-response may be substantial but differ considerably among surveys (Lemmens 1988). They are influenced by the mode and type of assessment and by the type of respondents (Rehm 1998). High non-response rates may attenuate the association between alcohol use and the disease outcome. As a result, associations that are really present cannot be demonstrated. Non-response may seriously influence

Table 3
Possible sources, types and assessment of errors

Source of error	Type of error	Assessment of error
Non-coverage of the target population	Overestimation or underestimation of mean intake	Assessment in sub-samples not covered
Selection bias	Non-drinkers may be ex-drinkers or lifetime abstainers	Assessment of drinking history
Non-response	Selective non-response: underestimation	Follow-up of non-response
Incomplete time sampling	Under- or overestimation	Spreading of self-reports over the reference period
Use of standard units	Probably underestimation	Conversion into a standard glass; assessment of the deviation from a standard glass
Recall bias	Under- or overestimation	Assessment of the length of the recall period by a diary method; comparison with collateral reports
Temporal variation of individual drinking	Underestimation	Questions about incidental, heavy drinking

the outcome of life-style surveys when the tendency to respond is related either to drinking behaviour or to the health risk. This could occur when a large proportion of non-responders consists of heavy drinkers. When the relation is equivalent in both responders and non-responders, then the non-response only affects the precision of the estimate (Lemmens 1988).

Item non-response is another type of non-response error. In this case, some items in the questionnaires are not filled in or answered by a number of respondents. When specific groups of responders are more likely than others not to respond to a given item, this may be a serious form of bias.

To find out whether error is introduced by non-response it is recommended to perform a follow-up in the group of non-responders. Although it is not clear whether non-response rates affect the outcome of surveys seriously, it is advisable to keep non-response rates as low as possible and to collepct information on characteristics of non-responders.

It may be difficult to determine the appropriate reference period, but it is necessary to do this because temporal variation in drinking affects the estimates of alcohol use (Lemmens et al. 1993, Istvan et al. 1995). Often the reference period chosen is too short. In studies with a limited time frame, serious bias can be expected to occur due to, for example, seasonal variation (Lemmens et al. 1993, Fitzgerald et al. 1987, Uitenbroek 1996). The extent of bias depends on the drinking pattern of the population (Duffy et al. 1992). A problem is that it is not always clear from the purpose of the study how long the reference period needs to be. Is it, for example, always necessary to assess lifetime intake when investigating the relationship of alcohol use with disease? When the behaviour is very stable over a lifetime or when, in other words, the correlations with alcohol intake over the years are invariably high, then it is not necessary to pry into the subject's past. However, data such as the age at onset of drinking will still be important for assessing lifetime alcohol exposure. Therefore, before starting a study, it is important to consider carefully whether it is sufficient to rely on assessment of short-term measurement of alcohol use only or if possible changes in drinking pattern over time have to be included (Lemmens et al. 1997).

Use of Unit-Standard Drink Size (Lemmens 1994a, b, Stockwell 1994)

Total alcohol use derived from self-reports is calculated as the alcohol concentration of the beverages multiplied by the capacity of the glass or container summed for all drinks. Alcohol concentration and volume may vary considerably in terms of time, region and individuals.

There is often a discrepancy between the presumed and actual alcohol content of a beverage. Therefore, it is important to check or add the alcohol content of the beverages in the composition table before starting a survey. For this purpose, it would be helpful if food composition tables included more detailed information about the types and sources of beverages and the analytical methods used.

An even larger and more stubborn problem is the error introduced by the use of unit-standard drink sizes. An important aspect is self-reported drinks consumed at home which contain more alcohol than the presumed standard of 10–15 g per drink. Often the respondent is asked to convert the size of their glasses to standardized units, which is not a good idea because it introduces new errors.

The magnitude of error introduced by the use of standard units probably depends on the type of beverage consumed: it appears to be larger for spirits than for fortified wine and is smallest for wine. This finding is supported by studies comparing self-reports with sales figures which show that spirits show the lowest coverage.

Simply asking people about the number of drinks they consume will thus lead to biased estimates of alcohol use. The researcher needs to get acquainted with the units commonly used in the population under survey. These units are mainly culturally determined. However, even within cultures or populations, respondents are not always consistent in their use of a glass or container. For example, in the Netherlands bottled beer is mostly drunk at home but draught beer in a bar. Thus, for a Dutch survey the best solution is probably to assess the capacity of the glasses most frequently used at home and to use standardized units for out of home drinks.

To avoid this type of error, the number of bottles, cans and glasses should be carefully converted into standard units, or the mean deviation from the standard sizes of the most habitually consumed drinks should be measured.

RECALL BIAS

Several social and psychological factors (Single et al. 1994) could introduce recall bias. Self-reports may be inaccurate either because the intoxicating properties of alcohol influence a subject's memory or because it is difficult to report actual alcohol intake. Respondents may intentionally leave out drinks, underestimate amounts consumed, change their drinking pattern on reporting days or provide socially desirable answers. A specific problem of recall bias occurs when respondents do not mention their actual drinking level since their drinking behaviour changed prior to the assessment, for example, because of the presence of disease (Lemmens et al. 1995). To avoid serious recall bias, it is recommended to limit the recall period to a maximum of 1 week.

In some studies recall bias from self-reports could be assessed by comparison with collateral reports. However, this is hard to achieve in case-control studies in which subjects know that alcohol use is related to their disease.

To develop questionnaires in different cultures or circumstances, it is important to assure beforehand that questions are clear and that the wording is optimal. One way to do this is to ask people to think aloud about the questions asked. Combinations of frequency and quantity used have to be adapted to the cultural usage of alcohol. At the simplest level, it has to be possible to identify and classify the different beverages drunk by various population groups in different countries.

Men and women appear to report their intake equally well (Lemmens 1991), although better agreement between different methods has been reported in men (Grönbæk et al. 1996, Romelsjö et al. 1995). It has been suggested that women are more comfortable with answering questions about alcohol use in an anonymous questionnaire. In general, there seems to be little reason to treat men and women in a methodologically different fashion.

TEMPORAL VARIATION IN INDIVIDUAL DRINKING

If temporal variation in drinking behaviour is not taken into account, alcohol use is likely to be underestimated because periods of heavy drinking are likely to be excluded. To avoid this type of error, it is necessary to ask questions about incidental heavy drinking.

Inaccurate assessments of alcohol intake are a serious problem because they affect the estimates of alcohol-related health risks (Lemmens 1998a, Lemmens et al. 1995). If random error is large or, in other words, if precision is low, risk will be underestimated. If systematic errors occur, interpretation of the results becomes even more complex because these may result in over- or underestimation of risk or protection. The consequences of a specific error may vary for different types of research questions.

Biological Markers of Alcohol Intake (Litten en al. 1992)

Several biological markers have been reported to be related to alcohol consumption (Table 4). However, none of these markers is suitable for assessing the actual level of intake, and therefore they can only be used to rank individuals according to their intake. Suitable markers for ranking have to be specific and sensitive to consumption of alcohol intake over the whole range of intake (Willett 1998).

Table 4
Characteristics of biological markers of alcohol use

Marker	Purpose	Estimated sensitivity (sens.) and specificity (spec.)	Source
Ethanol in serum, breath or urine	recent intake (2–6 h)	sens. 25%, spec. 100%	Litten et al. 1992, Hellander et al. 1996
Methanol in body fluids or breath	recent (5–15 h) and chronic intake	higher sensitivity than ethanol	Litten et al. 1992
MCV of erythrocytes	chronic intake	sens. 35%, spec. 40–90%	Litten et al. 1992, van Pelt et al. 1997
Erythrocyte acetaldehyde in plasma	recent intake (several days)	low sensitivity	Litten en al. 1992, Rosman et al. 1994
Transferases (GGT, ASAT, ALAT) in serum	chronic intake, screening	GGT: sens. 45%, spec. 75%; ASAT and ALAT: lower than for GGT	van Pelt et al. 1997, Rosman et al. 1994
5-Hydroxytryptophol in urine	recent intake (6–15 h)	sens. 70%, spec. 95%	Helander et al. 1996
HDL in serum	recent and chronic, moderate and high intake	sens. 30%	Litten et al. 1992, Rosman et al. 1994
FAEE in serum	recent intake (24 h)	higher sensitivity than ethanol	Doyle et al. 1996, Laposata et al. 1997
CDT in serum	chronic excessive intake, screening	sens. 75%, spec. 90%	van Pelt et al. 1997, Stibler et al. 1991
AANB in serum	chronic intake, monitoring	low sensitivity	Litten et al. 1992

MCV: mean corpuscular volume   GGT: γ-glutamyltransferase
ASAT: aspartate aminotranferase   ALAT: alanine aminotransferase
HDL: high-density lipo-protein   FAEE: fatty acid ethyl esters
CDT: carbohydrate-deficient transferrin   AANB: α-amino-N-butyric acid

An overview of markers presented in the literature for assessment of alcohol intake is discussed below. The markers will now be evaluated on their suitability to assess recent, habitual or chronic consumption.

TYPES OF MARKERS

Concentration of ethanol in serum, breath or urine (Levine et al. 1997, Laposata 1997)

Ethanol concentrations can only be used as markers for recent alcohol use, i.e. within the last 4–6 h, because ethanol is eliminated rapidly from the body. In urine, ethanol can be detected some hours longer than in breath or serum because urine remains in the bladder for some time.

Methanol in body fluids or breath

During ethanol metabolism, methanol increases in the body and its level remains higher for 2–6 h once ethanol in blood is no longer detectable. Thus, the sensitivity of this marker is somewhat higher than that of ethanol. Because the concentration of methanol in the body builds up slowly, higher levels may reflect chronic drinking.

Mean corpuscular volume (MCV) of red blood cells (Levine 1990)

MCV reflects dysfunctional production of red blood cells. It is used as a marker of chronic alcohol use, but its specificity is low.

Erythrocyte acetaldehyde (Rosman et al. 1994)

Acetaldehyde is the first metabolite of ethanol oxidation, and a significant amount may be bound to red blood cells for several days. Therefore, tests detecting erythrocyte acetaldehyde may be useful as screening markers of alcoholism.

γ-glutamyltransferase (GGT), alanine aminotransferase (ALAT) and aspartate aminotransferase (ASAT) in serum

These are markers of liver injury, caused by alcohol abuse. The specificity and sensitivity of GGT is relatively good, better than that of ASAT or ALAT (Levine 1990). One problem is that the concentrations of these enzymes are influenced by age, gender and body weight. Nevertheless, they are not only suitable to assess heavy drinking but also moderate drinking as was shown in a survey where increased concentrations of these enzymes could demonstrate lower drinking levels (40 g/day in men, 20 g/day in women) (Steffensen et al. 1997).

5-Hydroxytryptophol

Alcohol consumption can lead to increased production of 5-hydroxytryptophol and decreased values of 5-hydroxyindole-3-acetic acid, components of serotonin metabolism. The ratio between these two components increases with alcohol use and remains elevated for 6–15 h (Helander et al. 1996). 5-Hydroxytryptophol is more specific and sensitive to detect recent drinking than ethanol in blood, breath or urine. It is suitable for determining recent but not chronic alcohol use (Helander et al. 1996).

High-density lipoproteins (HDL) in serum

HDL-cholesterol levels are sensitive to alcohol intake (Haskell et al., 1984) and can, for example, be used to identify heavy drinkers in a clinical population. They also have been applied in some studies to validate self-reports of alcohol use (Giovanucci et al. 1998, Willett et al. 1987). In these studies, serum HDL levels appeared to be associated with alcohol use as estimated from food questionnaires and dietary records. A problem in using HDL-cholesterol as a marker of intake is that it is not only influenced by alcohol but also by other factors. Therefore, this marker can only be used as a qualitative, not as a quantitative measure of validity. Thus, if HDL-cholesterol is correlated with a questionnaire estimate of alcohol use, qualitative evidence is provided that alcohol use is being measured with at least some degree of validity.

Fatty acid ethyl esters (FAEE) in serum

FAEE are esterification products of alcohol and fatty acids. These components are still present in the blood long after ethanol has been eliminated (Laposata 1997). Therefore, this test is more sensitive to alcohol intake than tests of ethanol in serum or breath. Thus, FAEE are not only useful as a short-term confirmatory test for alcohol intake but also as a marker to prove that alcohol has been ingested in the previous 24 h (Doyle et al. 1996).

Carbohydrate-deficient transferrin (CDT) in serum (Rosman et al. 1994, Laposata 1997, Stibler 1991)

This component is seen as one of the most promising markers in alcohol assessment methodology. Chronic drinking may affect the metabolism of several glycoconjugates including transferrin. After regular heavy drinking, isoforms of serum transferrin appear that are reduced in their carbohydrate moiety. Daily alcohol use of more than 50–80 g for at least a week will result in an increased concentration of CDT in plasma. During a period of abstinence the value normalizes with a mean half-life of about 15 days. CDT is more sensitive to chronic alcohol abuse than mean corpuscular volume and transferase enzymes.

Also, CDT is relatively specific for excessive alcohol use (Rosman et al. 1994, van Pelt 1997). When CDT was combined with γ-glutamyltransferase, the predictive value of positive results in men was further increased (van Pelt 1997). It has also been suggested for use as a screening instrument to assess alcohol use in general practice patients (Meerkerk et al. 1998). Thus, CDT appears to be a very promising marker but, until now, it is only suitable as a marker for long-term heavy drinking, not for moderate drinking.

α-Amino-N-butyric acid (AANB) in serum

AANB relative to leucine appears to be a useful test for the detection of chronic drinking, especially when combined with GGT (Shaw et al. 1978).

Finally, other combinations of tests with different biomarkers might be useful. For example, GGT and CDT can identify a greater number of subjects with alcohol problems than either of them separately (Romelsjö et al. 1995, Levine 1990).

ADVANTAGES AND DISADVANTAGES OF BIOLOGICAL MARKERS

Biological markers of alcohol use could be used for clinical studies of alcoholics, to monitor change in drinking patterns of patients or to check abstinence. In addition, they can be applied as an additional objective measurement to validate assessment methods based on self-reports.

A great advantage of a marker is that it is an objective measure. Markers are not affected by socially desirable answers or interviewer effects. Moreover, it is possible to follow standard procedures for sampling and chemical analyses.

In general, biological markers have a low sensitivity due to a large between-individual variation in responsiveness, a large day-to-day within-person variability and interference with other factors. However, combining two or more markers can improve either their sensitivity or specificity. As yet, markers of alcohol intake can only be used to assess recent or chronic use or to detect alcohol abuse (Table 4). Thus, they are not suitable for assessing habitual moderate drinking. Moreover, they cannot be used to assess the actual level of use, and hence they can only be used to classify individuals according to their drinking level.

In addition, because biological markers are often expensive, they cannot be used in large-scale studies. For most of the measurements blood samples are necessary which could, for use in specific populations, cause ethical problems. The higher load put on subjects by using biological measurements, for example if sampling of urine is necessary, could lead to a low response rate. Finally, markers do not provide information about drinking patterns and beverage preferences, which is required for some research purposes.

Except for specific purposes, current biological measurements do not seem suitable for population studies.

Summary and Conclusions

It is obvious that methods for assessing alcohol use have serious limitations. It is not easy to say which method approximates most closely real intake because a gold standard is lacking. Studies evaluating reproducibility and relative validity report that the accuracy of different methods of self-reports appears to be very similar. Among self-reports, which can be seen as the nearest to a gold standard at present, the quantity-frequency method or the prospective diary method is probably the best choice, provided they ask separately for different types of alcoholic beverages and deal with the problem of standard units. Questionnaires must also be devised with regard to variation in drinking pattern and diverse patterns of alcohol use such as frequent but light drinking or sporadic but heavy drinking. In addition, the time frame must be appropriate for the goal of the study and the usual pattern of use of alcoholic beverage types must be taken into account.

Self-reports are not suitable for all types of data analysis, as classified by Beaton into the four approaches described in the introduction to this chapter. Most self-reports probably underestimate mean alcohol use, as needed for Beaton's first approach. Probably, they are also not accurate enough to perform distributional analyses, the second approach, which are needed when sensible limits for acceptable alcohol intake have to be set. However, self-reports appear to be suitable for carrying out the third approach, correlation and regression analyses, and the fourth approach, categorical analyses, for which subjects have to be classified correctly according to their drinking level.

Errors in the assessment of alcohol use will influence the outcome of epidemiological surveys. Random error will lead to attenuation of the regression factor. This means that the actual relationship between alcohol intake and disease outcome will be stronger than the association measured in the study. It is possible to correct for attenuation if the reliability of the technique used is known. For this, it is important to develop and use standard techniques of known reliability. Systematic error is more serious than random error because this type of error may yield false associations between alcohol use and the disease outcome.

When the time window taken for assessment of alcohol use is limited, the actual relationship may also be stronger than the association found in the study if actual consumption of alcohol is not highly associated with measured intake. A simulation study by Lemmens et al. (1997) showed that dose-response relationships between alcohol use and risk assessment is affected when current intake is assessed instead of lifetime use, and that the correlation between both measurements drops below 0.50. In general, error, either random or systematic, will affect assessment of dose-response curves depending on the shape of that curve. Estimates of risk for rare diseases are more prone to error than more prevalent diseases, such as heart disease, as the assessment of risk for rare diseases is based on fewer observations. The results of future simulation studies could provide more insight into the impact of different errors in measurement and the robustness of current outcomes.

Biological markers of alcohol use are as yet not an appropriate choice for surveys because they are not suitable for assessing low or moderate intakes. Research would benefit from a good marker of alcohol use in this range of consumption. Although such markers are not yet available, it could be possible to work creatively with repeated measurements of short-term intake markers such as ethanol in breath. The use of markers could help solve the problem of whether underreporting is proportional to actual intake at very low and very high levels and could also be used as a gold standard in testing of methods. There are some new promising markers, such as serum carbohydrate-deficient transferrin, which should be investigated further. In order to directly translate the results of questions combined with laboratory tests to drinking levels, markers should be tested in a controlled study in which subjects drink a specific amount of alcohol over a long period.

In addition, existing methods can be improved when researchers apply them carefully with respect to the aim of their study. One very important aspect to consider is the meaning of drinking (Caetano 1998). Cultural norms determine in what way and how accurately alcohol use can be assessed with survey methods. Also the context in which alcohol is drunk is important.

Researchers must also take different subgroups into account, such as ethnic minorities, adolescents or the elderly. Moreover, ex-drinkers and lifelong abstainers should be considered as two distinct groups.

This overview shows that it is very difficult to assess alcohol use accurately, and therefore the possible presence of errors should be borne in mind when interpreting results of studies. It is obvious that further research is needed to improve existing techniques and to develop new and more accurate techniques to assess alcohol use. In the meantime, it is important to select and apply existing techniques carefully with a view on the aim of the survey.

References

Alanko T (1984) An overview of techniques and problems in the measurement of alcohol consumption. Rec Adv Alcohol Drug Probl 8: 209–26

Beaton GH (1994) Approaches to analysis of dietary data: relationship between planned analyses and choice of methodology. Am J Clin Nutr 59 (Suppl): 253S–61S

Bingham S, Nelson M, Paul AA et al. (1988) Methods for data collection at an individual level. In: Cameron ME. van Staveren WA. (eds.), Manual on methodology for food consumption studies, Oxford University Press, Oxford, pp. 53–105

Caetano R (1998) Cultural and subgroup issues in measuring consumption. Alcohol Clin Exp Res 22: 21S–28S

Cameron ME, van Staveren WA (1988) Manual on methodology for food consumption studies, Oxford University Press, Oxford

Chenet L, McKee M (1997) Alcohol policy in the Nordic countries. Why competition law must have a public health dimension. BMJ 314: 1142–43

Cohen BB, Vinson DC (1995) Retrospective self-report of alcohol consumption: test-retest reliability by telephone. Alcohol Clin Exp Res 19: 1156–61

de Leeuw ED (1992) Data quality in mail, telephone and face to face surveys, Thesis, Free University, Amsterdam

Doyle KM, Cluette-Brown JE, Dube DM et al. (1996) Fatty acid ethyl esters in the blood as markers for ethanol intake. JAMA 276: 1152–56

Duffy JC, Alanko T (1992) Self-reported consumption measures in sample surveys: a simulation study of alcohol consumption. J Off Stat 8: 327–50

Embree B, Whitehead P (1991) Validity and reliability of self-reported drinking behaviour: dealing with the problem of response bias. J Stud Alcohol 54: 334–44

Ferraroni M, Decarli A, Franceschi S et al. (1996) Validity and reproducibility of alcohol consumption in Italy. Int J Epidemiol 25: 775–82

Feunekes GIJ, van 't Veer P, van Staveren WA et al. (1999) Alcohol intake assessment: the sober facts. Am J Epidemiol, in press

Fitzgerald JL, Mulford HA (1987) Self-report validity issues. J Stud Alcohol 48: 207–11

Flegal KM (1990) Agreement between two dietary methods in the measurement of alcohol consumption. J Stud Alcohol 51: 408–14

Giovanucci EL, Colditz, GA, Stampfer M et al. (1998) The assessment of alcohol consumption by a simple self-administered questionnaire. Am J Epidemiol 133: 810–17

Göransson M, Hanson BS (1994) How much can data on days with heavy drinking decrease the underestimation of true alcohol consumption? J Stud Alcohol 55: 695–700

Grönbæk M, Heitmann BL (1996) Validity of self-reported intakes of wine, beer and spirits in population studies. Eur J Clin Nutr 50: 487–90

Haskell WL, Camargo C Jr, Williams PT et al. (1984) The effect of cessation and resumption of moderate alcohol intake on serum high-density-lipoprotein subfractions. A controlled study. N Engl J Med 310: 805–10

Helander A, Beck O, Wayne Jones A (1996) Laboratory testing for recent alcohol consumption: comparison of ethanol, methanol, and 5-hydroxytryptophol. Clin Chem 42: 618–24

Höyer G, Nillsen O, Brenn T et al. (1999) The Svalbard study 1988–89: an unique setting for validation of self-reported alcohol consumption. Addiction 90: 539–44

Hughes SP, Dodder RA (1988) Alcohol consumption indices. J Stud Alcohol 49: 100–03

Istvan J, Murray R, Voelker H et al. (1995) The relationship between patterns of alcohol consumption and body weight. Int J Epidemiol 24: 543–46

King AC (1994) Enhancing the self-report of alcohol consumption in the community: two questionnaire formats. Am J Publ Health 84: 294–296

Laposata M (1997) Fatty acid ethyl esters: short-term and long-term serum markers of ethanol intake. Clin Chem 43: 1527–34

Lemmens PHHM (1988) Bias due to non-response in a Dutch survey on alcohol consumption. Br J Addict 83: 1069–77

Lemmens PHHM (1991) Measurement and distribution of alcohol consumption, Thesis, Limburg University, Maastricht, Netherlands

Lemmens PHHM (1994a) Reply to Dr Stockwell. *Addiction* 89: 1704–06

Lemmens PHHM (1994b) The alcohol content of self-report and "standard" drinks. Addiction 89: 593–601

Lemmens PHHM (1998a) Beleid en praktijk: het beschermend effect van matig alcoholgebruik: implicaties voor beleid. Tijdschr Soc Gezondheidszorg 76: 233–35

Lemmens PHHM (1998b) Measuring lifetime drinking histories. Alcohol Clin Exp Res 22: 29S–36S

Lemmens PHHM, Tan ES, Knibbe RA (1992) Measuring quantity and frequency of drinking in a general population survey: a comparison of five indices. J Stud Alcohol 53: 476–86

Lemmens PHHM, Knibbe RA (1993) Seasonal variation in survey and sales estimates of alcohol consumption. J Stud Alcohol 54: 157–63

Lemmens PHHM, Drop MJ (1995) Op zoek naar de gezonde drinker. Tijdschr Alcohol Drugs 21: 226–34

Lemmens PHHM, Volovics L, de Haan Y (1997) Measurement of lifetime exposure to alcohol: data quality of a self-administered questionnaire and impact on risk assessment. Contemp Drug Prob 24: 581–600

Levine J (1990) The relative value of consultation, questionnaires and laboratory investigation in the identification of excessive alcohol consumption. Alcohol Alcoholism 25: 539–53

Litten RZ, Allen JP (1992) Measuring alcohol consumption: psychosocial and biochemical methods, Humana Press, Totowa, NJ

Longnecker MP, Newcomb PA, Mittendorf R et al. (1992) The reliability of self-reported alcohol consumption in the remote past. Epidemiology 3: 535–39

Mäkelä K (1971) Measuring the consumption of alcohol in the 1968–1969 Alcohol Consumption Study, Social Institute of Alcohol Studies, Helsinki

Meerkerk GJ, Njoo KH, Bongers IM et al. (1998) The specificity of the CDT assay in general practice: the influence of common chronic diseases and medication on the serum CDT concentration. Alcohol Clin Exp Res 22: 908–13

Midanik L (1982) The validity of self-reported alcohol consumption and alcohol problems: a literature review. Br J Addict 77: 357–82

Midanik LT (1988) Validity of self-reported alcohol use: a literature review and assessment. Br J Addict 83: 1019–29

Midanik LT (1994) Comparing usual quantity/frequency and graduated frequency scales to assess yearly alcohol consumption: results from the 1990 US National Alcohol Survey. Addiction 89: 407–12

Midanik LT, Klatsky AL, Armstrong MA (1989) A comparison of a 7-day recall with two summary measures of alcohol use. Drug Alcohol Depend 24: 127–34

Midanik LT, Hines AM (1991) "Unstandard" ways of answering standard questions: protocol analysis in alcohol survey research. Drug Alcohol Depend 27: 245–52

Moreiras O, van Staveren WA, Amorim Cruz JA et al. (1996) Longitudinal changes in the intake of energy and macronutrients of elderly Europeans. Eur J Clin Nutr 50 (Suppl 2): S67–S76

Munger RG, Folsom AR, Kushi LH et al. (1992) Dietary assessment of older Iowa women with a food frequency questionnaire: nutrient intake, reproducibility, and comparison with 24-hour dietary recall interviews. Am J Epidemiol 136: 192–200

Ocké M, Bueno-de-Mesquita B, Pols M et al. (1996) The Dutch EPIC food frequency questionnaire. II. Relative validity and reproducibility for nutrients. Int J Epidemiol 26 Suppl: S49–58

Parker DR, Derby CA, Usner DW et al. (1996) Self-reported alcohol intake using two different question formats in southeastern New England. Int J Epidemiol 25: 770–74

Pietinen P, Hartman AM, Haapa E (1988) Reproducibility and validity of dietary assessment instruments. I. A self-administered food use questionnaire with a portion size picture booklet. Am J Epidemiol 128: 655–66

Rehm J (1998) Measuring quantity, frequency, and volume of drinking. Alcohol Clin Exp Res 22: 4S–14S

Rimm EB, Klatsky A, Grobbee D et al. (1996) Review of moderate alcohol consumption and reduced risk of coronary heart disease: is the effect due to beer, wine, or spirits? BMJ 312: 731–36

Romelsjö A, Leifman H, Nyström S (1995) A comparative study of two methods for the measurement of alcohol consumption in the general population. Int J Epidemiol 24: 929–36

Room R (1998) Measuring drinking practices: how far we've come and how far we need to go. Alcohol Clin Exp Res 22: 70S–75S

Rosman AS, Lieber CS (1994) Diagnostic utility of laboratory tests in alcoholic liver disease. Clin Chem 40: 1641–51

Ruchlin HS (1997) Prevalence and correlates of alcohol use among older adults. Prev Med 26: 651–57

Russell M, Marshall JR, Trevisan M (1997) Test-retest reliability of the cognitive lifetime drinking history. Am J Epidemiol 146: 975–81

Schoeller DA (1990) How accurate is self-reported dietary energy intake? Nutr Rev 48: 373–79

Searles JS, Perrine MW, Mundt JC et al. (1995) Self-report of drinking using touch-tone telephone: extending the limits of reliable daily contact. J Stud Alcohol 56: 375–82

Shaw S, Lue SL, Lieber CS (1978) Biochemical tests for the detection of alcoholism: comparison of plasma α-amino-n-butyric acid with other available tests. Alcohol Clin Exp Res 2: 3–7

Single E, Wortley S (1994) A comparison of alternative measures of alcohol consumption in the Canadian National Survey of alcohol and drug use. Addiction 89: 395–99

Steffensen FH, Sörensen HT, Brock A et al. (1997) Alcohol consumption and serum liver-derived enzymes in a Danish population aged 30–50 years. Int J Epidemiol 26: 92–99

Stibler H (1991) Carbohydrate-deficient transferrin in serum: a new marker of potentially harmful alcohol consumption reviewed. Clin Chem 37: 2029–37

Stockwell T (1994) Would standard drink labelling result in more accurate self-reports of alcohol consumption? Addiction 89: 1703–04

Swanson CA, Coates RJ, Malone KE et al. (1997) Alcohol consumption and breast cancer risk among women under age 45 years. Epidemiology 8: 231–37

Uitenbroek DG (1996) Seasonal variation in alcohol use. J Stud Alcohol 57: 47–52

van Pelt J (1997) Koolhydraat-deficiënt transferrine: een nieuwe biochemische marker voor chronisch overmatig alcoholgebruik. Ned Tijdschr Geneeskd 141: 773–77

van Staveren WA, Burema J, Livingstone MBE (1996) Evaluation of the dietary history method used in the SENECA study. Eur J Clin Nutr 50 (Suppl 2): S47–S55

Webb GR, Redman S, Gibberd RW et al. (1991) The reliability and stability of a quantity-frequency method and a diary method of measuring alcohol consumption. Drug Alcohol Depend 27: 223–31

Willett W (1998) Nutrition epidemiology. Monographs in epidemiology and biostatistics, Vol. 30, 2nd ed, Oxford University Press, Oxford

Willett WC, Reynolds RD, Cottrell-Hoehner S et al. (1987) Validation of a semi-quantitative food frequency questionnaire: comparison with a 1-year diet record. J Am Diet Ass 87: 43–47

Williams GD, Aitken SS & Malin H (1985) Reliability of self-reported alcohol consumption in a general population survey. J Stud Alcohol 46: 223–27

Williams GD, Proudfit AH, Quinn EA et al. (1994) Variations in quantity-frequency measures of alcohol consumption from a general population survey. Addiction 89: 413–20

Chapter 3

Alcohol and Genetics

P. Couzigou
University Victor Segalen, Bordeaux, France

H. Begleiter
SUNY Health Sciences Center, New York, USA

K. Kiianmaa
Alko Ltd., Helsinki, Finland

Abstract

Epidemiological and experimental studies provide substantial evidence for the role of heredity in alcoholism and alcohol-related end-organ disease. They also shed light on some of the problems to be expected in attempting to assess the interaction between genetic and environmental effects. Research on the genetics of alcoholism is still in the formative stage, despite the greater use of molecular biology and considerably more experimental studies being carried out. Family studies such as the Collaborative Study on the Genetics of Alcoholism (COGA) are of tremendous importance. Genotypic as well as phenotypic studies are necessary. Electrophysiological studies suggest that there are underlying genetic mechanisms in the pathogenesis of alcoholism, but searches for an association between neuromediators, polymorphism and alcoholism are not conclusive. Polymorphisms at the alcohol dehydrogenase and the aldehyde dehydrogenase level are associated with alcohol use and alcoholism, especially in oriental populations.

In the future, it seems that studies on polymorphisms at the end-organ metabolic level will contribute more than studies on polymorphism of alcohol metabolism to furthering our knowledge of the role of genetics in drinking problems. In this way, the gene candidate approach could be very helpful, probably in quantitative trait loci studies, both in animal and human populations. Areas needing further research include twin and family studies in order to measure heredity and the tendency for alcoholism and end-organ damage to co-aggregate in families. Also, linkage analysis is required, which scans substantial well mapped regions of the human genome to find markers of alcoholism or alcohol-related end-organ disease. The complexity of alcoholism and alcohol-related end-organ damage suggests that there is a strong interaction between multiple polymorphisms and environmental factors.

Introduction

It has long been observed that alcoholism runs in families. This well-established observation does not provide compelling evidence for a genetic or an environmental influence. The first solid evidence for a potential genetic influence came from the now famous twin study by Kaij (1960) and later from the Danish Adoption study by Goodwin et al. (1973). The Danish adoption study suggested that genetic factors might be of fundamental influence on the pathogenesis of alcohol dependence. The classic adoption studies by Goodwin and his colleagues provided a major impetus to delineate the specific genetic influence. The Swedish Adoption studies (Cloninger et al. 1981) provided strong support for the clinical impression that there are several types of alcoholism, and offered the additional insight that genetic factors might exert a greater influence in some types of alcoholism than in others. Thus, epidemiological studies (reviewed by Hesselbrock 1995) not only provided substantial evidence for the role of heredity in the transmission of a predisposition to develop alcoholism but also shed light on some problems to be expected in attempting to assess the interaction of genetic and environmental effects. While research on the genetics of alcoholism is still in its formative stages, in the past decade the advent of important animal models and the initiation and implementation of major human studies have yielded early results leading to tentative conclusions which appear not only possible but quite reasonable.

It is now widely accepted that a substantial proportion of alcoholic patients have a genetic predisposition to develop alcohol dependence. In contrast to a large number of so-called genetic disorders such as cystic fibrosis, sickle cell anaemia or Huntington's chorea, the development of alcoholism depends strongly on the interaction of genetically determined predisposing factors with environmentally determined precipitating factors. While the search for genes predisposing individuals to develop alcoholism is a compelling endeavour there are a number of caveats which must be heeded. Alcoholism is a complex disorder with a number of characteristic features common to complex diseases.

1. Clinical heterogeneity. Alcoholism has a variable onset and can involve a combination of different symptoms.
2. Reduced penetrance. Because of unknown genetic or environmental effects, not every individual who inherits the genes will develop the disorder.
3. Genetic heterogeneity. Single mutations at different genetic loci may result in clinically indistinguishable disease states.
4. Polygenic inheritance. The disorder might not be caused by a single gene, but could develop from additive effects of multiple genes.
5. Epistatic effects. The disorder might reflect the complex interactions between alleles at several loci.
6. Phenocopies. A substantial proportion of individuals without a disease genotype manifest alcoholism resulting from non-genetic causes.

In 1993, an update was published on the topic (Couzigou et al. 1993) with a review of the clinical and experimental published data, both neurophysiological and biological, on genetic trait markers of alcoholism and also on alcohol-related end-organ damage. During the past few years, a number of relevant papers have addressed these aspects, generally reinforcing the review and the conclusions expressed in 1993, but sometimes modifing views on specific points.

Twin and Adoption Studies

No recent publication is in conflict with previous papers on twin and adoption studies pointing to a genetic factor in alcoholism (Heath 1995, Schuckit 1995). Recent papers have focused on alcohol and other drug abuse, alcohol sensitivity and severity of alcoholism. Contradictory twin studies have been published on a common genetic factor (Koopmans et al. 1997b) or not (Swan et al. 1997) for tobacco and alcohol abuse. Log linear modelling of the data from one adoption study reveal two genetic pathways to drug abuse and dependence (Cadoret et al. 1995). Comorbidity between antisocial personality and drug use disorders may be the result of shared genetic influences, shared environmental influences or a combination of the two. In future twin and adoption studies a distinction should be made between alcohol and drug abuse and between juvenile and adult antisocial symptoms (van den Bree 1998). In a Dutch twin study, initiation of alcohol use in men was mainly due to shared environmental influences. For women, shared environmental influences contributed slightly more than genetic influences to variance in initiation of alcohol use (Koopmans et al. 1997a, 1997b). The pattern of twin pair concordance for alcohol reactions suggests that heritability and alcohol reaction in subjects of European descent are not caused by a single gene of high penetrance of the type found in the Asian alcohol flush reaction (Whitfield et al. 1996). One adoption study suggests that genetic factors influence the risk for alcohol and drug dependence at different thresholds of severity as determined by DSM-III-R symptom severity scores (Yates et al. 1996). One twin study raises the possibility of assessing the relative influence of genetic and environmental factors in individual cases of alcohol dependence (Johnson et al. 1996). From a national survey, a model providing an alternative to standard twin and adoption studies as a way to separate genetic and environmental risk factors has been proposed (Light 1996)

Animal Studies

Studies on alcohol intake in animals and the development of animal models of alcohol drinking are made possible and meaningful by the fact that a variety of animals including many laboratory species voluntarily consume ethanol (Fuller 1985, Fuller et al. 1985). Primates and rodents self-administering alcohol have been widely used in research. Different strains of laboratory rats differ in their level of alcohol drinking, as do individuals within each strain. Therefore, the researcher can choose the strain showing the highest alcohol intake and/or select the individuals consuming the highest amount of ethanol.

Such mouse strains have had an important role in studies on the heritability of alcohol consumption. Inbred strains represent populations of genetically identical individuals that have been produced by more than 20 generations of mating of closely related animals, such as siblings. Theoretically, this has resulted in random fixation of homozygous genes.

It is now well established that various inbred strains of mice vary widely in alcohol intake. When the alcohol intake of several inbred strains of mice was compared, C57Bl mice voluntarily drank large amounts of alcohol while C3H/2, A/2, BALB/c and DBA/2N strains preferred water (McClearn et al. 1959, Rodgers et al. 1962, Yoshimoto et al. 1987). The demonstration of significant strain differences is itself presumptive evidence for the involvement of genotypes in alcohol preference. Studies with inbred rat strains have also shown differences in alcohol preference (Brewster 1968, Satinder 1970) and provided further evidence for the inheritance of alcohol preference.

In basic research the selection is usually performed bidirectionally, i.e. by selecting for high and low extremes. This was done with rats almost 30 years ago (Eriksson 1990) at Alko Research Laboratories in Helsinki and resulted in the establishment of the AA (Alko Alcohol) line that voluntarily consumes large amounts of alcohol and the ANA (Alko Non-Alcohol) line that chooses water to the virtual exclusion of alcohol. Similar programmes have been started elsewhere and led to the ACE and UCHB rat lines at the University of Chile (Mardones 1972) and to the P and NP lines as well as the HAD and LAD lines at the University of Indiana (Li et al. 1981, 1987, Lumeng et al. 1986). The results of these selection programmes clearly indicate that genetic factors influence the animals' alcohol drinking; otherwise, it would not have been possible to separate the traits.

Animal Models in Studies on Alcohol Abuse

Human and animal studies have not revealed (1) what are the biological factors that are inherited and (2) what are the biological factors underlying susceptibility to alcohol abuse, i.e. the mechanisms of alcohol abuse. Since studies have demonstrated that what occurs in human individuals can also be found in animal studies, this justifies an approach where the questions raised may be studied with animal models. In particular, an animal model is ideal for studying a genetically transmitted trait, since it allows for studying both genetic and environmental influences through controlled manipulation of both the genotype and the environment.

The development of an animal model of alcohol abuse, however, raises questions about the criteria for such a model (Couzigou et al. 1993). Animal models of alcohol abuse should focus on the different biological factors that may contribute to the problem and to test hypotheses. An animal model makes it possible to separate different variables such as alcohol-seeking behaviour and voluntary alcohol consumption, sensitivity, tolerance and dependence, for genetic analysis and pharmacological investigations.

Selected lines are useful in studies on the mechanisms of alcohol abuse and the effects of alcohol. Since the lines are produced by selectively breeding animals from a heterogeneous base population for a specific ethanol-related trait, the selected lines should theoretically differ from each other only in the trait upon which selection has been applied, and in traits that are related to the selected trait. Therefore selected lines are a valuable tool to search for the existence of a genetic correlation between the selected trait and a specific biochemical, neurochemical or behavioural trait, and to test hypotheses regarding the underlying causes of alcohol abuse (Deitrich et al. 1984, Schuckit et al. 1985, Crabbe et al. 1985a, 1985b, 1990, Deitrich 1990).

The first studies with selected lines examined voluntary alcohol consumption. Subsequently selective breeding has been done with various other factors including the sensitivity to alcohol, the capacity to develop tolerance, the liability to develop physical dependence and withdrawal severity after chronic alcohol administration. Consequently, several sets of selected lines based on different alcohol-related traits have been developed to produce animal models for testing specific hypotheses concerning the basis for the genetic differences and their role in the effects of alcohol. The lines and related work have been discussed widely elsewhere (McClearn et al. 1981, Deitrich et al. 1984, Li et al. 1987, Crabbe 1989, Kiianmaa et al. 1989, Phillips 1997, Deitrich 1990, Sinclair et al. 1996) and listed by Couzigou (1993). The new lines selected for alcohol-related traits are listed below.

VOLUNTARY ALCOHOL CONSUMPTION

UCHA and UCHB rats are the oldest lines selected for differential voluntary alcohol intake. They have been developed by Mardones (1960, 1972) in Santiago, Chile.

AA (Alko, Alcohol) and ANA (Alko, Non-Alcohol) rats have been selectively outbred for their voluntary intake of a 10% alcohol solution in a free-choice situation (Eriksson 1968, Sinclair et al. 1989).

P (Preferring) and NP (Non-Preferring) rats are inbred lines. They were also developed for differences in their preference for a 10% alcohol solution (Li et al. 1981, 1987).

HAD (High Alcohol-Drinking) and LAD (Low Alcohol-Drinking) rats are the result of replicating the development work for the P and NP lines through outbreeding (Lumeng et al. 1986).

SP (Sardinia preferring) and SNP (Sardinia Non-Preferring) rats, differing in their preference for a 10% alcohol solution, were recently developed in Cagliari, Italy (Fadda et al 1989).

HARF, LARF and CARF lines were selectively bred for differences in alcohol consumption in a limited-access paradigm with alcohol being available for 20 min a day (Sinclair et al. 1996).

SENSITIVITY TO ALCOHOL

LS (Long-Sleep) and SS (Short-Sleep) mice have been selectively outbred for the duration of alcohol-induced loss of righting reflex ("sleep time") at the Institute for Behavioral Genetics in Boulder, Colorado (McClearn et al 1981, Philips et al. 1989, Deitrich 1990).

FAST and SLOW mice differ in the stimulatory effect of alcohol (2 g/kg) in the open field (Crabbe et al. 1987b, 1990a, Philips et al. 1989, 1991). HOT and COLD mice have been produced by selecting the hypothermic effect of an acute dose of alcohol (3 g/kg) (Crabbe et al. 1987a, 1990, Philips et al. 1989). Both FAST/SLOW and HOT/COLD mice are outbred lines.

AT (Alcohol-Tolerant) and ANT (Alcohol-Non-Tolerant) rats are outbred lines selected for differential alcohol-induced (2 g/kg) motor impairment on the tilting plane (Eriksson et al. 1981, Eriksson 1990).

HAFT (High Acute Functional Tolerance) and LAFT (Low Acute Functional Tolerance) mice differ in their acquisition of acute functional alcohol tolerance. They have been selected on the basis of the recovery of balance on a stationary dowel rod after two consecutive doses of alcohol, 1.75 g/kg followed by 2 g/kg (Erwin et al. 1996).

ALCOHOL WITHDRAWAL

SEW (Severe Ethanol Withdrawal) and MEW (Mild Ethanol Withdrawal) mice have been selectively outbred for their severity of alcohol withdrawal syndrome (McClearn et al. 1982, Philips et al. 1989). Physical dependence is produced by administration of an alcohol-containing liquid diet for nine days, and the withdrawal severity is scored on a battery of tests.

WSP (Withdrawal Seizure Prone) and WSR (Withdrawal Seizure Resistant) outbred mice have been selected for severe and mild signs of withdrawal induced by handling after three days of chronic inhalation of ethanol vapour (Crabbe et al. 1985b, Crabbe 1989, Philips et al. 1989).

LINES SELECTED FOR ALCOHOL-UNRELATED TRAITS

Lines selected for alcohol-unrelated traits, such as the Maudsley Reactive and Non-Reactive, the Roman high-avoidance and low-avoidance, as well as the Wistar-Kyoto spontaneously hypertensive and normotensive, the Wistar-Kyoto hyperactive and normoactive rat strains, have also been widely used to study the mechanisms of alcohol abuse and alcohol's effects. They can be valuable in studies on the contribution of alcohol-unrelated traits, such as behavioural or emotional reactivity (Satinder 1975, Satinder et al. 1986, Waller et al. 1986, Adams et al. 1991, Adams. 1995, Knapp et al. 1997, Mormède et al. 1998), consummatory behaviour, gustatory factors (Kampov-Polevoy et al. 1996, Razafimanalina et al. 1997, Velley et al. 1998) and other factors (Khanna et al. 1985, 1990, Crabbe et al. 1985) in the development of alcohol dependence.

Mapping of Quantitative Trait Loci

The use of a new statistical and molecular technique called quantitative trait loci (QTL) mapping applied to genetic animal models has greatly extended the understanding of the particular genes involved in the expression of alcohol-related traits and can be used eventually to identify the genes themselves (Crabbe et al. 1994, Crabbe 1996, Phillips 1997). A QTL is a small section on a chromosome thought to influence a specific trait. QTL analysis provides a means of localizing and measuring the effects of a single QTL on alcohol-related behavioural traits, and it probably is the most promising technique for identifying genes influencing alcohol-related traits.

QTL mapping can use selected animal lines or recombinant inbred (RI) mouse strains derived from crossbreeding the offspring of two genetically distinct parent strains. QTL mapping involves comparing alcohol-related behaviours in these lines and identifying patterns of known genetic markers shared by lines or strains with the same behaviours. The markers also identify the probable regions of chromosomes that influence specific alcohol-related traits.

Researchers are now extensively using BXD RI strains to investigate the genes that influence alcohol-related behaviours (Crabbe et al. 1994, Crabbe 1996). The BXD RI strains have been derived from F_2 offspring of the C57BL/6J and DBA/2J inbred mouse strains. Currently there are 26 strains. The RI strains have been used to perform QTL analysis to identify loci contributing to alcohol self-administration (Phillips et al. 1995a, Rodriguez et al. 1995, Belknap et al. 1997), locomotor activity and conditioned place preference (Cunningham 1995, Phillips et al. 1995b, 1998), alcohol sensitization and tolerance (Phillips et al. 1996), hypothermia and motor impairment (Crabbe et al. 1996b), and the severity of alcohol withdrawal symptoms (Belknap et al. 1993). Using these experimental approaches, researchers have mapped two QTLs that are associated with increased withdrawal severity, and one that confers protection against withdrawal (Crabbe 1996b). They also found a probable QTL affecting alcohol preference (Belknap et al. 1997). The specific genes still remain to be identified (Table 1).

RIs have also been developed from the Long-Sleep and Short-Sleep mice bred for differential alcohol sensitivity in order to identify the QTLs related to hypothermic and hypnotic sensitivity to alcohol (Erwin et al. 1990, Erwin et al. 1993). In these studies several provisional QTLs have been detected for alcohol sensitivity (Markel et al. 1996), two common QTLs for neurotensin immunoreactivity levels and alcohol-induced hypothermia, and two common QTLs for neurotensin receptor levels and the hypnotic effect of alcohol (Erwin et al. 1997).

Table 1
Probable QTLs affecting alcohol-related behaviours

Mouse model	Trait	Reference
BXD RI strains	self-administration	Philips et al. 1995a, Rodriguez et al. 1995, Belknap et al.1997
	conditioned place preference	Cunningham 1995, Philips et al. 1995b
	locomotor activity	Cunningham 1995, Philips et al. 1995b
	tolerance	Philips et al. 1996
	hypothermia	Crabbe et al. 1996b
	sensitization	Philips et al. 1996
	motor impairment	Belknap et al. 1993, Crabbe 1996
	withdrawal symptoms	Belknap et al. 1993, Crabbe 1996
Long-Sleep / Short-Sleep mice	sensitivity	Markel et al. 1996, Erwin et al. 1997
	hypothermia	Erwin et al. 1997
	neurotensin immuno-reactivity, neurotensin receptor levels	Erwin et al. 1997

Rat lines, such as the P and NP, HAD and LAD, and AA and ANA lines, selected for differential ethanol intake have also been used in the identification of QTLs, in this case for voluntary ethanol consumption (Ballas et al 1997, Bice et al 1998).

Genetic Engineering in Animal Models

The development of genetic engineering techniques has allowed progress to be made in identifying specific genes involved in the aetiology of alcoholism. These techniques include making transgenic mice in which foreign genes are inserted permanently into the animal's genetic material and knockout mice in which a gene is permanently inactivated, and using antisense RNA treatment that allows the temporary inactivation of individual genes (Hiller-Sturmhöfel et al. 1995, Phillips 1997).

The foreign gene in transgenic animals is expressed in future genera-tions. This technique could be used to study, in animal models, specific genes suspected of contributing to alcoholism, but it has not yet been used for this purpose.

The phenotype of knockout mice with one of their own genes eliminated is then compared with that of normal mice. Although the creation of knockout mice is a powerful tool, there are some limitations to its usefulness (Hiller-Sturmhöfel et al. 1995).

Knockout technology has already been used in alcohol research to study genes suspected to mediate alcohol's effects. An obvious place to start looking is with neurotransmitter receptor knockouts. Such studies have shown that mice lacking the 5-HT$_{1B}$ receptor gene consume more ethanol and are less sensitive to its ataxic effects than wild-type mice (Crabbe et al. 1996a). Furthermore, studies with GABA$_A$ receptor 6 subunit knockout mice have revealed that the subunit exerts little influence on alcohol sensitivity, functional tolerance or withdrawal hyperexcitability (Homanics et al. 1997, 1998). Although the information derived from investigations of this kind is still very limited, the results have demonstrated the power of the knockout technology in studies on the contribution of candidate genes to alcohol-related behaviours.

The Benefits of Animal Models

From the viewpoint of society, genetic studies in animals are important (1) for demonstrating that genetics has an influence, and as a precursor and a guide to studies testing whether genetics affects the characteristic in man, and (2) for providing an animal model with a particular genetic disorder in order to conduct further research aimed at finding better treatments.

Animals may be used in the search for predisposition markers. This has, however, its limitations. Markers may have only an accidental relationship to a factor affecting alcohol use, or the factor may be altered in several ways. For instance, the low drinking of ANA rats and some Orientals is caused apparently by a genetic alteration reducing aldehyde dehydrogenase activity, but at least preliminary results suggest that the specific enzymatic alterations in rats are different from those in man. In other words, animal models are better for discovering critical, essential factors directly causing overt differences than for discovering factors further removed from the phenotypic characteristic.

Specific features of animal lines may in some cases make them especially useful in the search for the "primary sites" where genes first produce an influence. For example, a particular type of line difference between the AT and ANT lines (Hellevuo et al. 1987) led to the prediction that the GABA system would contain a primary site (Sinclair 1992). An independent study a year later found a point mutation in the GABA system of the ANT line (Korpi et al. 1993). Furthermore, the application of genetic mapping and molecular techniques to genetic animal models will greatly extend the understanding of particular genes involved in the expression of alcohol-related traits and can be used eventually to identify the genes themselves. Most importantly, it points the way toward treatments for alcoholism based on genetic predisposition and provides a basis for testing them.

REINFORCEMENT

Animal studies show that alcohol is a reinforcer and that AA and P lines of rats, developed for high alcohol consumption, get more reinforcement from alcohol than do ANA and NP rats or unselected Wistar rats. Furthermore, P rats get reinforcement from alcohol directly into the brain. Thus genetics can alter the amount of reinforcement produced pharmacologically by alcohol in the brain.

BLOCKING REINFORCEMENT

Blocking the reinforcement from alcohol in the brain should be a useful addition to the treatment of alcoholism. It should be noted, however, that punishment for alcohol drinking is not the same as blocking re-inforcement. A large body of animal studies, amply supported by work with alcoholics, illustrates that punishment is not an effective method for treating alcoholism. What is needed instead is a pharmacological method for blocking the reinforcement from alcohol in the brain. This could then be used as a treatment for alcohol drinking, or as a preventative to stop the progressive development of alcoholism (Sinclair 1998).

A particularly useful form of animal genetics research is that which searches for genetic factors affecting reinforcement from alcohol and then for pharmacological means for blocking the high level of reinforcement found in lines selected for high drinking. This is likely to be relevant for humans with a genetic predisposition to high drinking and thus help in their treatment.

LEARNED BEHAVIOURAL DISORDER

Alcoholism in man is suspected to be a learned behavioural disorder. Some individuals receive so much reinforcement so often from alcohol that the responses involved in obtaining and drinking alcohol come to dominate their behaviour and cannot be controlled by normal social incentives and pressures. Culture, society, peer pressure and alcohol laws influence how often a person gets reinforcement from alcohol. Genetics may also influence this by helping to direct some individuals toward gangs and groups that drink more heavily. The amount of reinforcement per drinking experience, however, is almost certainly under strong genetic control. This is illustrated by animal studies and can be studied best with animal models.

PHYSICAL DEPENDENCE

After stopping drinking an alcohol-dependent individual will experience alcohol withdrawal symptoms, which are characterized by hyperactivity of the nervous system. Genetic animal models are being used to trace the pathways from complex drug responses in neuronal pathways to specific genes responsible for alterations in the sensitivity of neuronal systems during alcohol withdrawal. Understanding the genetic and biochemical correlates of the syndrome may yield improved treatments for withdrawal and other aspects of alcohol dependence.

ALCOHOL SENSITIVITY

Some animals have a genetically determined elevated susceptibility to motor impairment from alcohol. Recent work in human populations also suggests that genes influence the severity of intoxication. It seems likely that individuals who are more sensitive to alcohol-induced motor impairment and/or less able to counteract alcohol's effects are responsible for a large proportion of alcohol-related accidents.

One of the traditional goals in alcohol research has been to find drugs or other means to reverse alcohol intoxication. Research on animal lines with an inherent high resistance to intoxication might be particularly useful for reaching this goal.

PREDISPOSITION TO RELAPSE AND BINGE INTOXICATION

Most animals, including man, increase alcohol drinking temporarily after a period of forced abstinence. The heavy drinking level at that time often leads to severe intoxication, increased risk of accidents, alcohol poisoning, and perhaps some adverse medical consequences. This alcohol deprivation effect is also a factor promoting relapse. There is increasing evidence that the time course for the alcohol deprivation effect and its magnitude are influenced by genetics.

Important new work would be the development of lines differing in their alcohol deprivation effect and finding drug treatments for suppressing the alcohol deprivation effect or more specifically for suppressing excessively large alcohol deprivation effects.

In conclusion, selective breeding studies have made significant contributions to identifying genetic neurobiological mechanisms underlying the behavioural effects of alcohol. They are likely to continue to have an important role in this area of research. Future research will increasingly use genetic animal models for identification, mapping and cloning of the genes influencing alcohol-related traits by combining behavioural and molecular genetics. QTL mapping offers probably the most promising new tool for identifying risk and protective genes influencing alcohol-related traits in animals and subsequently for extrapolation to man.

Genetic Heterogeneity: Biological Markers

Alcoholism is clinically and genetically heterogeneous. Recent studies have tried to subgroup alcoholics into more homogeneous diagnostic categories using a variety of classification schemes such as type 1/type 2, primary versus secondary and type A/type B alcoholism (Anthenelli et al. 1994, 1998, Schuckit 1995, Johnson et al. 1996, Hall et al. 1996). No single method of phenotyping alcoholics is yet universally accepted (Hall et al. 1996, Bucholz et al. 1996, Anthenelli et al. 1998). This approach is however important: definition of more homogeneous subtypes of alcoholics should eliminate some of the variance and increase the likelihood of finding biological factors that, in part, mediate the risk of developing that subtype of alcoholism. In addition, identifying heritable biological trait markers associated with risk for alcoholism would help to focus the search for potential candidate genes amenable to more formal genotypic analysis (Anthenelli et al. 1997).

Neurophysiological Processes Involved in the Genetics of Alcoholism

A very large collaborative study known as the Collaborative Study on the Genetics of Alcoholism (COGA) has been implemented, whose specific purpose is to identify genes predisposing to the development of alcoholism. This large genetic study is entirely funded by the National

Institute of Alcohol Abuse and Alcoholism (NIAAA) which is part of the US National Institutes of Health. Because alcoholism is a complex disease, it was decided that an appropriate linkage analysis would require a very large sample. This rather large undertaking could not be accomplished by one investigator but would require the close collaboration of multiple sites to collect large samples of alcoholic families. The COGA study involves six sites: Indiana University, State University of New York, University of California at San Diego and the Scripps Institute, University of Connecticut, University of Iowa and Washington University. Great care was used in the development of an ascertainment scheme, which necessitates the recruitment of alcoholic probands from treatment facilities. The probands were either male or female and were diagnosed using DSM-III-R criteria for alcohol dependence as well as Feighner criteria for alcoholism at the definite level. In order to establish a comprehensive clinical instrument, the COGA group developed the Semi-Structured Assessment for the Genetics of Alcoholism (SSAGA). Families were enrolled in the study only if they included a sibship or at least three first-degree relatives and that the parents were available. The final inclusion of families requires that, in addition to the alcohol-dependent proband, two additional first-degree relatives are also diagnosed as alcohol-dependent by the COGA criteria. The reliability of the COGA data across the six sites has already been published (Bucholz et al. 1995). To date 348 alcoholic families (10,500 individuals) and 236 control families (1273 individuals) have been enrolled. In all families data have already been collected on over 1200 children. An extensive neurophysiological protocol has been implemented which collects electroencephalographic (EEG) results and brain event-related potentials (ERP). Couzigou et al. (1993) suggest that data obtained with EEG/ERP in abstinent alcoholics and offspring at risk for developing alcoholism might provide a novel quantitative phenotype for the genetic study of alcoholism.

ERP in subjects at risk for alcoholism have been studied for over a decade. In the first study, the high-risk (HR) group consisted of sons of alcoholic fathers between the ages of 7 and 13 years who had no prior exposure to alcohol (Begleiter et al. 1984). Their fathers had been diagnosed with alcoholism (DSM-III) and had been treated for alcoholism. Boys whose mothers had either drunk during pregnancy or had drunk excessively after birth were excluded. Only boys with neither medical problems nor exposure to alcohol or other substances of abuse were included. The low-risk (LR) group consisted of healthy normal boys matched for age and socio-economic status to the HR subjects. They were included only if they had no prior exposure to alcohol or other substances of abuse and if they had no first- or second-degree relatives with a history of alcoholism or psychiatric disorders. With the exception of family history of alcoholism, the same exclusion criteria were used in both the LR and HR groups. A complex visual head-orientation paradigm was used to elicit the P3 ERP component. Principal component analysis with varimax rotation (PCAV) performed on the data indicated that only the factor representing the P3 component was significantly different between the high-risk and the low-risk group. This study was the first in the field to indicate that the P3 amplitude is significantly reduced in boys at risk for alcoholism but without exposure to alcohol. Since this original study, several laboratories have replicated these findings using the same head-orientation paradigm, both in post-pubescent (O'Connor et al. 1986) and in prepubescent (Hill et al. 1993) boys at risk for alcoholism. In addition, these results have been replicated with other visual paradigms, namely in a continuous performance task (Whipple et al. 1988, 1991, Noble 1990, Berman et al. 1993) and a line discrimination task (Porjesz et al. 1990). Furthermore, reduced P3 amplitudes have been seen in pre- and post-pubescent male adolescents at risk for alcoholism using auditory tasks (Begleiter et al. 1987, Ramachandrun et al. 1996).

Begleiter et al. (1987) studied another group of sons of alcoholics to demonstrate that the reduced P3 amplitude observed in high-risk subjects was not modality- or task-specific. Another laboratory (Whipple et al. 1988, 1991) used a Continuous Performance Test (CPT) to examine ERPs in prepubescent boys at high risk for alcoholism. In agreement with both Begleiter et al. (1984, 1987) and O'Connor et al. (1986, 1987), a reduction in the amplitude of the late positive complex (LPC), including a P3 component, was observed. Later studies in the same laboratory replicated these original findings (Noble 1990, Whipple et al. 1991, Berman et al. 1993). An interesting study by Berman et al. (1993) indicates that P3 amplitude in prepubescent boys predicts later substance abuse in adolescence. These findings provide strong evidence that P3 amplitude in prepubescent boys may provide a vulnerability marker for the development of later substance abuse disorders.

The original findings of reduced visual P3 voltages have been recently replicated without the administration of alcohol in an older sample (18–23 years) of sons of alcoholic fathers (Porjesz et al. 1990). The results indicated that, prior to alcohol ingestion, P3 amplitude was significantly lower in HR subjects than in controls. The largest differences in P3 amplitude between groups was seen in the easy target to which LR subjects manifested extremely high voltages. These results are similar to those obtained in alcoholics with the same paradigm where the easy target elicited the greatest difference in P3 amplitude between groups (Porjesz et al. 1987). Most studies dealing with electrophysiological measures in subjects at risk for alcoholism have focused on male subjects. The results on female offspring have been less consistent. Hill et al. (1993b) studied P3 responses in both male and female pre- and post-pubertal offspring of male alcoholics. They replicated the P3 amplitude findings of Begleiter et al. (1987) in the pre-pubescent boys, but did not find that pre- or post-pubescent girls manifested lower P3 amplitudes, nor did post-pubescent boys. While lower P3 amplitudes were not reported in female offspring of male alcoholics using the visual paradigm (Hill et al. 1993), they were reported in female offspring of female alcoholics in a more recent report using an auditory paradigm (Hill et al. 1995). Recently, the national COGA study with a very large sample size has found reduced P3 amplitudes in female offspring of male alcoholics from high-density alcoholic families, albeit not to the same extent as in male offspring (Porjesz et al. 1996).

Taken together, the data reviewed indicate that the low P3 amplitude seems to be a robust finding which characterizes individuals at risk for alcoholism prior to any alcohol exposure. Low P3 amplitudes are not due to the neurotoxic effects of alcohol on the brain, and they do not recover with prolonged abstinence. Low P3 amplitude in young boys has been found to predict substance abuse in adolescence (Berman et al. 1993, Hill et al. 1995). P3 amplitude in alcoholics and high-risk individuals has been found to be directly related to the number of affected relatives in the family (Pfefferbaum et al. 1991, Benegal et al. 1995). Therefore, family history of alcoholism, rather than alcohol history, correlates with P3 amplitude. In order for this finding to be considered as a phenotypic marker for alcoholism, however, certain criteria must be met. The most important criterion is that it is heritable: there is a growing body of evidence indicating that the P3 component amplitude is a heritable property of this ERP component. There is a good deal of evidence indicating that characteristics of both the EEG and ERP are genetically determined (van Beijsterveldt et al. 1994). The production of fast EEG activity has been demonstrated to be genetically transmitted (Vogel 1970, Young et al. 1972, Propping 1977). The hereditary nature of several EEG variants (monomorphic α, low-voltage EEG, EEG with α and β diffusely mixed,

EEG with fronto-precentral β) has been reported (Vogel 1970, Vogel et al. 1986). Spectral analyses of EEG have revealed higher correlations for monozygotic than dizygotic twin pairs (Dumermuth 1968, Lykken et al. 1974, 1982, Stassen et al. 1987). In the study by Stassen et al. (1987), the spectral patterns of monozygotic twins were almost as similar as for the same individual tested twice, while the dizygotic twin patterns were significantly more similar to each other than were patterns in unrelated individuals. These findings were confirmed in a later study (Stassen et al. 1988) examining EEGs of monozygotic and dizygotic twin pairs reared apart.

In addition to this strong evidence that EEG patterns are genetically determined, there is also evidence that ERP are under genetic control. Monozygotic twins manifest ERP waveforms that are as concordant with each other as ERP obtained from the same individual tested twice (Dustman et al. 1965, Surwillo 1980). ERP recorded to flashes of light of different intensities have been reported to be under genetic control (Buchsbaum et al. 1971). Higher heritabilities have been reported for the endogenous ERP components compared to the exogenous components (van Beijsterveldt et al. 1994). The P3 component of the ERP is more similar in identical twins than in unrelated controls (Polich et al. 1987) and fraternal twins (Rogers et al. 1991, O'Connor et al. 1994, van Beijsterveldt 1996, Katsanis et al. 1997). Evidence that the P3 amplitude is genetically transmitted comes from both twin studies and family studies. (O'Connor et al. 1994, van Beijsterveldt 1996, Katsanis et al. 1997, Daw et al. 1995). Almasy et al. (in press) have estimated the heritability of P3 amplitude in 604 individuals from 100 pedigrees ascertained as part of the COGA project. They report significant heritabilities for both visual and auditory P3 amplitudes to target stimuli; heritabilities were higher for visual than for auditory P3 amplitudes. Most recently, the COGA project has undertaken various linkage analyses, including studies to identify the genetic basis of ERP (Begleiter et al. 1998). Two "hotspots" of significant linkage were identified, one on chromosome 6 and the other on chromosome 2 related posterior leads. A recent doctoral study in the Netherlands (van Beijsterveldt 1996) examined the visual P3 in a large sample of twins using a multivariate genetic analysis approach. Two independent factors account for visual P3 amplitude: one influences all the electrodes, and a second one influences occipital leads. Possibly, these chromosome 2 findings for the posterior leads represent this second occipital factor. A genetic linkage analysis has been performed joining analysis of the disease trait and the quantitative neuroelectric features: a chromosome 4 region strongly influenced liability to alcoholism, with pleiotropic effects on P3. Understanding the genetic control of brain electrical activity may provide clues about cerebral function and shed light on pathogenic mechanisms of neurological and psychiatric disorders where impairment of brain electrical activity is apparent (e.g. low P3 amplitudes observed in alcoholism). The endophenotypic QTLs obtained from the COGA project suggest that alcohol dependence is mediated by CNS disinhibition. The normal CNS homeostatic balance between excitation (NMDA) and inhibition (GABA) is disrupted in individuals at risk for developing alcoholism. The study of elementary or intermediary quantitative phenotypes, such as neuroelectric features, in combination with qualitative phenotypes, such as diagnosis, represents the appropriate method of the future for elucidating the genetics of complex traits.

The A1 Allele of the D2 Dopamine Receptor

The dopamine system has been considered a candidate for involvement in alcoholism with postulated links to novelty seeking and CNS reward. An association between the *Taq*1 A1 polymorphism in the DRD2 gene (mapped to chromosome 11) and alcoholism was first reported by Blum et al. (1990). Shortly after, the first non-replication study was reported. This polymorphism has subsequently been examined by many groups with varying results, some suggesting that the A1 allele could aggravate susceptibility to the medical complications of alcoholism (Couzigou et al. 1993). Recent papers are again conflicting: a link between dopamine receptor D2 (DRD2) polymorphism and early-onset alcoholism has been found (Kono et al. 1997) in a general Japanese population. The group of Noble has published new data in favour of the association (Lawford et al. 1997). Another group first found no association (Heinz et al. 1996) and later an association between DRD2 polymorphism, anxiety and depression scores has been reported (Finck et al. 1997). However, the quality of the control group is crucial as pointed out in a study that found different frequencies in control groups screened or unscreened to exclude alcoholism and heavy drinking (Turner et al. 1997). Studies in homogeneous Indian or Taiwanese populations found negative results (Goldman et al. 1997, Chen et al. 1997) as reported in a recent paper from the COGA study group testing the association between DRD2 polymorphism and alcohol dependence in a large family-based sample

(Edenberg et al. 1998). Association between the DRD2 gene and alcoholism is not supported by most of the recently published papers with good methodology. Similarly, no association has been found with the DRD4 gene (Geijer et al. 1997b, Chang et al. 1997, Roman et al. 1998). However, polymorphism in the promoter region of the DRD2 gene may affect the vulnerability for alcoholism in the Japanese (Ishiguro et al. 1998).

Monoamine Oxidase (MAO) Activity in Platelets

Decreased platelet MAO activity levels have been proposed as a potential marker for the predisposition to alcoholism. However, a number of intrinsic characteristics and extrinsic factors appear to influence MAO activity results. Chief among these appears to be smoking (Berlin et al. 1995). Few studies in alcoholism have considered this important variable (Anthenelli et al. 1995). Confusing findings have led some authors to conclude that lower MAO activity may be better considered as a more general marker for the risk of developing psychopathology (Devor et al. 1994). Others omit to take into account gender (Suarez et al. 1995) or sample collection at various lengths of abstinence (Rommelspacher et al. 1994). A recent paper from the COGA study group shows that variance of platelet MAO activity is explained by gender, smoking status and the site at which the platelet preparation was prepared. After univariate and multivariate analysis the authors concluded that decreased platelet MAO activity is not a trait marker of alcoholism or one of its subtypes but rather a state marker of cigarette smoking (Anthenelli et al. 1998).

Lymphocyte and Platelet Adenylate Cyclase Activities

The adenylate cyclase signal transduction system, a ubiquitous second messenger system, has been identified as a potential marker for genetic risk of alcohol and drug dependence. Male alcoholics with a positive family history have been described to have lower adenylate cyclase activity than male alcoholics with a negative family history (Anthenelli et al. 1995b, Parsian et al. 1996).

Recent unpublished data from the WHO ISBRA international project show decreasing levels of platelet adenylate cyclase activity during abstinence.

No association has been found with exon 13 polymorphism of the GS α gene (Kranzler et al. 1997).

Serotonin Transporter and Receptor Polymorphisms

Low serotonergic activity has been suggested to increase vulnerability to alcohol dependence in part by affecting harm avoidance. Thus, genes relating to serotonergic function are reasonable candidate genes for involvement with alcoholism. Abstinent alcoholics have been reported to have an enhanced uptake of serotonin (5-hydroxytryptamine, 5-HT) into lymphocytes which express the serotonin transporter HTT (mapped to chromosome 17). A functional polymorphism has been reported in the HTT promoter. A population-based association study suggested that the phenotype of severe alcoholism marked by withdrawal seizure or delirium or with antisocial personality was weakly associated with 5 HTTLPR promoter polymorphism (Sander et al. 1997, 1998), data also found by another group (Hammoumi et al. 1998). However, in a robust family-based study from COGA, no evidence of linkage or association of the HTT gene with alcohol dependence has been found (Edenberg et al. 1998b).

Allele frequencies of the human $5HT_{2C}$ gene did not differ between controls and alcoholics with severe dependence (Samochowiec et al. 1998).

Other Putative Trait Markers

- Gamma-aminobutyric acid (GABA) is the major inhibitory neuro-transmitter in the brain. GABA antagonists reduce some ethanol-induced behaviours. However, human GABA receptor α1 and α3 allele frequencies are similar in controls, alcoholics and subtypes of alcoholics (Parsian et al. 1997).
- Tyrosine hydrolase receptor polymorphism has not been found to be associated with alcoholism (Geijer et al. 1997b).
- Prodynorphin (related to opioid metabolism) allele distribution was similar in controls and chronic alcoholics (Geijer et al. 1997a).
- Cholecystokinin (CCK) plays a role in anxiety and nociception and modulates the release of dopamine and dopamine-related behaviours. An association between CCK promoter polymorphism and alcoholism has been described in Japan (Harada et al. 1998).
- In a genetic linkage analysis of sibling pairs in the COGA study, evidence for a locus on chromosome 16 was found, associated with the risk of alcoholism. The same COGA study group has reported suggestions of linkage (Foroud et al. 1998) with susceptibility loci for alcohol dependence on chromosomes 1 and 7 and evidence for a

protective locus on chromosome 4 near the alcohol dehydrogenase genes (Reich et al. 1998).

Alcohol and Acetaldehyde Metabolism, Alcohol Sensitivity and Alcoholism

During the past few years, several papers have been published on the relationship between alcohol dehydrogenase (ADH) and aldehyde dehydrogenase (ALDH) polymorphisms and alcohol sensitivity, drinking behaviour and alcoholism. An update was made in 1994 (Couzigou et al. 1994). As a whole, the data published after 1994 have confirmed the concept of a protective effect of the more active isozymes, especially the isozyme encoded by *ALDH2*2* and, to a lesser extent, *ADH2*2* with accumulation of acetaldehyde as a consequence. The *ADH2*2* allele has been found in a Jewish population to be associated with reduced alcohol consumption (Neumark et al1998). *ADH2*3* encodes a more active isoenzyme β3 with a faster alcohol elimination rate in man (Thomasson et al. 1995). Epidemiological data about drinking behaviour and its link with the *ADH2*3* allele in an African population would be worthwhile. The role of the *ADH3*1* allele encoding γ1 and *ADH3*2* encoding the γ2 isozyme is less impressive, and is probably related to the V_{max} for γ1 increasing only 2.5-fold relative to V_{max} for the γ2 isozyme. The few data favouring an effect of the *ADH3*1* allele are to be discussed in view of a linkage disequilibrium with the *ADH2*2* allele (Pares et al. 1998, Yin 1998).

Epidemiological data give little new information. The *ALDH2*2* allele has only been described in an Asian population. The *ADH2*3* allele found in African populations has also been found in native Indian Americans (Wall et al. 1997a). ALDH polymorphism is implicated in drinking behaviour (Wall et al. 1997b), and subjects heterozygous for *ALDH2*2* drink less and less frequently (Tanaka et al. 1997, Higuchi 1994, Higuchi et al. 1994b, 1995, 1996a). Subjects heterozygous for *ALDH2*2* experienced each stage or event in their drinking history 1 to 5 years later in life than subjects with the *ALDH2*1/2*1* genotype (Murayama et al. 1998). However, it is worthwhile noting that 33% of those heterozygous for *ALDH2*2* never flushed after alcohol ingestion. Intake of nutrients such as niacin could affect steady-state ALDH2 protein and contribute to between-individual variability in the alcohol flush reaction (Crabb et al. 1998). 15% of *ALDH2*1* homozygous subjects always flushed, suggesting the existence of factors other than ALDH2 polymorphism (Murayama et al. 1998).

Polymorphism of cytochrome P450 2E1 (CYP2E1) did not differ between flushers and non-flushers and was similar for moderate and heavy drinkers (Tanaka et al. 1997).

For alcohol dependence and alcoholism, all the recent data confirm previous findings (Couzigou et al. 1994). No case of alcoholism has been found in homozygous ALDH2-deficient subjects. The *ALDH2*2* allele is a protective factor against alcohol dependence (Tanaka et al. 1996, 1997, Nakamura et al. 1996, Murayama et al. 1998, Chao et al. 1997, Takeshita et al. 1998, Yin 1998). A clear interaction exists between a genetic factor (*ALDH2*2* polymorphism) and environmental factors (Higuchi et al. 1994). Very recently, a mutation in the promoter region of the *ALDH2* gene has been found and associated with a lower frequency of alcoholism. This mutation has been described in Asian and also in Caucasian population, but more extensive studies would be very worthwhile (Ishikawa et al. 1998). At the ADH polymorphism level, new data confirmed the protective role of the *ADH2*2* allele against alcohol dependence (Shen et al. 1997, Tanaka et al. 1996, Chao et al. 1997, Whitfield 1997, Yin et al. 1998, Nakamura et al. 1996). A recent European collaborative study has proved for the first time the existence of a genetic factor associated with alcohol dependence in a Caucasian population, with a lower frequency of the *ADH2*2* allele in alcoholics (Pares et al. 1998).

Recent studies on the relation between CYP2E1 polymorphism (C1 and C2 alleles) and alcoholism found no association (Carr et al. 1996, Nakamura et al. 1996, Tanaka et al. 1997, Pirmohamed et al. 1995). Conflicting data have been published (association with C1 allele or with C2 allele) but the functional significance of this polymorphism was not demonstrated and the bulk of published papers point to the probable absence of an association with alcohol dependence.

Thus, in alcohol dependence a protective role of the *ALDH2*2* allele and the *ADH2*2* allele is strongly supported. The role of ADH3 polymorphism seems very weak and is probably absent. No implication of CYP2E1, at the level of the alleles C1 and C2, has been demonstrated.

Genetics and Alcoholic Liver Disease

Only 20–30% of chronic alcoholics develop alcoholic cirrhosis (Couzigou 1993). A recent epidemiological study gave similar results with 15–20% cirrhosis in patients with chronic excessive alcohol use. The relative risk is higher for women for a given level of reported alcohol use (Becker et al. 1996). A twin study found a higher concordance rate of alcoholic cirrhosis in monozygous subjects even after taking into account the concordance rate due to alcoholism by itself. This study of more than 15,000 male twin pairs was reanalysed 16 years later with more cases of alcoholism and cirrhosis (Reed et al. 1996). Again, 50% of overall variance was due to genetic effects. Most, but not all, of the genetic liability to the organ-specific end-point of cirrhosis was due to the shared genetic liability to alcoholism. Once the shared variance with alcoholism was considered, there was no further shared genetic liability to psychosis and cirrhosis (Reed et al. 1996). The genetic factor could be at the alcohol metabolism level or related to hepatic cellular biology. For alcohol metabolism, it is important to stress the probable opposite effects of acetaldehyde accumulation on drinking behaviour and hepatic lesions. Thus, a genetic factor implicated in alcohol metabolism probably would act differently for alcoholism and cirrhosis (Couzigou et al. 1994). This tendency is observed for the *ALDH2*2* allele with a less striking difference in allele frequencies between alcoholic cirrhotic patients and controls than between controls and alcoholics without alcoholic liver disease (ALD) (Chao et al. 1997, Tanaka et al. 1996, Higuchi et al. 1996b). The same tendency is observed for ADH2 polymorphism: the difference between controls and alcoholic cirrhotic patients for the *ADH2*2* allele was less striking than for alcoholics without ALD (Yamauchi et al. 1995, Tanaka et al. 1996). A recent meta-analysis points in the same direction (Whitfield 1997). For ADH3 polymorphism recent findings confirm earlier data (Couzigou et al. 1993) suggesting that ADH3 has little or no effect on ALD (Ceni et al. 1997, Whitfield 1997). A recent European collaborative study from Spain, France, Germany, Poland and Sweden found no association between ADH3 polymorphism and alcoholic cirrhosis (Pares et al. 1998)

A number of studies have focused on ALD and CYP2E1 polymorphism. The mutation so far identified indicates no change in the protein but could be associated with a different inducibility (Ingelman Sundberg 1996). The data published are confusing, with an association between the C1 allele and ALD (Maezawa et al. 1995) and between the C2 allele and ALD (Pirmohamed et al. 1995) and without any association in Caucasian or Oriental populations (Ball et al. 1995, Carr et al. 1995, 1996, Agundez et al. 1996, Lucas et al. 1996, Chao et al. 1995, Savolainen et al. 1997). Overall, data do not favour a role for CYP2E1 polymorphism in ALD at least for the mutations reported. A very recent study again found no substantial role of the CYP2E1 gene in susceptibility to alcoholic cirrhosis and alcoholism (Parsian et al. 1998).

Other polymorphisms have also been studied in recent years. A new study again found negative results for a possible association between HLA antigens and ALD (Couzigou et al. 1993, Llop et al. 1995).

One study, in contrast with previous data (Couzigou et al. 1993), found an association between glutathione transferase (GST) M1 "null" and ALD (Savolainen et al. 1996). An association between ALD and apolipoprotein E polymorphism was not confirmed (de Ledinghen 1997). In the past few years, no new study has explored the tentative association between collagen polymorphism and ALD (Couzigou et al. 1993).

The most stimulating recent data were on cytokine polymorphisms: two studies found an association of a tumour necrosis factor (TNF) promoter polymorphism, linked with increased TNFα expression, and increased risk of ALD (Allott et al. 1996, Grove et al. 1997). Cytokine interleukin 1 (IL1) receptor antagonist (IL1RA) is a potent anti-inflammatory protein, and genetic polymorphism with differential expression of IL1RA has been described. A correlation of IL1RA polymorphism with hepatic fibrosis has been found in Japanese alcoholics (Takamatsu et al. 1998).

Hepatocellular carcinoma (HCC) is associated with ALD. In a short study, ALDH2 polymorphism has not been found to be associated with HCC (Ohhira et al. 1996). CYP2E1 polymorphism could be implicated in hepatocellular carcinogenesis through differential oxidation of carcinogens. Its implication has been found in one study (Ladero et al. 1996) but has not been confirmed (Kerjean et al. 1997).

The knowledge of genetic factors in ALD is slowly growing but without enough data to be precise about its role and to predict ALD in alcoholics.

Genetics and Other End-Organ Alcohol-Related Disease

First studies on alcoholic pancreatitis and ADH polymorphism observed a trend for an association (Couzigou et al. 1993). Recent data found a significant association between a lower *ADH2*1* allele frequency and pancreatitis. Patients with alcoholic cirrhosis and those with alcoholic pancreatitis could be from two distinct populations (Chao et al. 1997, Yamauchi 1998). In the same way, it is worthwhile remembering that a mutation in the trypsinogen gene has been described in hereditary pancreatitis but its association with alcoholic pancreatitis is not clear (Le Bodic et al. 1996, Gorry et al. 1997).

The correlation between ADH2 genotype and other alcohol-related organ injury (myopathy, cerebral atrophy, hyperuricaemia) has been studied with no convincing results (Yamauchi 1998).

Two studies found an association between ADH3 genotype and oropharyngeal cancer (Coutelle et al. 1997, Harty et al. 1997) and also one with a link with GST M1 polymorphism (Coutelle et al. 1997). Thus, the *ADH3*1* allele could substantially increase the risk of alcohol-related oropharyngeal cancer. These interesting data require confirmation in more extensive studies.

In oesophageal cancer, the inactive ALDH2 genotype is significantly more frequent but this association could be essentially a link with excessive drinking and not with carcinogenesis itself (Yokoyama et al. 1996).

Genetic factors linked to alcohol metabolism could modulate the risk of ischaemic heart disease. The protective effect of alcohol on ischaemic heart disease could be especially relevant for patients with the Lewis phenotype Le (a-b-) (Hein et al. 1993) and also in the case of B2 homozygotes at the level of the cholesteryl ester transfer protein gene (Fumeron et al. 1995).

General Conclusion

For the future, animal models, especially transgenic models, are needed for answering questions related to alcoholism and alcohol-related disease, even if no animal model of alcoholism exists. Family studies with several members presenting alcoholism or alcohol-related disease could help from a phenotypic and genotypic point of view, using the QTL approach. However, the candidate gene approach remains promising. Studies on polymorphism in alcohol metabolism are worthwhile, but the genetic approach at polymorphism of end-organ metabolism seems the most important. Genetic determination of high-risk individuals, and pharmacogenetic therapeutic approaches, remain a long way off.

References

Adams N (1995) Sex differences and the effects of tail pinch on ethanol drinking in Maudsley rats. Alcohol 12: 463–68
Adams N, Shihabi ZK, Blizard DA (1991) Ethanol preference in the Harrington derivation of the Maudsley Reactive and Non-Reactive strains. Alcohol Clin Exp Res 15: 170–74
Agundez J, Ladero J, Diaz-Rubio, et al (1996) Rsa I polymorphism at the cytochrome P450IIE1, locus is not related to the risk of alcohol-related severe liver disease. Liver 16: 380–83.

Allott RL, Quest LJ, Pirmohamed M, et al. (1996) Investigation of the role of the TNF α gene polymorphism in alcoholic liver disease ALD. Hepatology 24: 443A

Almasy L, Porjesz B, Blangero, et al. (1999) Heritability of the P300 and N100 components of the event-related brain potential in families with a history of alcoholism. Behav Genet (in press)

Anthenelli RM, Smith TL, Irwin MR, et al (1994) A comparative study of criteria for subgrouping alcoholics. The primary/secondary diagnostic scheme versus variations of the type 1/type 2 criteria. Am J Psychiatry 10: 1468–74

Anthenelli RM, Tabakoff B (1995a) The search for biochemical markers. Alcohol Health Res World 19: 176–80

Anthenelli RM, Smith TL, Craig CE et al. (1995b) Platelet monoamine oxidase activity levels in subgroups of alcoholics: diagnostic, temporal, and clinical correlates. Biol Psychiatry 38: 361–68

Anthenelli RM, Schuckit MA (1997) Genetics. In: Lowinson JH, Ruiz P, Millman RB (eds.), Substance abuse: a comprehensive textbook, 3nd ed. Williams & Wilkins, Baltimore, pp. 41–51

Anthenelli RM, Tipp J, Li TK, et al. (1998) Platelet monoamine oxidase activity in subgroups of alcoholics and controls: results from the Collaborative Study on the Genetics of Alcoholism. Alcohol Clin Exp Res 22: 598–604

Ball DM, Sherman D, Gibb R, et al. (1995). No association between the c2 allele at the cytochrome P450IIE1 gene and alcohol induced liver disease, alcohol Korsakoff's syndrome or alcohol dependence syndrome. Drug Alcohol Depend 39: 181–84

Ballas C, Golden G, Haley C, et al. (1997) Quantitative trait loci study of alcoholism in AA/ANA rats. Soc Neurosci Abstr 23: 2389

Becker U, Deis A, Sørensen TIA (1996) Prediction of risk of liver disease by alcohol intake, sex, and age: a prospective population study. Hepatology 23: 1025–29

Begleiter H, Porjesz B, Bihari B, et al. (1984) Event-related potentials in boys at risk for alcoholism. Science 225:1493–96

Begleiter H, Porjesz B, Rawlings R, et al. (1987) Auditory recovery function and P3 in boys at high risk for alcoholism. Alcohol 4: 315–21

Begleiter H, Porjesz B, Reich T, et al. (1998) Quantitative trait loci analysis of human event-related brain potentials: P3 voltage. Electroencephalogr Clin Neurophysiol 108: 244–50

Belknap JK, Metten P, Helms ML, et al. (1993) Quantitative trait loci (QTL) applications to substances of abuse: physical dependence studies with nitrous oxide and ethanol in BXD mice. Behav Genet 23: 213–22

Belknap JK, Rickhards SP, O'Toole, et al. (1997) Short-term selective breeding as a tool for QTL mapping: ethanol preference drinking in mice. Behav Genet 27: 55–66

Benegal V, Jain S, Subbukrishna DK, et al. (1995) P300 amplitudes vary inversely with continuum of risk in first degree male relatives of alcoholics. Psychiatric Genet 5: 1–8

Berlin I, Said S, Spreuz-Varoquaux O, et al. (1995) Monoamine oxidase A and B activities in heavy smokers. Biol Psychiatry 38: 756–61

Berman M.S, Whipple SC, Fitch RJ, et al. (1993) P3 in young boys as a predictor of adolescent substance abuse. Alcohol 10: 69–76

Bice P, Foroud T, Bo R, et al. (1998) A QTL for alcohol consumption identified in the P and NP rat lines confirmed in the HAD1 and LAD1 rat lines. Alcohol Clin Exp Res 22: 159A

Blum K, Noble EP, Sheridan PJ, et al. (1990) Allelic association of human dopamine D2 receptor gene in alcoholism. JAMA 263: 2055–60

Brewster DJ (1968) Genetic analysis of ethanol preference in rats selected for emotional reactivity. J Hered 59: 283–86

Bucholz KK, Hesselbrock VM, Shayka JH, et al. (1995) Reliability of individual diagnostic criterion items for psychoactive substance dependence and the impact on diagnosis. J Stud Alcohol 56: 500–05

Bucholz KK, Heath AC, Reich T, et al. (1996) Can we subtype alcoholism? A latent class analysis of data from relatives of alcoholics in a multicenter family study of alcoholism. Alcohol Clin Exp Res 20: 1462–71

Buchsbaum, MS, Pfefferbaum A (1971) Individual differences in stimulus intensity response. Psychophysiology 8: 600–11

Cadoret RJ, Yates WR, Troughton E, et al. (1995) Adoption studies demonstrating two genetic pathways to drug abuse. Arch Gen Psychiatry 52: 42–52

Carr LG, Hartleroad JY, Liang Y, et al. (1995) Polymorphism at the P450IIE1 locus is not associated with alcoholic liver disease in Caucasian men. Alcohol Clin Exp Res 19: 182–84

Carr LG, Yi IS, Li TK, et al. (1996) Cytochrome P4502E1 genotypes, alcoholism, and alcoholic cirrhosis in Han Chinese and Atayal Natives of Taiwan. Alcohol Clin Exp Res 20: 43–46

Ceni E, Galli A, Casini A (1997) Genetics, alcohol, and cirrhosis. Ann Intern Med 126: 1000

Chang FM, Ko HC, Lu RB, et al. (1997) The dopamine D4 receptor gene (DRD4) is not associated with alcoholism in three Taiwanese populations: six polymorphisms tested separately and as haplotypes. Biol Psychiatry 41: 394–405

Chao YC, Young TH, Chang WK, et al. (1995) An investigation of whether polymorphisms of cytochrome P4502E1 are genetic markers of susceptibility to alcoholic end-stage organ damage in a Chinese population. Hepatology 22: 1409–14

Chao YC, Young TH, Tang HS, et al. (1997) Alcoholism and alcoholic organ damage and genetic polymorphisms of alcohol metabolizing enzymes in Chinese patients. Hepatology 25: 112–17

Chen WJ, Lu ML, Hsu YPP, et al. (1997) Dopamine D2 receptor gene and alcoholism among four aboriginal groups and han in Taiwan. Am J Med Genet 74: 129–36

Cloninger CR, Bohnan M, Sigvardsson S (1981) Inheritance of alcohol abuse. Arch Gen Psychiatry 38: 861–68

Coutelle C, Ward PJ, Fleury B, et al. (1997) A laryngeal and oropharyngeal cancer and alcohol dehydrogenase 3 and glutathione S-transferase M$_1$ polymorphisms. Hum Genet 99: 319–25

Couzigou P, Begleiter H, Kiianmaa K, et al. (1993) Genetics and alcohol. In: Verschuren PM (ed.), Health issues related to alcohol consumption. ILSI Europe, Brussels, pp. 281–329

Couzigou P, Coutelle C, Fleury B, et al. (1994) Alcohol and aldehyde dehydrogenase genotypes, alcoholism and alcohol related disease. Alcohol Alcoholism suppl 2: 21–27

Crabb D, Xiao Q (1998) Studies on the enzymology of aldehyde dehydrogenase 2 in genetically modified hela cells. Alcohol Clin Exp Res 22: 780–81

Crabbe JC (1989) Genetic animal models in the study of alcoholism. Alcohol Clin Exp Res 13: 120–27

Crabbe JC (1996) Quantitative trait locus gene mapping: A new method for locating alcohol response genes. Addict Biol 1: 229–35

Crabbe JC, Rigter H (1985) Vasopressin and ethanol preference. II. Altered preference in two strains of diabetes insipidus rats and nephrogenic diabetes insipidus mice. Peptides 6: 677–83

Crabbe JC, McSwigan JD, Belknap JK (1985a) The role of genetics in substance abuse. In: Galizio M, Maisto SA (eds) Determinants of substance abuse. Plenum, New York, pp. 13–64

Crabbe JC, Kosobud A, Young ER, et al. (1985b) Bidirectional selection for susceptibility to ethanol withdrawal seizures in *Mus musculus*. Behav Genet 15: 521–36

Crabbe JC, Kosobud A, Tam BR, et al. (1987a) Genetic selection of mouse lines sensitive (COLD) and resistant (HOT) to acute ethanol hypodermia. Alcohol Drug Res 7: 163–74

Crabbe JC, Young ER, Deutsch CM, et al. (1987b) Mice genetically selected for differences in open-field activity after ethanol. Pharmacol Biochem Behav 27: 577–81

Crabbe JC, Phillips TJ, Kosobud A, et al. (1990) Estimation of genetic correlation of experiments using selectively bred and inbred animals. Alcohol Clin Exp Res 14: 141–51

Crabbe JC, Belknap JK, Buck KJ, et al. (1994) Genetic animal models of alcohol and drug abuse. Science 264: 1715–23

Crabbe JC, Phillips TJ, Feller DJ, et al. (1996a) Elevated alcohol consumption in null mutant mice lacking 5-HT1B serotonin receptors. Nat Genet 14: 98–101

Crabbe JC, Phillips TJ, Gallaher EJ, et al. (1996b) Common genetic determinants of the ataxic and hypothermic effects of ethanol in BXD/Ty recombinant inbred mice: genetic correlations and quantitative trait loci. J Pharmacol Exp Ther 277: 624–32

Cunningham CL (1995) Localization of genes influencing ethanol-induced conditioned place preference and locomotor activity in BXD recombinant inbred mice. Psychopharmacology 120: 28–41

Daw EW, Rice JP, Reich T, et al. (1995) Relationship of ERPs in COGA control families. Psychiatric Genet 5 (suppl 1): S78

Deitrich RA (1990) Selective breeding of mice and rats for initial sensitivity to ethanol: contributions to understanding of ethanol's actions. In: Deitrich RA, Pawlowski AA (eds.), Initial sensitivity to alcohol. NIAAA Research Monograph 20. US Government Printing Office, Rockville, MD, pp. 7–59

Deitrich RA, Spuhler K (1984) Genetics of alcoholism and alcohol actions. In: Smart K, Sellers EM (eds), Research advances in alcohol and drug problems. Plenum, New York, vol. 8, pp. 47–98

De Ledinghen V, Grimaldi S, Iron A, et al. (1997) Genetic polymorphism of apoproteins E in alcoholic cirrhosis. Gastroenterology 112: 1254A

Devor EJ, Abell CW, Hoffman PL, et al. (1994) Platelet MAO activity in type I and type II alcoholism. Ann NY Acad Sci 708: 119–28

Dumermuth G (1968) Variance spectra of electroencephalograms in twins. In: Kellaway P, Petersen I (eds.), Clinical Electroencephalography of Children.. Grune & Stratton, New York, pp. 119–54

Dustman RE, Beck EC (1965) The visually evoked potentials in twins. Electroencephalogr Clin Neurophysiol 19: 541–638

Edenberg HJ, Foroud T, Koller DL, et al. (1998a) A family-based analysis of the association of the dopamine D2 receptor (DRD2) with alcoholism. Alcohol Clin Exp Res 22: 505–12

Edenberg HJ, Reynolds J, Koller DL, et al. (1998b) A family-based analysis of whether the functional promoter alleles of the serotonin transporter gene HTT affect the risk for alcohol dependence. Alcohol Clin Exp Res 22: 1080–85

Eriksson CJP (1990) Finnish selective breeding studies for initial sensitivity to ethanol: update 1988 on the AT and ANT rat lines. In: Deitrich RA, Pawlowski AA (eds.), Initial sensitivity to alcohol. NIAAA Research Monograph 20. US Government Printing Office, Rockville, MD, pp. 61–86

Eriksson K (1968) Genetic selection for voluntary alcohol sonsumption in the albino rat. Science 159: 739–41

Eriksson K, Rusi M (1981) Finnish selection studies on alcohol-related behaviors: general outline. In: McClearn GE, Deitrich RA, Erwin G (eds.), Development of animal models as pharmacogenetic tools. NIAAA Research Monograph 6. US Government Printing Office, Rockville, MD, pp. 87–117

Erwin VG, Jones BC, Radcliffe RJ (1990) Further characterization of LS*SS recombinant inbred strains of mice: activating and hypothermic effects of ethanol. Alcohol Clin Exp Res 14: 200–04

Erwin VG, Jones BC (1993) Genetic correlations among ethanol-related behaviors and neurotensin receptors in Long Sleep (LS) × Short Sleep (SS) recombinant inbred strains of mice. Behav Genet 23: 191–96

Erwin VG, Deitrich RA (1996) Genetic selection and characterization of mouse lines for acute functional tolerance to ethanol. J Pharmacol Exp Ther 279: 1310–17

Erwin VG, Markel PD, Johnson TE, et al. (1997) Common quantitative trait loci for alcohol-related behaviors and central nervous system neurotensin measures: hypnotic and hypothermic effects. J Pharmacol Exp Ther 280: 211–218

Fadda F, Mosca E, Colombo G, et al. (1989) Effect of spontaneous ingestion of ethanol on brain dopamine metabolism. Life Sci 44: 281–87

Finck U, Rommelspacher H, Kuhns S, et al. (1997) Influence of dopamine D2 receptor (DRD2) genotype on neuroadaptative effects to alcohol and the clinical outcome of alcoholism. Pharmacogenetics 7: 271–81

Foroud T, Bucholz KK, Edenberg HJ, et al (1998) Linkage of an alcoholism-related severity phenotype to chromosome 16. Alcohol Clin Exp Res 22: 2035–42

Fuller JL (1985) The genetics of alcohol consumption in animals. Social Biol 32: 210–21

Fuller JL, McClearn GE, Wilson JR, et al. (1985) Genetics and human encounter with alcohol. Social Biol 32: 327

Fumeron F, Betoulle D, Luc C, et al. (1995) Alcohol intake modulates the effect of a polymorphism of the cholesteryl ester transfer protein gene on the plasma high density lipoprotein and the risk of myocardial infarction. J Clin Invest 96: 1664–71

Geijer T, Jönsson E, Neiman J, et al. (1997a) Prodynorphin allelic distributions in Scandinavian chronic alcoholics. Alcohol Clin Exp Res 21: 1333–-36

Geijer T, Jönsson E, Neiman J, et al (1997b). Tyrosine hydroxylase and dopamine D4 receptor allelic distribution in Scandinavian chronic alcoholic. Alcohol Clin Exp Res 21: 35–39

Goldman D, Urbanek M, Guenther R, et al. (1997) Linkage and association of a functional DRD2 variant (Ser 311 Cys) and DRD2 markers to alcoholism, substance abuse and schizophrenia in southwestern American Indians. Am J Med Genet 74: 386–94

Goodwin DW, Schulsinger F, Hermansen L, et al. (1973) Alcohol problems in adoptees raised a part from alcoholic biological parents. Arch Gen Psychiatry 28: 238–43

Gorry MC, Gabbaizedeh D, Furey W, et al. (1997) Mutations in the cationic trypsinogen gene are associated with recurrent acute and chronic pancreatitis. Gastroenterology 113: 1062–68

Grove J, Daly AK, Bassendine MF, et al. (1997) Association of a tumor necrosis factor promoter polymorphism with susceptibility to alcoholic steatohepatitis. Hepatology 26: 143–46

Hall W, Sannibale C (1996) Are there two types of alcoholism? Lancet 348: 1258

Hammoumi S, Payen A, Favre JD, et al. (1998) The serotonin transporter linked polymorphism region constitute a marker of alcohol dependence. Alcohol Clin Exp Res 22: 176A

Harada S, Okubo T, Tsutsumi M, et al. (1996) Investigation of genetic risk factors associated with alcoholism. Alcohol Clin Exp Res 20: 293A–96A

Harada S, Okubo T, Tsutsumi M, et al. (1998) A new genetic variant in the Sp1 binding cis-element of cholecystokinin gene promoter region and relationship to alcoholism. Alcohol Clin Exp Res 22: 93S–96S

Harty LC, Caporaso NE, Hakes RB, et al. (1997) Alcohol dehydrogenase 3 genotype and risk of oral cavity and pharyngeal cancers. J Natl Cancer Inst 89: 1698–1705

Heath AC (1995) Genetic influences on alcoholism risk: a review of adoption and twin studies Alcohol Health Res World 19: 166–70

Hein HO, Sørensen H, Suadicani P, et al. (1993) Alcohol consumption, lewis phenotypes and risk of ischaemic heart disease. Lancet 341: 392–96

Heinz A, Sander T, Harms H, et al. (1996) Lack of allelic association of dopamine D_1 and D2 (Taq 1A) receptor gene polymorphisms with reduced dopaminergic sensitivity in alcoholism. Alcohol Clin Exp Res 20: 1109–13

Hellevuo K, Kiianmaa K, Juhakoski A, et al. (1987) Intoxicating effects of lorazepam and barbital in rat lines selected for differential sensitivity to ethanol. Psychopharmacology 91: 263–67

Hesselbrock VM (1995) The genetic epidemiology of alcoholism. In: Begleiter H, Kissin B (eds.), Alcohol and alcoholism, vol. 1. Oxford University Press, New York, pp. 17–39

Higuchi S (1994) Polymorphisms of ethanol metabolizing enzyme genes and alcoholism. Alcohol Alcoholism 28 (suppl.2): 29–34

Higuchi S, Matsushita S, Imaseki H, et al. (1994a) Aldehyde dehydrogenase genotypes in Japanese alcoholics. Lancet 343: 741–42

Higuchi S, Parrish KM, Dufour MC, et al. (1994b) Relationship between age and drinking patterns and drinking problems among Japanese, Japanese-Americans, and Caucasians. Alcohol Clin Exp Res 18: 305–10

Higuchi S, Matsushita S, Murayama M, et al. (1995) Alcohol and aldehyde dehydrogenase polymorphisms and the risk for alcoholism. Am J Psychiatry 152: 1219–21

Higuchi S, Matsushita S, Muramatsu T, et al. (1996a) Alcohol and aldehyde dehydrogenase genotypes and drinking behavior in Japanese. Alcohol Clin Exp Res 20: 493–97

Higuchi S, Muramatsu T, Matsushita S, et al. (1996b). Polymorphisms of ethanol-oxidizing enzymes in alcoholics with inactive ALDH2. Hum Genet 97: 431–34

Hill SY, Steinhauer SR (1993) Assess boys and girls at risk for developing alcoholism with P300 from a visual discrimination task. J Stud Alcohol 54: 350–58

Hill SY, Steinhauer S, Lowers L, et al. (1995) Eight-year longitudinal follow-up of P300 and clinical outcome in children from high-risk for alcoholism families. Biol Psychiatry 37: 823–27

Hiller-Sturmhöfel S, Bowers BJ, Wehner JM (1995) Genetic engineering in animal models. Alcohol Health Res World 19: 206–13

Homanics GE, Ferguson C, Quinlan JJ, et al. (1997) Gene knockout of the alpha 6 subunit of the γ-aminobutyric acid type A receptor: lack of effect on responses to ethanol, pentobarbital, and general anesthetics. Mol Pharmacol 51: 588–96

Homanics GE, Le NQ, Kist F, et al. (1998) Ethanol tolerance and withdrawal responses in $GABA_A$ receptor α6 subunit null allele mice in inbred C57BL/6J and strain 129/SvJ mice. Alcohol Clin Exp Res 22: 259–65

Ingelman Sundberg M (1996) Ethanol inducible cytochrome P450 ($CYP2E_1$) biochemistry, molecular biology and clinical relevance: 1996 update. Alcohol Clin Exp Res 20 (suppl): 138A–46A

Ishiguro H, Arinami T, Saito T, et al. (1998) Association study between the 141 ins/del and TaqIA polymorphism of the dopamine D2 receptor gene and alcoholism. Alcohol Clin Exp Res 22: 845–48

Ishikawa Y, Harada S, Okubo T, et al. (1998) A mutation in the promoter region of ALDH2 gene. Alcohol Clin Exp Res 22 (suppl.3): 164A

Johnson EO, Vandenbree MB, Pickens RW (1996) Indicators of genetic and environmental influences in alcohol dependent individuals. Alcohol Clin Exp Res 20: 67–74

Kaij L (1960) Studies on the etiology and sequels of abuse of alcohol. Department of Psychiatry, University of Lund, Sweden

Kampov-Polevoy AB, Kasheffskaya OP, Overstreet DH, et al. (1996) Pain sensitivity and saccharin intake in alcohol-preferring and -nonpreferring rat strains. Physiol Behav 59: 683–88

Katsanis J, Jacono W.G, McGue MK, et al. (1997). P300 event-related potential heritability in monozygotic and dizygotic twins. Psychophysiology 34: 47–58

Kerjean A, De Ledinghen V, Lucas D, et al. (1997). Hepatocellular carcinoma developed on alcoholic cirrhosis and cytochrome P450IIE$_1$ polymorphism. Gastroenterol Clin Biol 21: A198

Khanna JM, Le AD, Kalant H, et al. (1985) Differential sensitivity to ethanol, pentobarbital, and barbital in spontaneously hypertensive and normotensive Wistar-Kyoto rats. Psychopharmacology 86: 296–301

Khanna JM, Kalant H, Chau AK, et al. (1990) Initial sensitivity, acute tolerance and alcohol consumption in four inbed strains of rats. Psychopharmacology 101: 390–95

Kiianmaa K, Tabakoff B, Saito T (eds.) (1989) Genetic Aspects of Alcoholism. Finnish Foundation for Alcohol Studies 37, Helsinki, 264 pp.

Knapp DJ, Kampov-Polevoy AB, Overstreet DH, et al. (1997) Ultrasonic vocalization behavior differs between lines of ethanol-preferring and non-preferring rats. Alcohol Clin Exp Res 21: 1232–40

Kono Y, Yoneda H, Sakai T, et al. (1997). Association between early onset alcoholism and the dopamine D2 receptor gene. Am J Med Genet 74: 179–82

Koopmans JR, Heath AC, Neale, MC et al. (1997a) The genetics of initiation and quantity of alcohol and tobacco use. In: Koopmans J (ed.), The genetics of health related behaviors: a study of adolescent twins and their parents, pp. 89–108

Koopmans JR, van Doormen LJP, Boomsma DI (1997b) Association between alcohol use and smoking in adolescent and young adult twins a bivariate genetic analysis. Alcohol Clin Exp Res 2: 537–46

Korpi ER, Kleingoor C, Kettenmann H, et al. (1993) Benzodiazepine-induced motor impairment linked to point mutation in cerebellar GABA$_A$ receptor. Nature 361: 356–59

Kranzler HR, McCaul ME, Gelernter J, et al. (1997) No allelic association of an exon 13 polymorphism of the GSα gene to alcohol and/or drug dependence. Addiction Biol 2: 309–15

Ladero JM, Agundez JAG, Rodriguez-Lescure A, et al. (1996) RsaI polymorphism at the cytochrome P450IIE$_1$ locus and risk of hepatocellular carcinoma. Gut 39: 330–33.

Lawford BR, Young RMcD, Rowell JA, et al. (1997) Association of the D2 dopamine receptor A1 allele with alcoholism: medical severity of alcoholism and type of controls. Biol Psychiatry 41: 386–93

Lebodic L, Bignon JL, Raguenes O, et al. (1996) The hereditary pancreatitis gene maps to long arm of chromosome 7 Hum Mol Genet 5: 549–54

Li TK, Lumeng L, McBride WJ, et al. (1981) Indiana selection studies on alcohol-related behaviors. In McClearn GE, Deitrich RA, Erwin G (eds.), Development of animal models as pharmacogenetic tools. NIAAA Resarch Monograph 6, US Government Printing Office, Rockville, MD, pp. 171–91

Li TK, Lumeng L, McBride WJ, et al. (1987) Rodent lines selected for factors affecting alcohol consumption. In: Lindros KO, Ylikahri R, Kiianmaa K (eds.), Advances in biomedical alcohol research. Alcohol Alcoholism Suppl 1: 91–96

Light JR, Irvine KM, Kjerulf L (1996) Estimating genetic and environmental effects of alcohol use and dependence from a national survey: a "quasi adoption" study. J Stud Alcohol 57: 507–20

Llop E, Hirsch S, De La Maza MP, et al. (1995) Major histocompatibility system as a risk factor for alcoholic liver disease. Rev Med Chil 123: 687–93

Lucas D, Menez C, Floch F, et al. (1996) Cytochromes P4502E1 and P4501A1 genotypes and susceptibility to cirrhosis or upper aerodigestive tract cancer in alcoholic caucasians. Alcohol Clin Exp Res 20: 1033–37

Lumeng L, Doolittle DP, Li TK (1986) New duplicate lines of rats that differ in voluntary alcohol consumption. Alcohol Alcoholism 21: A125

Lykken D, Tellegen A, Thorkelson K (1974) Genetic determination of EEG frequency spectra. Biol Psychol 1: 245–59

Lykken D, Tellegen A, Iacono W (1982) EEG spectra in twins: evidence for a neglected mechanism of genetic determination. Physiol Psychol 10: 60–65

Maezawa Y, Yamauchi M, Toda G, et al. (1995) Alcohol-metabolizing enzyme polymorphisms and alcoholism in Japan. Alcohol Clin Exp Res 19: 951–54

Mardones J (1960) Experimentally induced changes in the free selection of ethanol. Int Rev Neurobiol 2: 41–76

Mardones J (1972) Experimentally induced changes in alcohol appetite. In: Forsander O, Eriksson K (eds), Biological aspects of alcohol consumption, vol. 20. Finnish Foundation for Alcohol Studies, Helsinki, pp. 15–23

Markel PD, Fulker DW, Bennett B, et al. (1996) Quantitative trait loci for ethanol sensitivity in the LS × SS recombinant inbred strains interval mapping. Behav Genet 26: 447–58

McClearn GE, Rodgers DA (1959) Differences in alcohol preference among inbred strains of mice. Q J Stud Alcohol 20: 691–95

McClearn GE, Deitrich RA, Erwin G (eds.) (1981a) Development of animal models as pharmacogenetic tools. NIAAA Research Monograph 6. US Government Printing Office, Rockville, MD, 302 pp.

McClearn GE, Kakihana R (1981b) Selective breeding for ethanol sensitivity: short-sleep and long-sleep mice. In: McClearn GE, Deitrich RA, Erwin G (eds), Development of animal models as pharmacogenetic tools. NIAAA Research Monograph 6. US Government Printing Office, Rockville, MD, pp. 147–59

McClearn E, Wilson JR, Petersen DR, et al. (1982) Selective breeding in mice for severity of ethanol withdrawal syndrome. Subst Alcohol Actions/Misuse 3: 135–43

Mormède P, Razafimanalina N, Courvoisier H. et al. (1998) QTLs for temperament traits in rats: relevance for alcohol drinking. Alcohol Clin Exp Res 22: 151A

Murayama M, Matsushita S, Muramatsu T, et al. (1998). Clinical characteristics and disease course of alcoholics with inactive aldehyde dehydrogenase-2. Alcohol Clin Exp Res 22: 524–27

Nakamura K, Iwahashi K, Matsuo Y, et al. (1996) Characteristics of Japanese alcoholism with the atypical aldehyde dehydrogenase 2*2-1. A comparison of the genotype of ALDH2, ADH2, ADH3 and cytochrome P4502E1 between alcoholics and non alcoholics. Alcohol Clin Exp Res 20: 52–55

Neumark YD, Friedlanger Y, Thomasson, HR et al. (1998) Association of the ADH 2-2 allele with reduced ethanol consumption in Jewish men in Israel: a pilot study. J Stud Alcohol 59: 133–39

Noble EP (1990) Alcoholic fathers and their sons: neurophysiological, electrophysiological, personality, and family correlates. Banbury Report 33. In: Cloninger CR, Begleiter H (eds.) Genetics and biology of alcoholism. Cold Spring Harbor Laboratory Press, Cold Spring Harbor, NY, pp. 159–74.

O'Connor SJ, Hesselbrock V, Tasman A (1986) Correlates of increased risk for alcoholism in young men. Prog Neuropsychopharmacol Biol Psychiatry 10: 211–18

O'Connor SJ, Hesselbrock V, Tasman A, et al. (1987) P3 amplitude in two distinct tasks are decreased in young men with a history of paternal alcoholism. Alcohol 4: 323–30

O'Connor SJ, Morzorati S, Christian JC, et al. (1994) Heritable features of the auditory oddball event-related potentials: peaks, latencies, morphology and topography. Electroencephalogr Clin Neurophysiol 92: 115–25

Ohhira M, Fujimoto Y, Matsumoto A, et al. (1996) Hepatocellular carcinoma associated with alcoholic liver disease: a clinicopathological study and genetic polymorphism of aldehyde dehydrogenase 2. Alcohol Clin Exp Res 20: 378A–82A

Pares X, Farres J, Crosas B, et al. (1998) Alcohol dehydrogenase genotypes in Europeans. Alcohol Clin Exp Res 22 (suppl.3): 140A

Parsian A, Todd RD, Cloninger CR, et al. (1996) Platelet adenylyl cyclase activity in alcoholics and subtypes of alcoholics. Alcohol Clin Exp Res 20: 745–51

Parsian A, Cloninger CR (1997) Human $GABA_A$ receptor α_1 and α_2 subunits genes and alcoholism. Alcohol Clin Exp Res 21: 430–33

Parsian X, Cloninger R, Zhang ZH (1998) Association studies of polymorphisms of CYP2E1 gene in alcoholics with cirrhosis, antisocial personality and normal controls. Alcohol Clin Exp Res 22: 888–91

Pfefferbaum A, Ford JM, White PM, et al. (1991) Event-related potentials in alcoholic men: P3 amplitude reflects family history but notalcohol consumption. Alcohol Clin Exp Res 15: 839–50

98   Health Issues Related to Alcohol Consumption

Philips TJ, Feller DJ, Crabbe JC (1989) Selected mouse lines, alcohol and behavior. Experimentia 45: 805–27

Philips TJ, Burkhart-Kasch S, Terdal ES, et al. (1991) Response to selection for ethanol-induced locomotor activation: genetic analyses and selection response characterization. Psychopharmacology 103: 557–66

Phillips TJ, Crabbe JC, Matten P, et al. (1995a) Localization of genes affecting alcohol drinking in mice. Alcohol Clin Exp Res 18: 931–41

Phillips TJ, Huson M, Gwiazdon C, et al. (1995b) Effects of acute and repeated ethanol exposures on the locomotor activity of BXD recombinant inbred mice. Alcohol Clin Exp Res 19: 269–78

Phillips TJ, Lessov CN, Harland RD, et al. (1996) Evaluation of potential genetic associations between ethanol tolerance and sensitization in BXD/Ty recombinant inbred mice. J Pharmacol Exp Ther 277: 613–23

Phillips, TJ (1997) Behavioral genetics of drug sensitization. Crit Rev Neurobiol 11: 21–33

Phillips TJ, Huson MG, McKinnon CS (1998) Localization of genes mediating acute and sensitized locomotor responses to cocaine in BDX/Ty recombinant inbred mice. J Neurosci 18: 3023–34

Pirmohamed M, Kitteringham NR, Quest LJ, et al. (1995) Genetic polymorphism of cytochrome P4502E1 and risk of alcoholic liver disease in Caucasians. Pharmacogenetics 5: 351–57

Polich J, Burns T (1987) P300 from identical twins. Neuropsychologia 25: 299–304

Porjesz B, Begleiter H, Bihari B, et al. (1987) The N2 component of the event-related brain potential in abstinent alcoholics. Electroencephalogr Clin Neurophysiol 66: 121–31

Porjesz B, Begleiter H (1990) Event-related potentials in individuals at risk for alcoholism. Alcohol 7: 465–69

Porjesz B, Begleiter H, Litke A, et al. (1996) Visual P3 as a potential phenotypic marker for alcoholism: evidence from the COGA national project. In: Ogura C, Koga Y, Shimokochi M (eds.), Recent advances in event-related brain potential research. Elsevier, Amsterdam, pp. 539–49

Propping P (1977) Genetic control of ethanol action in the central nervous system: an EEG study in twins. Hum Genet 35: 309–34

Ramachandran G, Porjesz B, Begleiter H, et al. (1996) A simple auditory oddball task in young adult males at high risk for alcoholism. Alcohol Clin Exp Res 20: 9–15

Razafimanalina N, Mormède P, Velley L (1997) Alcohol consumption and gustatory hedonic profiles in Wistar-Kyoto hyper- and normoactive rat strains. Alcohol Alcoholism 32: 485–91

Reed T, Page WF, Viken RJ, et al. (1996) Genetic predisposition to organ specific endpoints of alcoholism. Alcohol Clin Exp Res 20: 1528–33

Reich T, Edenberg HJ, Goate A, et al (in press) A genome-wide search for genes affecting the risk for alcohol dependence. Neuropsychiatric Genet

Rodgers DA, McClearn GE (1962) Mouse strain differences in preference for various concentrations of alcohol. Q J Stud Alcohol 23: 26–33

Rodriguez LA, Plomin R, Blizard DA, et al. (1995) Alcohol acceptance, preference and sensitivity in mice. II. Quantitative trait loci mapping analysis using BXD recombinant inbred strains. Alcohol Clin Exp Res 19: 367–73

Rogers TD, Deary I (1991) The P300 component of the auditory event-related potential in monozygotic and dizygotic twins. Acta Psychiatrica Scand 83: 412–16

Roman T, Bau CHD, Hutz HM (1998). No association between alcoholism and a variable number of tandem repeat polymorphism at the dopamine D4 receptor gene. Alcohol Clin Exp Res 22: 967A

Rommelspacher H, May T, Dufeu P, et al. (1994) Longitudinal observations of monoamine oxidase b in alcoholics: differentiation of marker characteristics. Alcohol Clin Exp Res 18: 1322–29

Samochowiec J, Sander T, Smolka M, et al. (1998) Association analysis of Cys23 Ser substitution polymorphism with in the 5HT2c receptor gene with neuronal hyperexcitability and personality traits in alcohol-dependent patients. Alcohol Clin Exp Res 22: 176A

Sander T, Harms H, Lesch KP, et al. (1997) Association analysis of regulatory variations of the serotonin transporter gene with severe alcohol dependence Alcohol Clin Exp Res 21: 1356–59

Sander T, Harms H, Dufeu P, et al. (1998) Serotonin transporter gene variants in alcohol dependent subjects with dissocial personality disorder. Biol Psychiatry 43: 908–12

Satinder KP (1970) Behavior-genetic-dependent self-selection of alcohol in rats. J Comp Physiol Psychol 80: 422–34

Satinder KP (1975) Interactions of age, sex and long-term alcohol intake in selectively bred strains of rats. J Stud Alcohol 36: 1493–1507

Satinder KP, Wooldridge GE (1986) Emotional reactivity and alcohol preference among genetic crosses of the Maudsley and Roman rats. Pharmacol Biochem Behav 24: 879–81

Savolainen VT, Pajarinen J, Perola M, et al. (1996) Glutathione S transferase GST M1 "null" genotype and the risk of alcoholic liver disease. Alcohol Clin Exp Res 20: 1340–45

Savolainen VT, Pajarinen J, Perola M, et al. (1997) Polymorphism in the cytochrome P450 2E1 gene and the risk of alcoholic liver disease. J Hepatol 26: 55–61

Schuckit MA (1995) A long term study of sons of alcoholics. Alcohol Health Res World 19: 172–75

Schuckit MA, Li TK, Cloninger CR, et al. (1985) Genetics of alcoholism. Alcohol Clin Exp Res 9: 475–92

Schuckit MA, Tipp J, Smith TL, et al. (1995) An evaluation of type A and B alcoholics. Addiction 90: 1189–1203

Shen YC, Fan JH, Edenberg HJ (1997). Polymorphism of ADH and ALDH genes among four ethnic groups in China and effects upon the risk of alcoholism. Alcohol Clin Exp Res 21: 1272–77

Sinclair JD (1992) Localization of the primary sites of genetic influence. Behav Genet 22: 1–10

Sinclair JD (1998) From optimal complexity to the naltrexone extinction of alcoholism. In: Hoffman R, Sherrick MF, Warm JS (eds.), Viewing psychology as a chole: the integrative science of William N. Dember. American Psychological Association, Washington, D.C., pp. 491–508

Sinclair JD, Lê AD, Kiianmaa K (1989) The AA and ANA rat lines, selected for differences in alcohol consumption. Experimentia 45: 798–805

Sinclair JD, Li TK (1996) High and low drinking rat lines: contributions to current understanding and future development. Alcohol Clin Exp Res 20: 109A–12A

Spuhler K, Deitrich RA, Baker RC (1990) Selective breeding of rats differing in sensitivity to the hypnotic effects of acute ethanol administration. In: Deitrich RA, Pawlowski AA (eds.), Initial sensitivity to alcohol. NIAAA Research Monograph 20. US Government Printing Office, Rockville, MD, pp. 87–102.

Stassen H, Bomben G, Propping P (1987) Genetic aspects of the EEG: an investigation into the within-pair similarity of monozygotic and dizygotic twins with a new method of analysis. Electroencephalogr Clin Neurophysiol 66: 489–501

Stassen H, Lykken D, Bomben G (1988) The within-pair EEG similarity of twins reared apart. Eur Arch Neurol Sci 237: 244–52

Suarez BK, Hampe CL, Parsian A, et al. (1995). Monoamine oxidases and alcoholism. II. Studies in alcoholic families. Am J Med Genet 60: 417–23

Surwillo WW (1980) Cortical evoked potentials in monozygotic twins and unrelated subjects: comparisons of exogenous and endogenous components. Behav Genet 10: 201–09

Swan GE, Carmelli D, Cardon LR (1997). Heavy consumption of cigarettes, alcohol and coffee in male twins. J Stud Alcohol 58: 182–90

Takamatsu M, Yamauchi M, Maezawa Y, et al. (1998) Correlation of a polymorphism in the interleukin-1 receptor antagonist gene with hepatic fibrosis in Japanese alcoholics. Alcohol Clin Exp Res 22: 141S–44S

Takeshita T, Maruyama S, Morimoto K (1998) Relevance of both daily hassles and the ALDH2 genotype to problem drinking among Japanese male workers. Alcohol Clin Exp Res 22: 115–20

Tanaka F, Shiratori Y, Yokosuka O, et al. (1996) High incidence of ADH2*1/ALDH2*1 genes among Japanese alcohol dependents and patients with alcoholic liver disease. Hepatology 23: 234–39

Tanaka F, Shiratori Y, Yokosuka O, et al. (1997) Polymorphism of alcohol-metabolizing genes affects drinking behavior and alcoholic liver disease in Japanese men. Alcohol Clin Exp Res 21: 596–601

Thomasson HR, Beard JD, Li TK (1995). ADH2 gene polymorphisms are determinants of alcohol pharmaco kinetics. Alcohol Clin Exp Res 19: 1494–99

Turner A, Lawrence J, Chih-Huichen A, et al. (1997) Frequency of the A1/A2 alleles of the dopamine receptor (DRD2) gene in a british caucasian control group screening to exclude alcoholism and heavy drinking. Addiction Biol 2: 207–13

van Beijsterveldt CEM, Boomsma DI (1994) Genetics of the human electroencephalogram (EEG) and event-related brain potentials (ERPs): a review. Hum Genet 94: 319–30 van Beijsterveldt T (1996) The genetics of electrophysiological indices of brain activity: an EEG study in adolescent twins. University of Amsterdam

Vandenbree MB, Svikis DS, Pickens RW (1998) Genetic influences in antisocial personality and drug use disorders. Drug Alcohol Depend 49: 177–87

Velley L, Pujol H, Mormède P (1998) Initial alcohol consumption in three inbred strains deriving from wistar rats: gustarory and post-ingestional factors? Alcohol Clin Exp Res 22: 167A

Vogel F (1970) The genetic basis of the normal human electroencephalogram (EEG). Humangenetik 10: 91–114

Vogel F, Kruger J, Hopp HP, et al. (1986) Visually and auditory evoked EEG potentials in carriers of four hereditary EEG variants. Hum Neurobiol 5: 49–58

Wall TL, Garcia AS, Thomasson HR, et al. (1997a) Alcohol dehydrogenase polymorphisms in native Americans: identification of the ADH2-3 allele. Alcohol Alcoholism 32: 129–32

Wall TL, Peterson CM, Peterson KP, et al. (1997b) Alcohol metabolism in Asian-American men with genetic polymorphisms of aldehyde dehydrogenase. Ann Intern Med 127: 376–79

Waller MB, Murphy JM, McBride WJ, et al. (1986) Effect of low dose ethanol on spontaneous motor activity in alcohol-preferring and non preferring lines of rats. Pharmacol Biochem Behav 24: 617–23

Whipple SC., Parker ES, Noble EP (1988) An atypical neurocognitive profile in alcoholic fathers and their sons. J Stud Alcohol 49: 240–44

Whipple SC, Berman SM, Noble EP (1991) Event-related potentials in alcoholic fathers and their sons. Alcohol 8: 321–27

Whitfield JB (1994) ADH and ALDH genotypes in relation to alcohol metabolic rate and sensitivity. Alcohol Alcoholism (suppl 2): 59–65

Whitfield JB, Martin NG (1996) Alcohol reactions in subjects of European descent: effects on alcohol abuse and on physical and psychomotor responses to alcohol. Alcohol Clin Exp Res 20: 81–87

Whitfield JB (1997) Meta-analysis of the effects of alcohol dehydrogenase genotype on alcohol dependence and alcoholic liver disease. Alcohol Alcohol 32: 613–19

Yamauchi M (1998) Association of polymorphism in the alcohol dehydrogenase 2 gene with alcohol-related organ injuries, especially liver cirrhosis. Addict Biol 3: 151–57

Yamauchi M, Maezawa Y, Mizuhara Y, et al. (1995a) Polymorphisms in alcohol metabolizing enzyme gene and alcoholic cirrhosis in Japanese patients: a multivariate analysis. Hepatology 22: 1136–42

Yamauchi M, Maezawa Y, Toda G, et al. (1995b) Association of a restriction fragment lenght polymorphism in the alcohol deshydrogenase 2 gene with Japanese alcoholic liver cirrhosis. J Hepatol 23: 519–23

Yates WR, Cadoret RJ, Troughton, E et al. (1996) An adoption study of DSM III R alcohol and drug dependence severity. Drug Alcohol Depend 41: 9–15

Yin SJ (1998) Allelic variations of the alcohol dehydrogenase genes and alcoholism in Asians. Alcohol Clin Exp Res 22 (Suppl.3): 140A

Yokoyama A, Muramatsu T, Ohmori T, et al. (1996) Esophageal cancer and aldehyde dehydrogenase 2 genotypes in Japanese males. Cancer Epidemiol Biomarkers Prev 5: 99–102

Yoshimoto K, Komura S (1987) Reexamination of the relationship between alcohol preference and brain monoamines in inbred strains of mice including senescence-accelerated mice. Pharmacol Biochem Behav 27: 317–22

Young YP, Lader MH, Fenton GW (1972). A twin study on the genetic influences on the electroencephalogram. J Med Genet 9: 13–16

Chapter *4*

Alcohol and Body Weight

K.R. Westerterp
Maastricht University, The Netherlands

A.M. Prentice
MRC International Nutrition Group, London, UK

E. Jéquier
University of Lausanne, Switzerland

Abstract

There is no consensus on the relationship between moderate alcohol use and body weight. In the literature there has been substantial controversy as to whether or not alcohol calories count. Studies on alcohol use and food consumption provide a remarkable level of consistency in demonstrating that alcohol use is associated with minimal compensatory down-regulation of energy intake from other foods. Thus, it is concluded that in most people alcohol energy is largely additive to the normal diet, and other explanations are sought for the paradoxical association between alcohol and body weight. However, studies on energy and nutrient balances clearly show that alcohol is a nutrient that is utilized efficiently by the body and that alcohol calories do count. Balance studies conducted over several weeks confirm this notion. The interpretation of (epidemiological) observations on alcohol consumption and body weight in daily life is complicated by many factors such as reporting errors and the confounding influence of other subject characteristics. Direct measurement of total daily energy expenditure without and with alcohol consumption is needed in normal daily living conditions. Alcohol could be associated with or induce a higher level of physical activity, the most variable component of daily energy expenditure.

Glossary

Cross-sectional study: the collection and analysis of information relating to persons in a population or group at a defined point in time, with particular reference to their individual characteristics and exposure to factors thought likely to predispose them to disease.

Doubly labelled water: water labelled with the stable isotopes ^2H (heavy hydrogen, deuterium) and ^{18}O (heavy oxygen); water labelled with ^2H and ^{18}O ($^2H^{18}O$) is used for the measurement of total daily energy expenditure. Subjects receive a weighed dose of $^2H_2^{18}O$ which equilibrates with the body water. Subsequently, ^2H is eliminated as water while ^{18}O is eliminated as both water and carbon dioxide. The difference between the two elimination rates is therefore a measure of carbon dioxide production. Carbon dioxide production is converted to energy expenditure with an energy equivalent based on the substrate mixture used.

Epidemiological studies: studies of epidemic diseases, aimed at finding means of control and future prevention. They include all forms of diseases that relate to the environment and the way of life.

NAD: nicotinamide adenine dinucleotide.

NADH: the reduced form of NAD.

Placebo: a medicine that is ineffective but may help to relieve a condition, because the patient has faith in its powers. New drugs are tested against placebos in clinical trials.

Pre-load: an accurately prepared sample of food or drink which is presented to a subject at a specified time, often one hour before a test of consumption. It can vary in volume, energy content and all other parameters which may influence satiation.

Introduction

Alcohol is a significant component of the diet in many countries. Nation-wide studies indicate an average per capita consumption of about 10–30 g per day or about 3–9% of daily energy intake. The efficiency with which alcohol energy is used in the body has not yet been clearly established. In an overview of 38 studies (Macdonald et al. 1993), 12 reported a positive correlation between alcohol intake and body weight, 12 a negative correlation and 14 no correlation. Therefore it was not possible to draw a conclusion on the relation between moderate drinking and body weight from the epidemiological studies. Interestingly, in most of the studies reporting a positive correlation between alcohol intake and body weight the correlation was restricted to men while in most of the studies with a negative correlation it was restricted to women.

Alcohol seems to supplement rather than displace food-derived daily energy intake. Even in heavy drinkers the average energy intake excluding alcohol is the same as in non-drinkers, i.e. drinkers have a higher energy intake than non-drinkers and the difference in energy intake between drinkers and non-drinkers seems to be equivalent to the energy value of the alcohol consumed. In epidemiological studies drinkers have been shown to have a higher daily energy intake. Thus, the lack of a relationship between the apparent alcohol energy surplus and body mass index has led to the suggestion that alcohol energy has a low biological efficiency. Alcohol energy may count like other energy (Schutz 1995) or count otherwise (Westerterp 1995).

The effect of alcohol on energy balance will be discussed by a detailed analysis of the interaction between alcohol intake and food consumption and the interaction between alcohol intake and energy expenditure. Subsequently, the conclusions from the two analyses are combined with the epidemiological data on alcohol intake and body weight with suggestions for further research.

Alcohol and Food Consumption

The effects of alcohol on food consumption have been investigated in a number of different ways each of which provides strong evidence that alcohol energy is at least partly additive to food energy over a wide range of drinking patterns (but excluding alcoholics). The first method consists of an analysis of dietary survey data to test the extent to which alcohol energy substitutes for food energy. This can be done both by cross-sectional comparisons of drinkers versus non-drinkers and by analysis of dietary patterns on days with and without alcohol consumption. The second method provides direct measurements of appetite and food consumption in the presence or absence of alcohol pre-loads and supplements. The third method uses behavioural studies to analyse differences in eating behaviours between drinkers and abstainers, and between drinking days and dry days among the drinkers. The results from these studies are summarized below.

Dietary Studies of Free-Living People

In recent years it has become increasingly recognized that dietary studies of free-living people are very vulnerable to extensive errors and biases (Black et al. 1993). This holds in particularly for studies of alcohol use in which national estimates of alcohol purchases usually exceed estimates based on self-reports by a factor of about two (Lemmens et al. 1992). Such surveys must therefore be interpreted with due caution. In the light of these caveats the data on interactions between alcohol and other food are impressively consistent.

Table 1 summarizes 12 large studies each of which has investigated cross-sectional trends in energy and nutrient intake in population sub-groups identified according to their habitual alcohol intake. Total energy intake is expressed as a percentage of the intake of non-drinkers in the sample. Only one study (Hillers et al. 1985) showed similar records. All of the remaining studies showed that alcohol consumption was associated

Table 1
Effect of alcohol consumption on total energy intake in epidemiological studies

Source	Country	Drinking level	Total energy intake (%)[1]		
			men	women	both
Bebb et al. (1971)	USA	no alcohol	100	100	
		trace -4.9% energy	103	114	
		5.0–9.9% energy	115	128	
		>10.0% energy	119	128	
Jones et al. (1982)	USA	non-drinkers	100	100	
		0–24 g/d	109	106	
		25–49 g/d	102	111	
		50+ g/d	130	142	
Gruchow et al. (1985)	USA	non-drinkers	100	100	
		<6 g/d	102	101	
		6–24 g/d	104	105	
		>24 g/d	116	111	
Hillers et al. (1985)	USA	lowest tertile	100		
		middle tertile	98		
		upper tertile	102		
Herbeth et al. (1988)	France	controls	100		
		moderate drinkers	115		
		heavy drinkers	126		
De Castro et al. (1990)	USA	abstainers			100
		low intake			108
		moderate intake			116
Colditz et al. (1991)	USA	0 g/d	100	100	
		0.1–4.9 g/d	99	100	
		5.0–14.9 g/d	101	103	
		15.0–24.9 g/d	105	108	
		25.0–49.9 g/d	112	113	
		>50 g/d	135	130	
La Vecchia et al. (1992)	Italy	0 drinks/d	100	100	
		<3 drinks/d	104	110	
		>3 drinks/d	124	119	
Veenstra et al. (1993)	Netherlands	non-drinkers	100	100	
		moderate drinkers	107	105	
		heavy drinkers	120	116	
Liu et al. (1994)	USA	non-drinkers	100	100	
		<12 drinks/year	104	103	
		<1 drinks/week	111	111	
		1–6.9 drinks/week	114	111	
		1–1.9 drinks/day	120	114	
		>2 drinks/day	125	115	
Rose et al. (1995)	USA	none	100	100	
		light	100	100	
		moderate	109	113	
		heavy	120	120	
Tremblay et al. (1995)	Canada	lower quartile	100	100	
		upper quartile	117	111	

[1] Expressed relative to non-drinkers

with a raised total energy intake in both men and women. In most of these studies the non-alcohol food energy remained rather constant irrespective of the level of alcohol consumption thus yielding a linear trend between alcohol intake and overall energy consumption since the alcohol energy is essentially additive. There is some variation in this finding; for example, Colditz et al. (1991) report a slight compensation in men, Rose et al. (1995) report constant food energy, and Liu et al. (1994) actually show higher food energy intakes in drinkers. However, these differences are probably within the errors of the estimates. The mean increment in energy intake for men in the highest drinking category was 23% (range 16–35%, excluding Hillers et al. 1985) and for women 21% (range 11–42%). For more modest social drinkers the table indicates that the increment would be close to 10%.

Appetite Studies in Metabolic Laboratories

Alcohol has a reputation for its "aperitif" effect by which it is claimed to stimulate appetite in the short term. However, it is rapidly absorbed and highly metabolically active requiring oxidation as the only means of detoxification (Prentice 1995). According to some theories of appetite control this should give it a high satiety index (Friedman 1989, Stubbs 1995).

There have been surprisingly few direct studies of alcohol and appetite. Poppitt et al. (1996) used a classic short-term pre-load followed by test-meal paradigm to compare the satiating effects of an alcohol pre-load (0.91 MJ) against water, carbohydrate and alcohol-flavoured no-energy pre-loads, all with a volume of 392 ml, in 20 women. There was no difference in voluntary food consumption 30 min later, indicating either no physiological recognition or no compensatory down-regulation of intake in response to a liquid pre-load of less than 1 MJ. Similarly, there was no difference in subjective feelings of hunger assessed by visual analogue scores (VAS).

Tremblay et al. (1995) studied the effects of 0.72 MJ alcohol (341 ml beer) consumed with both lunch and supper during four 2-day protocols in 8 men (placebo low-fat; alcohol low-fat; placebo high-fat; alcohol high-fat). Again, there was no significant compensation so the alcohol energy was essentially additive. There were no detectable effects on VAS scores of hunger and fullness.

In contrast, Westerterp-Plantenga et al. (1999) investigated the effects of an alcohol aperitif (1 MJ, 300 ml) at lunch, in comparison with a fat, protein, carbohydrate and water aperitif, on energy intake in men and women (n = 52). The alcohol aperitif resulted in a higher subsequent energy intake (3.5±0.3 MJ) than the other iso-energetic iso-volumetric aperitifs (2.7±0.2 MJ, $P<0.001$), with no energy intake compensation during the rest of the day. After an alcohol aperitif eating rate was higher than after the other macronutrients (44±3 g/min vs. 38±3 g/min, $P<0.001$), and meal duration was prolonged (14 versus 12 min, $P<0.01$),

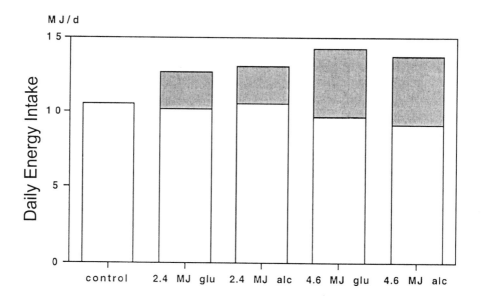

Figure 1
Effect of alcohol and glucose supplements on daily energy intake (MJ/day) in a metabolic ward setting

Open area, voluntary food energy intake; shaded area, obligatory supplement intake; glu, glucose; alc, alcohol. Redrawn from Foltin et al. (1993).

with satiation starting later (3.5 min versus 1.5 min, $P<0.01$) and with prolonged eating after satiation reached its maximum (2.5 min versus 0.6 min, $P<0.01$). Part of this may be explained by the disinhibition induced by alcohol.

Foltin et al. (1993) performed a similar study using five 2-day residential study periods in which dietary compensation was tested in response to energy supplements provided as alcohol or glucose at 2.4 and 4.6 MJ/d. Figure 1 illustrates that there was minimal compensation with the 2.4 MJ/d supplements, and greater, though still inadequate (ca. 37%), compensation with 4.6 MJ/d extra. There were no significant differences between alcohol and glucose. This was a study with a tight experimental design and larger alcohol supplements. The authors surmise that the low level of compensation may be due to the fact that the alcohol was provided at evening meals, thus minimizing opportunities for within-day compensation. Since most alcohol is consumed in the evening this represents a realistic simulation of real-life conditions.

Behavioural Studies in Free-Living People

Observational studies have the great advantage of addressing the effects of alcohol in the subjects' normal ecological setting in which disinhibition and social facilitation of eating are potent stimulators of energy intake. One of these studies was undertaken by de Castro et al. (1990) who investigated moderate alcohol intake and spontaneous eating patterns. Their key results are summarized in Figure 2 which, once again, shows that drinkers tend to have a higher energy intake than non-drinkers, and that among drinkers energy intake is higher on days when alcohol is consumed. De Castro et al. describe this as "unregulated supplementation". These data are included in Table 1 for sexes combined and amounts to an increment very similar to that in other studies (+16% in moderate drinkers). These socio-behavioural effects are partly caused by the fact that alcohol consumption often occurs at special meals and in company, each of which usually stimulates greater food intake.

Summary of Interactions between Alcohol and Food Energy Intake

The three different sources of information summarized above provide a remarkable level of consistency in demonstrating that alcohol consumption is associated with minimal compensatory down-regulation of energy intake from other foods. It can safely be concluded that in most people alcohol energy is largely additive to the normal diet. Thus other explanations must be sought for the paradoxical associations between alcohol and body weight.

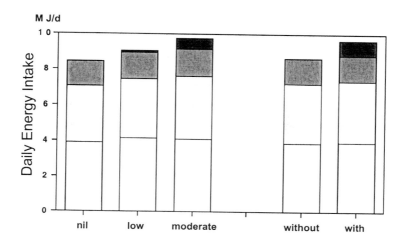

Figure 2
**Total daily energy intakes of free-living subjects in relation to alcohol
consumption**
The three left-hand columns compare low and moderate alcohol
drinkers against abstainers. The right-hand columns compare days
with and without alcohol in habitual consumers. Areas from bottom
to top: carbohydrate, fat, protein, and alcohol, respectively. Redrawn
from de Castro et al. (1990).

Alcohol and Energy Expenditure

The bioavailability of alcohol energy has been considered to be lower
than that of lipids and carbohydrates. The excretion of ethanol as a gas in
breath and sweat represents small proportions (0.7 and 0.1% respectively)
of ingested alcohol (Holford 1987). Ethanol is principally eliminated by
metabolism in the liver, urinary ethanol losses being negligible (0.3% of
the dose) (Holford 1987). A way to assess the efficiency of alcohol
utilization is to measure the thermogenic effects of alcohol. The aim of this
section is to review recent data on ethanol-induced thermogenesis (EIT).
The general conclusion is that no mysterious loss of energy results from
alcohol intake in healthy moderate drinkers. The hypothesis of a
stimulation of energy-wasting mechanisms, such as futile cycles, after
alcohol ingestion (Pirola et al. 1976, Lands et al. 1991, Lieber 1991) is not
supported by most recent studies (Suter et al. 1992, Sonko et al. 1994,

Suter et al. 1994, Murgatroyd et al. 1996).

The efficiency of energy utilization of a substrate can be studied in vivo by measuring the increase in energy expenditure resulting from its intake. The latter, called nutrient-induced thermogenesis or the thermic effect of a nutrient, results from the utilization of ATP due to absorption, processing and storage of the nutrient. This obligatory ATP utilization represents a loss of energy that is not available for other metabolic processes. Nutrient-induced thermogenesis is about 4%, 8% and 25% for fats, carbohydrates and proteins respectively (Jéquier 1995). This means, for proteins for instance, that the energy used for absorption, processing and storage accounts for 25% of the protein energy intake; therefore only 75% of this energy is available for other energy-requiring metabolic processes.

Alcohol-Induced Thermogenesis

In contrast to other macronutrients, the gross energy of ethanol (7.1 kcal/g or 29.7 kJ/g) is identical to its metabolizable energy because losses of ethanol in faeces or urine are negligible (Atwater et al. 1902). After alcohol ingestion, alcohol cannot be stored in the body and must be metabolized by the liver. The first step in alcohol metabolism is the irreversible conversion of alcohol to acetaldehyde. This reaction, catalysed by the enzyme alcohol dehydrogenase (ADH), requires NAD and produces NADH according to the formula:

$$CH_3CH_2OH + NAD^+ \xrightarrow{(ADH)} CH_3CHO + NADH + H^+$$

The synthesized NADH is further used and yields 3 ATPs per NADH oxidized. Complete oxidation of one acetaldehyde molecule yields 15 ATPs, but 2 ATPs are utilized at the step of activating free acetate to acetyl-CoA; therefore the net gain of the oxidation of one acetaldehyde molecule is 13 ATPs. The calculated ethanol-induced thermogenesis (EIT) based on the ratio of ATP used over ATP made is 2/18 or 11%.

A second pathway of hepatic alcohol metabolism is the microsomal ethanol oxidation system (MEOS) (Pirola et al. 1976). In this pathway, the irreversible conversion of alcohol to acetaldehyde is described by the formula:

$$CH_3CH_2OH + NADPH + H^+ + O_2 \xrightarrow{(MEOS)} CH_3CHO + NADP^+ + 2H_2O$$

In this pathway, there is a loss of reducing equivalents and, as a result, there is a consumption of 3 ATPs rather than a production of 3 ATPs. The calculated EIT by the MEOS pathway is 5/18 or 28%. As postulated by Pirola et al. (1976), this pathway represents a wastage of energy, and could account, at least in part, for the lack of a positive correlation between an excess alcohol energy intake and body mass index (BMI) in men and women (Colditz et al. 1991). Lieber also postulated that hepatic microsomal enzymes are induced by the repeated intake of alcohol, and these enzymes are known to be responsible for the oxidation of numerous endogenous substrates. Therefore, when alcohol intake is high, activation of MEOS could lower the efficiency of energy utilization of substrates other than alcohol.

Another possible explanation for an energy-wasting process induced by alcohol intake is the suggestion that alcohol energy is dissipated through an unregulated futile cycle that involves irreversible oxidation of alcohol (–3 ATP equivalents) and a reduction of acetaldehyde to alcohol (–3 ATP equivalents) (Lands et al. 1991). This cycle would dissipate 6 ATP equivalents for each turn, and the occurrence of two to three cycles for each net mole of alcohol metabolism would eliminate any net gain from alcohol. Isotopic measurements of labelled ethanol suggest that a fraction of ethanol can be formed from acetaldehyde, which suggests that this futile cycle can play a role in energy dissipation (Cronholm et al. 1988).

Human studies on EIT have been mainly carried out by using short-term ventilated hood measurements of energy expenditure after alcohol ingestion in healthy subjects (Table 2). Although significant increases in energy expenditure were observed, the periods of measurement were often not long enough to obtain the complete thermogenic response (Stock et al. 1974, Rosenberg et al. 1978, Weststrate et al. 1990, Klesges et al. 1994). Rosenberg et al. (1978) reported an increase in resting energy expenditure after alcohol intake without or with a meal, but the duration of measurements (165 min) was too short to assess EIT. Weststrate et al. (1990) reported an EIT of 3.8% of energy fed after ingestion of 20 g ethanol (594 kJ), but measurements were carried out during 90 min only, and no correction was made for unmetabolized alcohol. Klesges et al. (1994) reported an increase by 30 to 68 kJ in 16 women who consumed 29 ml pure ethanol (861 kJ), but the duration of the test (105 min) was too short to determine EIT.

Table 2
Published estimates of ethanol-induced thermogenesis (EIT) in man

Reference and treatment	Sub-jects	Alcohol dose g/kg BW	Duration	Outcome	EIT, % of alcohol energy
Rosenberg et al. (1978) 1.25 MJ alcohol	5 M	0.52-0.65	105 min	RMR+4%	1.5
Rosenberg et al. (1978) 1.5 MJ food + 0.8 MJ alcohol	10 F	0.30-0.40	165 min	RMR+27%	4.0
Weststrate et al. (1990) 0.6 MJ alcohol 1.96 MJ food + 0.6 MJ alcohol	10 M 12 M	0.26	90 min 4 h	RMR+4.7% RMR+17%	3.8 1.4
Suter et al. (1992) 11.4 MJ food + 2.8 MJ alcohol	8 M	1.30	24 h	TEE+7%	28.0
Suter et al. (1994) 0.95 MJ alcohol 11.2 MJ food + 2.85 MJ alcohol	6 M 6 M	0.43 1.30	4 h 24 h	RMR+7.4% TEE+5.3%	17.1 22.5
Sonko et al. (1994) 4.2 MJ food + 1.12 MJ alcohol	5 M	0.55	6 h	TEE+6.7%	14.0
Murgatroyd et al. 1996 10.4 MJ food + 1.15 MJ alcohol 8.2 MJ food + 1.15 MJ alcohol	5 M 6 F	0.53 0.63	6.5 h 6.5 h	REE+5.7% REE+5.7%	16.0 14.0

M, men; F, women; RMR, resting metabolic rate; REE, resting energy expenditure; TEE, total energy expenditure.

Suter et al. (1994) studied the thermogenic response induced by alcohol ingestion in six healthy male volunteers (aged 24 ± 0.7, body weight 73 ± 2 kg) who had their previous meal 13 h before the test. The subjects ingested 32 g alcohol and energy expenditure was continuously measured over 4 h. Their blood alcohol concentration (BAC) rose from 0 to 12 mmol/l within 45 min after alcohol ingestion and then gradually decreased to reach 3.5 mmol/l 4 h after alcohol ingestion. EIT was calculated as the difference between average energy expenditure during the

4 h after alcohol ingestion and energy expenditure at baseline. EIT was expressed as the percentage of the alcohol energy ingested minus the amount of unmetabolized ethanol. The latter was calculated from the BAC and the distribution volume of alcohol, which is known to be equal to total body water. The increase in energy expenditure during the 4 h study period corresponded to $17 \pm 2\%$ of the ethanol metabolized.

Sonko et al. (1994) studied five healthy male volunteers who received either a control meal (with an energy content calculated as 0.7 times the basal metabolic rate) or the same meal with the addition of 23% energy as alcohol. With the meal plus alcohol, energy expenditure increased by 7%, which amounted to 155 kJ, or 14% of the additional energy supplied by alcohol. This value of EIT (14%) is close to that reported by Suter et al. (1994), i.e. 17%. The slightly lower value found by Sonko et al. can be explained by the fact that these authors assumed complete oxidation of ethanol within 6 h after the meal, whereas Suter et al. (1994) corrected for unmetabolized alcohol. From these two studies, one can conclude that ethanol ingested either alone or with a meal has an EIT of about 15%. There is no evidence of a large increase in heat dissipation after alcohol use as a possible explanation for the apparent lack of weight gain when excess energy is consumed as alcohol (Pirola et al. 1976, Lands et al. 1991, Lieber 1991).

Several studies have been carried out by using whole-body indirect calorimeters to assess EIT in healthy volunteers (Suter et al. 1992, 1994, Murgatroyd et al. 1996). These studies are of longer duration than the previously described investigations, and therefore the complete EIT can be measured. Suter et al. (1994) studied EIT in six young male volunteers over 24 h by using a whole-body indirect calorimeter. In a first 24 h period, no ethanol was given and the measured 24 h energy expenditure served as a baseline when the subjects received a diet covering 1.5 times their basal metabolic rate to satisfy their energy requirements. During the second period, 25% of the calculated energy requirement was added as alcohol, and was given with each of the three meals as a 32 ± 0.6 g alcohol supplement per meal. On the alcohol addition day, energy expenditure rose by 629 ± 137 kJ/day, which corresponded to an increase of $5.3 \pm 1.2\%$. EIT was calculated as $22.5 \pm 4.7\%$ of the alcohol dose when measured over the 24 h period.

In another study with eight healthy volunteers in which a whole-body indirect calorimeter was used, Suter et al. (1992) also investigated EIT resulting from the addition of 25% of energy requirement as alcohol. The addition of alcohol (96 ± 4 g given as 3 portions of 32 g each) to the meals resulted in an increase of 24 h energy expenditure by 7 ± 1%, which corresponded to an EIT of 28%. More recently, Murgatroyd et al. (1996) studied 11 subjects (5 men and 6 women) using whole-body calorimetry for 15.5 h after a test meal which was served at 17:30 h. Alcohol addition (control plus 23% energy as alcohol) resulted in an EIT value of 16% for the men, and 14% for the women, when measured during 6.5 h after the meal with alcohol. These EIT values are similar to those reported for resting subjects (Sonko et al. 1994, Suter et al. 1994). The prescribed protocol in the Murgatroyd's study imposed sedentary activities with no unnecessary physical activity. By contrast, in the studies by Suter et al. (1992, 1994), the subjects were allowed to move as they wanted during the whole day. Therefore, part of the EIT measured by Suter et al. might have been attributable to an effect of alcohol on behaviour, with a stimulation of physical activity. Thus, EIT values in this latter study appear to result not only from metabolic but also from behavioural components.

In conclusion, EIT measured in resting healthy subjects represents about 15% of the energy contained in the alcohol ingested (Sonko et al. 1994, Suter et al. 1994, Murgatroyd et al. 1996). This value lies between the two calculated theoretical EIT values of 11% and 28% for the ADH and the MEOS pathway respectively. In non-alcoholic individuals, most ethanol is metabolized by the ADH pathway (Lieber 1991). The measured EIT value (15%), which is slightly greater than the theoretical value of EIT by the ADH pathway (11%), can be explained by the metabolism of the synthesized acetate. If the latter is completely oxidized to CO_2 and H_2O, the overall theoretical EIT value is 11%. However, if acetate is partially used for *de novo* lipogenesis, there is an increase in calculated EIT due to the fact that the lipogenic pathway is highly thermogenic.

The overall conclusion of the recent studies of EIT shows that the stimulation of energy expenditure resulting from alcohol ingestion can be entirely explained by the known energy-requiring processes of alcohol metabolism via the ADH pathway. There is no evidence of mysterious losses of energy due to futile cycles after alcohol ingestion. Alcohol energy is used in the body with an efficiency that is lower than that of fats, close to that of carbohydrates, and higher than that of proteins.

Alcohol Competition with Other Energetic Fuels

The influence of chronic alcohol use on body weight might more readily be explained by studying its effects on utilization of macronutrients than by its effects on energy expenditure. Therefore, several groups have recently studied the effect of alcohol ingestion on the oxidation of other fuels. Since ethanol is not stored in the body, it must be oxidized preferentially to other fuels (Sonko et al. 1994).

In order to study the competition between alcohol and other fuels for oxidation, protocols with alcohol substitution or alcohol addition were designed (Suter et al. 1992, Sonko et al. 1994, Murgatroyd et al. 1996). In the first of these studies (Suter et al. 1992), 25% of total energy requirement was added as alcohol to three meals (breakfast, lunch and dinner) in 8 normal men; in another study, 25% of energy requirement was replaced by ethanol, which was isocalorically substituted for lipids and carbohydrates. Both the addition of and the substitution by alcohol reduced lipid oxidation measured over 24 h whereas the oxidation of carbohydrate was slightly inhibited in the "replacement" protocol only. In both protocols, protein oxidation was not changed by alcohol use.

Other studies on the effect of alcohol ingestion on substrate oxidation confirm that fat oxidation is reduced, but inhibition of carbohydrate oxidation was also observed after alcohol intake (Sonko et al. 1994, Murgatroyd et al. 1996). In these studies, fat balances became positive when alcohol energy was added to the control diet. These positive balances observed when alcohol is added to a maintenance diet indicate that the extra energy provided by alcohol is accounted for as reasonably expected. In addition, these metabolic investigations show that habitual consumption of alcohol in excess of energy needs favours lipid storage and weight gain.

The acute effects of infused ethanol on the utilization of macro-nutrients were studied in six normal men before and after an intravenous glucose load (Shelmet et al. 1988). During the pre-glucose phase, ethanol infusion resulted in an 87% decrease in fat oxidation, whereas carbo-hydrate and protein oxidation were not altered. After glucose infusion, fat oxidation further decreased, and the rise in carbohydrate oxidation (seen in controls at 120 min) was mostly abolished. Thus, ethanol acts as a preferred fuel, almost totally replacing fat as substrate for oxidation during the basal period and preventing the glucose load from being oxidized.

In conclusion, these studies on energy and nutrient balances clearly show that alcohol is a nutrient that is efficiently utilized by the body and that alcohol calories do count. Balance studies conducted over several weeks confirm this notion. Contaldo et al. (1989) substituted 75 g per day alcohol iso-energetically for other nutrients during a two-week period in men, and did not find any change in body weight between the beginning and the end of the experimental period. Reinus et al. (1989) conducted 5-week balance experiments in eight chronically alcoholic men fed by nasogastric infusion. He concluded that the fuel value of an alcohol-containing diet relative to a glucose control formula varied between 95% and 99% depending on the plasma alcohol level. In a study on the energy value of moderate alcohol doses in 16 men and 32 women, Rumpler et al. (1996) showed that, on an energy basis, ethanol and carbohydrate were utilized in the diet with the same efficiency. Thus, all the evidence from metabolic controlled studies shows that alcohol calories do count, and these studies do not support Lieber's concept of energy wastage. As discussed by Prentice (1995), the low rates of weight gain in Lieber's human studies (Pirola et al. 1972) when carbohydrate was substituted by an excess of alcohol could possibly be explained by glycogen depletion, since glycogen binds three times its weight of water. Thus, a wastage of alcohol energy is not needed to explain the low rate of weight gain in the subjects overfed with alcohol, or the small weight loss in subjects with isocaloric substitution of alcohol for carbohydrate up to 50% of total energy for 16 days (Pirola et al. 1972).

Discussion

Studies of alcohol intake and food consumption have resulted in the conclusion that alcohol energy is largely additive to the normal diet. Studies on energy and nutrient balances show that alcohol is a nutrient that is efficiently utilized by the body and that alcohol calories do count. Thus, the analyses are in conflict with the epidemiological evidence of no clear correlation between alcohol intake and body weight. However, the interpretation of (epidemiological) observations on alcohol consumption and body weight in daily life is complicated by many factors like reporting errors and the confounding influence of other subject characteristics.

Studies with doubly labelled water have shown that measures of energy intake are often biased by underreporting. Alcohol intake is even more liable to underreporting. Nation-wide surveys on alcohol consumption show that only 40–60% of the sales are covered, indicating that the error in self-report data on alcohol use can be substantial (Lemmens et al. 1992). However, underreporting seems to be of a linear nature. The ranking of individuals according to their self-reports is relatively stable across methods. We only have to realize that the real intake level will be systematically higher. Consequently, in relationships between alcohol use and, for example, body weight, the real intake could be twice as high.

From studies on energy intake we could postulate one non-linear bias. Subjects who are overweight systematically under-report energy intake more than lean subjects. Thus, the absence of the expected positive relation between alcohol intake and body weight could be due to underreporting in overweight subjects. In a further step on the same line, even a negative correlation between alcohol use and body weight as often observed in women could be due to a high degree of underreporting in this weight-conscious gender.

Epidemiological studies are mainly cross-sectional, comparing subjects differing in their drinking levels. This type of study is not conclusive as to the consequences of alcohol use for energy intake and body weight regulation. Drinkers and abstainers probably do not differ only with respect to alcohol use. A well-known example of a confounding factor is smoking, which is often associated with drinking and counteracts the potential effect of alcohol on energy balance. Prentice et al. (1996) concluded that a large proportion of the paradoxical inverse association between alcohol intake and body mass index could be explained by such confounding variables as age, smoking, social class, education and physical activity.

Until now no direct measurement of total daily energy expenditure without and with alcohol has been undertaken in normal daily living conditions. Alcohol could be associated with or induce a higher level of physical activity, the most variable component of daily energy expenditure. The method with doubly labelled water allows assessment of daily energy expenditure under daily living conditions over intervals of 1–3 weeks. With this instrument we can meet several of the methodological objections mentioned. The method with doubly labelled water method is the method of choice to validate records of daily energy intake to see whether alcohol really supplements daily energy intake. Simultaneously measuring average daily metabolic rate and basal metabolic rate allows the assessment of energy expenditure for physical activity over intervals with and without alcohol "supplementation". Additionally, there are suggestions that the thermogenic effect of alcohol is higher in lean than in fat subjects (Clevidence et al. 1995, Lands, 1995). One explanation is that lean subjects can lose heat more readily than fat subjects. Another interesting experiment would be the measurement of the thermogenic effect as a function of physical activity. Subjects can lose heat more easily when they are active than when they are sedentary or even at complete rest as in a respiration chamber or under a ventilated hood, the methods adopted so far to quantify the thermogenic effect of alcohol.

The magnitude of the supplementation of alcohol to daily food intake of 10–30 g or 3–9% as mentioned above has dramatic consequences when food intake and energy expenditure remain unchanged. Converted to the equivalent of body fat this would mean an increase of 2.5–7.5 kg body fat per year. Obviously very few people gain weight so fast. On the other hand, intake and/or expenditure changes of this magnitude can be detected with present-day instruments. Thus the mechanism behind the relation between alcohol consumption and the maintenance of energy balance is open for future research.

References

Atwater WO, Benedict FG (1902) An experimental inquiry regarding the nutritive value of alcohol. Mem Natl Acad Sci 8: 235–95

Bebb HT, Houser HB, Witschi JC, et al. (1971) Calorie and nutrient contribution of alcoholic beverages to the usual diets of 155 adults. Am J Clin Nutr 24: 1042–52

Black AE, Prentice AM, Goldberg GR, et al. (1993) Measurements of total energy expenditure provide insights into the validity of dietary measurements of energy intake. J Am Diet Ass 93: 572–79

Clevidence BA, Taylor PR, Campbell WS, et al. (1995) Lean and heavy women may not use energy from alcohol with equal efficiency. J Nutr 125: 2536–40

Colditz GA, Giovannucci E, Rimm EB, et al. (1991) Alcohol intake in relation to diet and obesity in women and men. Am J Clin Nutr 54: 49–55

Contaldo F, D'Arrigo E, Carandente V, et al. (1989) Short-term effects of moderate alcohol consumption on lipid metabolism and energy balance in normal men. Metabolism 38: 166–71

Cronholm T, Jones AW, Skagerberg S (1988) Mechanism and regulation of ethanol elimination in humans: intermolecular hydrogen transfer and oxido reduction in vivo. Alcohol Clin Exp Res 12: 683–86

De Castro JM, Orozco S (1990) Moderate alcohol intake and spontaneous eating patterns of humans: evidence of unregulated supplementation. Am J Clin Nutr 52: 246–53

Foltin RW, Kelly TH, Fischman MW (1993) Ethanol as an energy source in humans: comparison with dextrose-containing beverages. Appetite 20: 95–110

Friedman MI (1989) Metabolic control of food intake. Biol Ass Med PR 81: 111-13

Gruchow HW, Sobocinski KA, Barboriak JJ, et al. (1985) Alcohol consumption, nutrient intake and relative body weight among US adults. Am J Clin Nutr 42: 289–95

Herbeth B, Didelot-Barthelemy L, Lemoine A, et al. (1988) Dietary behaviour of French men according to alcohol drinking pattern. J Stud Alcohol 49: 268–72

Hillers VN, Massey LK (1985) Interrelationships of moderate and high alcohol consumption with diet and health status. Am J Clin Nutr 41: 356–62

Holford NH (1987) Clinical pharmacokinetics of ethanol. Clin Pharmacokinet 13: 273–92

Jéquier E (1995) Nutrient effects : post-absorptive interactions. Proc Nutr Soc 54: 253–65

Jones BR, Barrett-Connor E, Criqui MH, et al. (1982). A community study of calorie and nutrient intake in drinkers and nondrinkers of alcohol. Am J Clin Nutr 35: 135–39

Klesges RC, Mealer CZ, Klesges LM (1994) Effects of alcohol intake on resting energy expenditure in young women social drinkers. Am J Clin Nutr 59: 805–09

Lands WEM (1995) Alcohol and energy intake. Am J Clin Nutr 62/Suppl.: S1101–06

Lands WE, Zakhari S (1991) The case of the missing calories. Am J Clin Nutr 54: 47–48

La Vecchia C, Negri E, Franceschi S et al. (1992) Differences in dietary intake with smoking, alcohol and education. Nutr Cancer 17: 297–304

Lemmens PHHM, Tan ES, Knibbe RA (1992) Measuring quantity and frequency of alcohol consumption. A comparison of 5 indices. J Stud Alcohol 53: 476–86

Lieber CS (1991) Perspectives: do alcohol calories count? Am J Clin Nutr 54: 976–82

Liu S, Serdula MK, Williamson DF, Mokdad AH, et al. (1994) A prospective study of alcohol intake and change in body weight among US adults. Am J Epidemiol 140: 912–20

Macdonald I, Debry G, Westerterp K (1993) Alcohol and overweight. In: Verschuren PM (ed.), Health issues related to alcohol consumption. ILSI Europe, Brussels, pp. 263–79

Murgatroyd PR, van de Ven MLHM, Goldberg GR, et al. (1996) Alcohol and the regulation of energy balance: overnight effects on diet-induced thermogenesis and fuel storage. Br J Nutr 75: 33–45

Pirola RC, Lieber CS (1972) The energy cost of the metabolism of drugs, including ethanol. Pharmacology 7: 185–96

Pirola RC, Lieber CS (1976) Hypothesis: energy wastage in alcoholism and drug abuse: possible role of hepatic microsomal enzymes. Am J Clin Nutr 29: 90–93

Poppitt SD, Eckhardt JW, McGonagle J et al. (1996). Short-term effects of alcohol consumption on appetite and energy intake. Physiol Behav 60: 1063–70

Poppitt SD, Prentice AM (1996) Energy density and its role in the control of food intake: evidence from metabolic and community studies. Appetite 26: 153–74

Prentice AM (1995) Alcohol and obesity. Int J Obes 19/Suppl. 5: S44–S50

Prentice AM, Jebb SA, Cole TJ (1996) Paradoxical associations between alcohol consumption and obesity in men and women. Int J Obes 20/Suppl. 4: S138

Reinus JF, Heymsfield SB, Wiskind R, et al. (1989) Ethanol: relative fuel value and metabolic effects in vivo. Metabolism 38: 125–35

Rosenberg K, Durnin JVGA (1978) The effect of alcohol on resting metabolic rate. Br J Nutr 40: 293–98

Rose D, Murphy SP, Hudes M, et al. (1995) Food energy remains constant with increasing alcohol intake. J Am Diet Ass 95: 698–700

Rumpler WV, Rhodes DG, Baer DJ, et al (1996) Energy value of moderate alcohol consumption by humans. Am J Clin Nutr 64: 108–14

Schutz Y (1995) Alcohol calories count the same as other calories. Int J Obes 19/Suppl. 2: S12–S13

Shelmet JJ, Reichard GA, Skutches CL, et al. (1988) Ethanol causes acute inhibition of carbohydrate, fat, and protein oxidation and insulin resistance. J Clin Invest 81: 1137–45

Sonko BJ, Prentice AM, Murgatroyd PR, et al. (1994) Effect of alcohol on postmeal fat storage. Am J Clin Nutr 59: 619–25

Stock MJ, Stuart JA (1974) Thermic effects of ethanol in the rat and man. Nature Med 17: 297–305

Stubbs RJ (1995) Macronutrient effects on appetite. Int J Obes 19/Suppl. 5: S11–S19

Suter PM, Jéquier E, Schutz Y (1994) Effect of ethanol on energy expenditure. Am J Physiol 266: R1204–12

Suter PM, Schutz Y, Jéquier E (1992) The effect of ethanol on fat storage in healthy subjects. N Engl J Med 326: 983–87

Tremblay A, Wouters E, Wenker M, et al. (1995) Alcohol and a high-fat diet: a combination favoring overfeeding. Am J Clin Nutr 62: 639–44

Veenstra J, Schenkel JAA, van Erp-Baart AMJ, et al. (1993) Alcohol consumption in relation to food intake and smoking habits in the Dutch National Food Consumption Survey. Eur J Clin Nutr 47: 482–89

Westerterp KR (1995) Alcohol calories do not count the same as other calories. Int J Obes 19/Suppl. 2: S14–S15

Westerterp-Plantenga MS, Verwege CRT (1999) The appetizing effect of an alcohol aperitif in overweight and normal weight humans. Am J Clin Nutr 69: 205–12.

Weststrate JA, Wunnink I, Deurenberg P, et al. (1990) Alcohol and its acute effects on resting metabolic rate and diet-induced thermogenesis. Br J Nutr 64: 413–25

Chapter 5

Alcohol and the Cardiovascular System

D.E. Grobbee
University Medical Centre, Utrecht, The Netherlands

E.B. Rimm
Harvard School of Public Health, Boston, MA, USA

U. Keil
University of Munster, Germany

S. Renaud
University of Bordeaux, France

Abstract

There is abundant epidemiological and clinical evidence to show that light to moderate alcohol consumption is associated with a reduced risk of CHD, total and ischaemic stroke and total mortality in middle-aged and elderly men and women. Although several alternative explanations for the findings have been proposed these do not appear to explain the observed inverse association. These findings are supported by evidence from animal, clinical and biochemical studies suggesting several plausible biological mechanisms whereby alcohol could reduce cardiovascular risk, notably through favourable modification of the serum lipid profile and a reduction of thrombotic tendency. There is little basis to expect one particular beverage to be more effective in reducing risk than another, and the effect appears largely due to alcohol itself although some discussion remains. Despite the absence of a randomized intervention trial, it is highly likely that the association is causal.

Alcohol use in moderation thus appears to promote cardiovascular health. However, from a public health point of view, the fear of stimulating alcohol overuse prevents us from advising individuals to start drinking if they have previously abstained. A formal assessment of benefits and risks on a population scale and the best way to achieve the positive effects of moderate drinking while preventing social and medical adverse consequences of changes in alcohol use by populations at large is clearly needed for rational recommendations. However, guidelines for moderation which have been adopted in the USA, the UK and elsewhere suggest that individuals who do consume alcohol responsibly may achieve some benefit if daily consumption is limited to 2 to 3 drinks.[1]

---

[1] In the literature definitions of units of alcohol have not been standardized. Commonly, the quantity of alcohol in a "glass" or a "drink" ranges from 10 to 20 g with 15 g as a good general estimate. Sometimes the alcohol content of drinks is expressed in volume with estimates ranging from 10 to 15 ml alcohol per glass. Alternatively, alcohol is expressed in "units" equal to 10 g of alcohol. These estimates are independent of the type of beverage. The assumption is that different beverages have a different alcohol content but that different sizes of glasses compensate for this.

Introduction

Alcohol drinking, especially in the form of wine, held a prominent place in many ancient cultures. Plato, the Greek philosopher who lived to the age of 80, wrote: "No thing more excellent nor more valuable than wine was ever granted mankind by God". This concept still prevailed in Mediterranean countries in the 19th century. The French microbiologist L. Pasteur wrote that "wine is the most healthful and hygienic of beverages".

Beneficial effects of alcohol on the cardiovascular system have been recognized since Heberden (1786), who was the first to describe angina pectoris, and who recommended wine or spirits for its treatment.

Paul D. White, in his famous textbook on heart disease published in the 1950s, noted that "the most effective drug after the nitrites is alcohol" for rapid relief from angina pectoris. Only in the second part of this century, however, has sound, indisputable scientific evidence been accumulating on the beneficial cardiovascular effects of moderate alcohol use.

Public Beliefs on the Relationship between Alcohol Drinking and Health

It is difficult to find information on public beliefs about alcohol and health in the international literature. These beliefs differ from country to country, but in general it is believed that binge drinking is harmful for health, predisposes to violence and accidents, and should be strictly avoided.

In Mediterranean countries, moderate drinking has been part of a healthy life-style for generations. Historically, in the USA, for fear of stimulating alcohol abuse, dietary guidelines either did not mention alcohol or recommended abstinence. However, the Dietary Guidelines and the Food Guide Pyramid have recently recognized the potential benefits of moderate drinking (Food and Nutrition Board 1989, USDA). Policies and legislation vary widely among countries and a general consensus is lacking.

Alcohol and Coronary Heart Disease

In almost all epidemiological studies, an inverse correlation between moderate drinking levels and coronary heart disease (CHD) incidence has been found. These studies can be classified as ecological studies, case-control studies and cohort studies.

Moore et al. (1986), Kannel (1988), Veenstra (1991), Marmot et al. (1991), Poikolainen (1991), Jackson et al. (1993), Maclure (1993) and Klatsky (1996) have produced extensive reviews and discussed the scientific evidence available.

Ecological Studies

A number of ecological studies (Brummer 1969, St Leger et al.1979, La Porte et al.1980, Hegsted et al. 1988, Renaud et al.1992b, Criqui et al. 1994, Rimm et al. 1996) have investigated the relationship between moderate alcohol consumption and CHD in various countries. A clear inverse relationship between average alcohol use and CHD mortality was found. Ecological studies are very suggestive but do not provide proof of a favourable effect of alcohol use on CHD development. Results suggest a relationship on a population level. However, differences among countries with regard to culture, living and working conditions, diet and other potential confounders cannot accurately be taken into account. A second drawback of these studies is that alcohol use is derived from alcohol sales data, uncorrected for sales to visitors from abroad or for self-produced alcoholic beverages. Finally, in some countries a small proportion of the population may consume a large proportion of the alcohol. In other countries, like France or Spain, average per capita consumption of alcohol may be more representative as a larger proportion of the population drinks.

Case-Control Studies

In the previous version of this report (van Gijn et al. 1993), results from eleven case-control studies were outlined. Studies included populations of men and of women and of young and old adults; they were undertaken mainly in the USA, but also in the UK, New Zealand and Japan. In general, the odds of confirmed CHD was higher among men and women who abstained than among those who drank 1–4 drinks/day. Only one case-control study (Kaufman et al. 1985) found no effect of moderate drinking.

In the past few years other case-control studies of CHD have examined the importance of alcohol on risk of disease. A recent large case-control study from Australia has provided new information on drinking patterns and risk of CHD (McElduff et al. 1997). In this study of over 11,500 acute myocardial infarctions (MI) the authors reported odds of MI by the number of days alcohol was consumed and the average number of drinks consumed on those days. After excluding men and women who were former moderate or heavy drinkers, they found the lowest odds of MI (OR 0.36, 95% CI 0.19–0.66) among men who consumed 1–2 drinks per day during 5–6 days per week. Consistent inverse associations were also reported among men who had 3 or 4 drinks per day on 3–6 days per week. Compared to abstainers the lowest odds of CHD among women was the group which consumed 1–2 drinks every other day. Women who consumed 3–4 drinks daily also had a significant reduction in MI (OR 0.40, 95% CI 0.16–0.98).

Cohort Studies

In prospective cohort studies, large study populations are classified into drinking categories at baseline. After several years of follow-up of an initially healthy population, the association between baseline alcohol use and occurrence of newly diagnosed CHD is analysed. Prospective cohort designs are generally preferable to case-control studies because results are less susceptible to bias caused by incomparability of controls or differential recall of past intake. In the past 35 years, the effect of alcohol use on CHD incidence has been investigated in more than 50 cohorts around the world in which participants report consuming different types of brewed, distilled or fermented alcohol-containing beverages.

Table 1 shows the results of several large cohort studies in which daily alcohol use was assessed. In most studies, participants drinking moderate amounts of alcohol had a significantly lower risk of developing CHD.

Particular confidence can be given to the results of the most recent studies, which considered very large cohorts from several geographic locations. For example, in a 7-year follow-up of 18,244 men from Shanghai, China, Yuan et al. (1997) reported that men who consumed 1–28 drinks/week had a 36% reduction in ischaemic heart disease mortality compared to abstainers. A similar reduction in CHD mortality (35%)

Table 1
Large cohort studies of alcohol use and coronary heart disease

Reference (country)	Population	Follow-up (yrs)	Alcohol measure	Relative risk (95% CI)	Adjusted for
Kono et al. 1986 (Japan)	5,477 men	19		**CHD mortality**	age, smoking
			non-drinkers	1.0	
			ex-drinkers	1.5 (1.0–2.4)	
			occasional drinkers	0.6 (0.4–0.9)	
			<54 ml/day	0.7 (0.5–1.1)	
			≥54 ml/day	0.7 (0.4–1.1)	
Rimm et al. 1991b USA	51,529 men (40-75 years)	2		**CAD mortality**	age, smoking, BMI, profession, family history of CHD, pre-existing conditions, dietary fibre, cholesterol, energy, mono- and polyunsa-turated and saturated fat
			0 g/day	1.0	
			0.1–5 g/day	0.99 (0.74–1.33)	
			5–10 g/day	0.79 (0.55–1.14)	
			10–15 g/day	0.68 (0.45–1.01)	
			15–30 g/day	0.73 (0.51–1.05)	
			30–50 g/day	0.57 (0.35–0.79)	
			>50 g/day	0.41 (0.20–0.84)	
Doll et al. 1994 UK	12,321 men (48–78 years)	13		**IHD mortality**	age, smoking, year of death, pre-existing disease
			0 units/day	1.0	
			1–7/week	0.81 (0.66–0.99)	
			8–14/week	0.69 (0.57–0.84)	
			15–21/week	0.58 (0.46–0.73)	
			22–28/week	0.63 (0.50–0.80)	
			29–42/week	0.75 (0.60–0.94)	
			43+/week	0.73 (0.56–0.95)	
Gronbæk et al. 1995 (Denmark)	13,285 men and women (30-79 years)	12		**CVD mortality** **Beer**	age, gender, smoking
			never	1.0	
			monthly	0.79 (069–0.91)	
			weekly	0.87 (0.75–0.99)	
			1–2 drinks per day	0.79 (0.68–0.91)	
			3–5/day	0.72 (0.61–0.88)	

Table 1 (continued)

Reference (country)	Population	Follow-up (yrs)	Alcohol measure	Relative risk (95% CI)	Adjusted for
Gronbæk et al. 1995 (Denmark) continued				**Wine**	
			never	1.0	
			monthly	0.69 (0.62–0.77)	
			weekly	0.53 (0.45–0.63)	
			1–2 drinks per day	0.47 (0.35–0.62)	
			3–5/day	0.44 (0.24–0.80)	
				Spirits	
			never	1.0	
			monthly	0.95 (0.85–1.06)	
			weekly	1.08 (0.93–1.26)	
			1–2 drinks per day	1.16 (0.98–1.39)	
			3–5/day	1.35 (1.00–1.83)	
Fuchs et al. 1995 (USA)	85,709 women (34-59 years)	12		**CHD mortality**	age, smoking, BMI, aspirin, exercise, family history of CHD, pre-existing conditions, hormone use, menopausal status, dietary intake of fibre, saturated fat and total energy
			0 g/day	1.0	
			<1.5 g/day	0.82 (0.59–1.15)	
			1.5–5 g/day	0.51 (0.36–0.73)	
			5–15 g/day	0.64 (0.46–0.89)	
			15–30 g/day	0.65 (0.43–0.99)	
			≥30 g/day	0.59 (0.35–0.99)	
Klatsky et al. 1997 (USA)	128,934 men and women (20-90 years)	13		**Incident CAD** **Men**	age, race, smoking, BMI, marital status, education, coffee, baseline CAD
			0 drinks/day	1.0	
			<1 drink/day	0.93 (0.80–.09)	
			1–2/day	0.77 (0.65–0.91)	
			3+/day	0.71 (0.59–0.86)	
				Women	
			0 drinks/day	1.0	
			<1 drink/day	0.83 (0.70–0.98)	
			1–2/day	0.64 (0.52–0.79)	
			3+/day	0.60 (0.42–0.85)	
Yuan et al. 1997 (China)	18,244 men (45-64 years)	6.7		**IHD mortality**	age, smoking, education
			non-drinker	1.0	
			1–28 drinks per week	0.64 ($P<0.05$)	
			≥29/week	0.88	

Table 1 (continued)

Reference (country)	Population	Follow-up (yrs)	Alcohol measure	Relative risk (95% CI)	Adjusted for
Thun et al. 1997 (USA)	490,000 men and women[*] (30-104 years)	9		**CHD mortality** **Men**	age, smoking, race, education, BMI, fat intake, exercise, marital status, aspirin, employment status, hormone therapy (women)
			0 drink/day	1.0	
			<1 drink/day	0.9 (0.80–1.00)	
			1 drink/day	0.8 (0.70–0.90)	
			2–3/day	0.7 (0.60–0.80)	
			≥4/day	0.8 (0.70–1.00)	
				Women	
			0	1.0	
			<1 drink/day	0.8 (0.70–1.00)	
			1 drink/day	0.8 (0.60–1.00)	
			2–3/ay	0.9 (0.70–1.10)	
			≥4/day	0.9 (0.60–1.20)	
Rehm et al. 1997 (USA)	6,788 men and women (25-75 years)	14.6		**Incident CHD** **Men**	age, smoking, BMI, physical activity, aspirin
			lifetime abstainers	1.0	
			current abstainers	0.87 (0.67–1.13)	
			<2 drinks/wk	0.76 (0.61–0.95)	
			2–7/week	0.62 (0.49–0.79)	
			8–14/week	0.65 (0.48–0.88)	
			15–28/week	0.66 (0.47–0.93)	
			29–42/week	0.51 (0.30–0.89)	
			>42/week	0.62 (0.36–1.07)	
				Women	
			lifetime abstainers	1.0	
			current abstainers	1.20 (0.95–1.55)	
			<2 drinks/wk	0.93 (0.78–1.10)	
			2–7/week	0.51 (0.37–0.70)	
			8–14/week	0.62 (0.35–1.09)	
			15–28/week	0.61 (0.31–1.19)	
			≥29/week	2.56 (1.19–5.48)	
Camargo et al. 1997 (USA)	22,071 men (40–84 years)	11		**MI**	age, smoking, family history of CHD, diabetes, and randomized arm of aspirin and/or β-carotene
			<1 drink/wk	1.0	
			1 drink/wk	1.08 (0.85–1.38)	
			2–4/week	0.96 (0.78–1.20)	
			5–6/week	0.82 (0.62–1.07)	
			1 drink/day	0.65 (0.52–0.81)	
			≥2/day	0.53 (0.32–0.88)	

Table 1 (continued)

Reference (country)	Population	Follow-up (yrs)	Alcohol measure	Relative risk (95% CI)	Adjusted for
Renaud et al. 1998 (France)	34,014 men (40–60 years)	10–15	occasional 1–21 g/day 22–32 g/day 33–54 g/day 55–76 g/day 77–128 g/day ≥128 g/day	**CHD mortality** 1.0 0.89 (0.54–1.44) 0.65 (0.41–1.03) 0.70 (0.47–1.04) 0.66 (0.40–1.11) 0.61 (0.41–0.92) 0.65 (0.37–1.15)	age, smoking, education, systolic blood pressure, serum cholesterol, BMI
Kitamura et al. 1998 (Japan)	8,476 men (40–59 years)	8.8	never-drinkers ex-drinkers 1–22 g/day 23–45 g/day 46–68 g/day ≥69 g/day	**Incident CHD** 1.0 0.83 (0.24–2.86) 0.69 (0.37–1.29) 0.55 (0.29–1.05) 0.41 (0.19–0.88) 0.59 (0.23–1.51)	age, smoking, serum cholesterol, BMI, left ventricular hypertrophy, diabetes

* Average subjects without pre-existing disease (i.e. stroke, hypertension, diabetes, CHD).
CI, confidence interval; CHD, coronary heart disease; CAD, coronary artery disease;
IHD, ischaemic heart disease; CVD, cardiovascular disease; MI, mycoardial infarction

was reported among women having 1–2 drinks daily (compared to abstainers) in the study of 85,709 women from the Nurses' Health Study (Fuchs, 1995). Other large studies from the UK, Japan, France, Denmark and Germany have reported similar reductions in CHD among men and women.

Is there a U-Shaped Curve for Alcohol and Coronary Heart Disease?

It is generally agreed that there is a J-shaped rather than a U-shaped relation between alcohol intake and total mortality, with increases in death from cirrhosis, accidents, violence and cancer in heavier drinkers (Thun 1997, Fuchs 1995). In addition, there is a general concurrence that there is a U-shaped curve for the association between alcohol and total cardiovascular disease (CVD) mortality, which includes stroke and non-CHD deaths (Kagan 1981, Klatsky et al. 1981a, Criqui et al. 1987, Shaper et al. 1988).

Some studies of the alcohol-CHD association address only mortality data, while others have reported both morbidity and mortality. The Lipid data, while others have reported both morbidity and mortality. The Lipid Research Clinics (LRC) Follow-up Study evaluated mortality only and showed a benefit limited to <3 drinks per day, beyond which CHD began to increase (Criqui et al. 1987). In the MRFIT the alcohol benefit for CHD mortality reached a maximum at 2–3 drinks per day (Suh et al. 1992). Similarly, in the recent American Cancer Society prospective study of 490,000 men and women, the maximum CHD benefit for men was achieved at 1–3 drinks/day, while among women the maximum benefit was at 1 drink/day (Thun 1997).

Several studies have evaluated both CHD morbidity and mortality. In general, the CHD benefit for moderate drinking has been reported for both fatal and non-fatal CHD. In the Honolulu Heart Study there was a similar benefit for both CHD morbidity and mortality up to intake levels of 3 drinks per day (Yano et al. 1977). However, a later publication showed some loss of benefit for mortality at 4 or more drinks per day (Kagan et al. 1981). By contrast, data from the Yugoslavia Cardiovascular Disease Study did not suggest a plateau of benefit at low levels of intake, but did indicate a stronger benefit for non-fatal MI than for CHD death (Kozarevic et al. 1980). Similarly, in the Health Professionals Follow-Up Study, the benefit for non-fatal MI and coronary artery bypass graft or percutaneous transluminal coronary angioplasty was somewhat greater than of fatal CHD. This was due to a

slightly smaller protective effect of alcohol for fatal CHD at >3 drinks/day compared to 1–2 drinks/day (Rimm et al. 1991). The Kaiser Permanente Study data show the biggest discrepancy between morbidity and mortality data. Both acute MI and all coronary disease are lower in the highest drinking category of ≥6 drinks/day (Klatsky et al. 1981b), whereas the lowest coronary mortality was in the group consuming 1–2 drinks/day (Klatsky et al. 1981a).

In summary, the evidence suggests that, similar to total mortality and all CVD, there is a U-shaped relationship between alcohol and CHD as well. The threshold at which the right side of the U begins to increase for all CVD and total mortality is about 2 drinks/day. However, the threshold for the right side of the U for fatal and non-fatal CHD is somewhat less clear, and could be as few as 2 or as many as 6 drinks/day.

Modifiers and Confounders

Although in almost all populations an inverse association between alcohol and CHD has been reported, it is still important to examine the independence of the observed association with regard to possible confounding or effect modification.

Gender

The majority of studies concern men, but there are also studies conducted among women only or of women and men together. Although a lower risk of CHD among drinkers has been reported for both sexes, the benefits are found at lower quantities for women. Differences in alcohol-metabolizing enzymes and body size may explain why women achieve reduction in CHD at lower intakes.

Length of Follow-Up

The study of Rimm et al. (1991) considered a follow-up of only 2 years and found a relative risk of 0.57 for 30–50 g alcohol per day. In the follow-up of the Framingham Heart Study, Gordon et al. (1983a) collected a single baseline measure of alcohol consumption and followed participants for 22 years. For a similar intake of alcohol, they found a relative risk of 0.58. In longitudinal studies, whatever the length of follow-up, the results are surprisingly similar. Studies among men and women in which alcohol use is repeatedly assessed during follow-up are still missing in the epidemiological literature. This would allow groups to study changes in drinking patterns and subsequent risk of CHD. There also have been no studies to show that individuals who begin consuming alcohol after age 40 have a lower risk of subsequent CHD than have lifelong abstainers.

Countries

There is a remarkable consistency in the findings even across diverse populations in different states of the USA, in different regions of the UK, Yugoslavia, Italy, Puerto Rico, Japan, Australia, New Zealand, France, China and many other countries. A study from Finland (Suhonen et al. 1987) did not report an inverse association between alcohol and CHD. This lack of association from Finland can probably be attributed to unusual drinking patterns (weekend only) or other confounding factors.

Other Possible Confounders

Although most studies adjust relative risks for age and smoking habits, many other factors have also been considered (Table 1). Interestingly, apart from age and smoking, few other factors substantially modify the strong and consistent inverse association between alcohol and CHD. Only a few studies have accounted for dietary intake other than alcohol. In the Health Professionals Follow-up Study, Rimm et al. (1991a) adjusted for coronary risk factors including dietary intake of cholesterol, fat and fibre, and aspirin use (Rimm et al. 1991b). Even after accounting for these potential confounders, alcohol intake was still inversely related to CHD incidence.

Uncritical inclusion of factors related to alcohol use as confounders in the analyses may, however, also result in over-adjustment. If there is a direct effect of alcohol on a biological variable, which is also included in the model, the risk or benefit associated with alcohol is attenuated. In several studies of alcohol and CHD in which baseline HDL cholesterol levels were simultaneously entered in a model the apparent protective effect of alcohol was reduced by about half (Criqui 1987, Langer et al. 1992, Suh et al. 1992, Gaziano et al. 1993, Marques-Vidal et al. 1996).

Type of Alcoholic Beverage

Several studies (Rosenberg et al. 1981, Yano et al. 1977, Stampfer et al. 1988, Klatsky et al. 1986, 1990, 1996, Rimm et al. 1991a, Friedman et al. 1986, Gronbæk et al. 1995, Rimm et al. 1996) have separately assessed consumption of wine, beer and spirits and presented beverage-specific relative risks. From these studies it can be inferred that there is no clear evidence that one type of beverage is more protective than the other. In a recent review of the literature, Rimm and colleagues summarized all the available literature from ecological, case-control and cohort studies (Rimm et al. 1996). Although most ecological studies support the hypothesis that wine consumption is most beneficial (Criqui, 1994), the methodological problems of these studies limit their usefulness in drawing conclusions. Results from observational studies, in which individual consumption can be assessed in detail and linked directly to CHD, provide strong evidence that a substantial proportion of the benefits of wine, beer or spirits is attributable to alcohol rather than other components of each beverage.

In specific studies where alcohol from one beverage appears to be more beneficial, it is likely that other unaccountable factors like occupation, diet and drinking pattern explain much of the beverage-specific differences in relative risks. In a report from the Kaiser Permanente Medical Center on 129,000 persons (Klatsky et al. 1990), wine preference was associated with significantly lower risk (RR 0.7) and beer drinking with greater risk (RR 1.2) of cardiovascular death. These differences were almost entirely eliminated after further adjustment for sex, race, smoking, coffee use and education. A further follow-up of this cohort (Klatsky et al. 1997) concluded that alcohol protects against CHD, and that there may be minor additional benefits from drinking beer or wine, but not especially red wine.

Some suggest that specific components in wine have antioxidant and anti-platelet effects (Frankel et al. 1993, Goldberg et al. 1995, Renaud et al. 1992a, b, Renaud et al., 1979). There is also clear evidence from prospective studies conducted among predominantly wine drinking populations that moderate wine use lowers CHD risk. However, even if wine is consumed through regular moderate use at meals, its superiority over other beverage alcohol still has not yet been satisfactorily established.

Drinking Pattern

Only a few studies have addressed the question of drinking pattern directly. Rimm et al. (1991b) found that the average number of days per week on which alcohol was consumed was also inversely associated with risk of coronary artery disease (CAD). Men who reported drinking, on average, on 3–4 days per week had a relative risk of 0.66 (95% CI 0.46–0.96) compared with men who drank on less than 1 day a week. Because total alcohol intake and average number of days per week on which alcohol was consumed were so highly correlated ($r = 0.89$), the two predictors were not modelled simulta-neously.

Kannel (1988) states that a small amount of alcohol taken weekly is beneficial only if it is spread out over the week. "Binge drinking" of the entire week's allocation is harmful. Other studies showing an increased risk of CHD with alcohol intake were the result of weekend drinking of spirits (Suhonen et al. 1987) or binge drinking of beer (Kauhanen et al. 1997).

As mentioned above, a recent study from Australia also reported drinking patterns (McElduff, 1997). Among both men and women, the strongest inverse association was reported among participants who consumed 1–2 drinks per day on 5–6 days per week. Those who had a similar average weekly consumption of alcohol, but consumed it on fewer days, had either less or no benefit at all.

Continuing Controversies

Each of the studies relating alcohol to CVD has its flaws. Although consistency of the finding is often cited as one of the criteria making an observed association more likely to be causal than artefactual, studies can be wrong consistently. Two main arguments concerning non-drinkers are questioned in the international literature and deal with "sick quitters" and "ill health in abstainers". These possible biases were first raised by Shaper et al. (1988). They found an inverse relationship between alcohol consumption and CVD mortality in their whole cohort, but the inverse relationship could no longer be found in the sub-cohort initially free from heart disorders and other related conditions.

The argument suggests that it is the inclusion of "sick quitters" in the group of non-drinkers that accounts for the high incidence of CHD in non-drinkers compared with moderate drinkers. Several studies (Jackson et al. 1991, Kono et al. 1986, 1991, Yano et al. 1977, Stampfer et al. 1988, Miller et al. 1988, Klatsky et al. 1990, Lazarus et al. 1991) have been able to separate lifetime abstainers from people who stopped drinking.

In addition, in the report from Klatsky et al. (1990), moderate alcohol use was associated with lower CHD mortality, even in the population remaining after exclusion of anyone who had one of 17 indicators of cardiovascular illness or risk factors. Similarly, in the Health Professionals Follow-up Study, Rimm et al. (1991a, b) reported an inverse association between moderate alcohol use and incidence of CHD, even after excluding 16,342 men (37% of the entire population) with previous conditions such as diabetes, hypertension and angina, which may have caused a change in their recent drinking behaviour.

Thus, it seems that the inclusion of former drinkers in the non-drinking group did not account for the higher incidence of CHD in non-drinkers in the studies that have the data to address this question directly.

Alcohol and Atherosclerosis

Autopsy Studies

In the autopsy studies by Moore et al. (1986), alcohol use was estimated by interviewing relatives instead of relying on cirrhosis as a marker. Five (Hirst et al. 1965, Viel et al. 1966, Sackett et al. 1968, Rissanen 1974, Rhoads et al. 1978) out of seven studies did not observe any significant lowering of atherosclerotic lesions in drinkers, especially after adjusting for age, smoking, cholesterol and blood pressure. The main difficulty of these studies is in the selection of adequate controls. They should not be patients dying from CHD or other chronic diseases known to be associated with a lesser degree of atherosclerosis. The controls should ideally be violent deaths as in the studies of Parrish et al. (1961), Viel et al. (1966), Rissanen (1974), and others. Under these conditions, significantly less atherosclerosis in drinkers has not been found. Nevertheless, it can be argued that, since alcohol drinking is frequently associated with violent death, reliable information on alcohol use by these people is hard to obtain.

In conclusion, the inhibitory effect of alcohol on atherosclerotic lesions has not been clearly demonstrated in autopsy studies or by clinical observation, especially for moderate intake of alcohol.

Clinical Studies

In a series of studies, Barboriak et al. (1982) observed, in more than 2500 patients undergoing diagnostic coronary arteriography, an inverse relationship between the extent of coronary occlusion and the amount of alcohol consumed, for both males and females. In further studies (Gruchow et al. 1982) it was found that a consumption of 5.7 to 17.1 g alcohol daily decreased the occlusion score by 3%. Interestingly, a similar intake of alcohol is associated, in prospective studies, with a 10–50% lower incidence of CHD (see Table 1). It was only with intakes higher than 34 g daily that a decrease of ca. 20% in the score could be observed. The more consistent the intake of alcohol, the lower the occlusion score. By contrast, drinkers with variable drinking patterns had higher occlusion scores, regardless of amounts consumed. As subsequent studies show, the authors suggested that the anti-atherogenic effect of alcohol on CHD was at least partially explained by the alcohol-induced rise of plasma HDL-cholesterol (Barboriak et al. 1979). However, drinkers with a variable pattern of drinking, and thus with a high occlusion score, had a high level of HDL-cholesterol similar to regular drinkers (Gruchow et al. 1982).

By contrast, in the Artherosclerosis Risk in Communities (ARIC) cross-sectional study of over 13,000 men and women, alcohol was not associated with the extent of carotid artery intimal-media thickness (Demirovic 1993). However, this population had a somewhat limited variation in alcohol consumption.

Those studies which use preclinical measures of atherosclerosis suggest a more complex association than results from epidemiological studies which have consistently reported an inverse relationship between alcohol intake and CHD. At a moderate intake, there is little or no protective effect, while a high daily intake of alcohol is associated with a substantial lessening of coronary lesions.

Alcohol and Lipids

HDL Cholesterol

Ethanol is oxidized almost exclusively in the liver. Since the liver also plays a central role in the metabolism of lipids, there are several interactions of ethanol with lipid metabolism. The main interest in the present review is the effect of alcohol, in human studies, on lipids and lipoprotein particles known to be associated with CHD.

In numerous epidemiological studies, a positive association has been found between alcohol use and the level of HDL cholesterol (Moore et al. 1986, Veenstra 1991, Rimm et al. 1999). In addition, in a number of experimental studies in human subjects, even moderate amounts of alcohol were shown to increase HDL cholesterol within a few weeks. Earlier studies have provided evidence that HDL_3 cholesterol is more sensitive to the alcohol-induced increase than the HDL_2 sub-fraction (Valimaki et al. 1988). However, a more recent study has not found this to be the case (Clevidence 1995). In epidemiological studies both HDL sub-fractions are associated with a reduced risk of CHD (Miller et al. 1988, Stampfer et al. 1991). Epidemiological and experimental studies that have included measurements of the HDL-associated apolipoproteins A1 and A2 confirm the positive association between alcohol consumption and HDL.

There is little doubt that alcohol, even at moderate levels of consumption, increases HDL cholesterol but before definite conclusions can be drawn as to whether the increased level of HDL cholesterol contributes to a reduction in CHD risk, it is necessary to have a better understanding of the mechanism underlying this increase. Also, definite evidence of an increase in the excretion of cholesterol and bile acids with moderate drinking is needed to support the reverse cholesterol transport hypothesis, as well as definite evidence that reverse cholesterol transport inhibits atherosclerosis.

Does the Effect of Alcohol on Lipoproteins Explain the Effect of Alcohol on Coronary Heart Disease?

Given the multiplicity of effects of alcohol on the cardiovascular system, it would appear that much of the benefit on the left side of the U-shaped curve is attributable to the increase in HDL cholesterol (HDL-C) and related apolipoproteins (Criqui et al. 1990, Rimm et al. 1999), a question first explored in the LRC Follow-Up Study. If moderate alcohol use lowers the risk of CHD incidence via an increase in HDL-C, adding HDL-C to a multivariate model predicting CHD incidence as a function of alcohol (and other variables) would reduce the strength of the inverse association for alcohol, since the only benefit remaining for alcohol would be that which is not through the HDL-C pathway. Among men and women, Criqui et al. (1987) reported a 50% reduction of the protective strength of the alcohol coefficient after the addition of HDL cholesterol to the model.

Since this initial study, other case-control and cohort studies have reported that 45–60% of the association between moderate alcohol use and risk of CHD is explained via the HDL-C pathway (Langer et al. 1992, Suh et al. 1992, Gaziano et al. 1993, Marquis-Vidal et al. 1996). In a case-control study from Boston a similar analysis was conducted where, for the first time, total energy intake and dietary intake of saturated fat was also considered. After controlling for HDL-C or other lipids, men who consumed 1–3 drinks per day had a 40% reduction in risk of MI. The inverse association was reduced by 60% after controlling for HDL-C. Other lipid fractions did not substantially alter the association. In all four studies, the effect attributable to HDL-C may actually be somewhat larger than estimated since misclassification due to measurement error will attenuate the degree to which HDL-C appears to mediate the effects of alcohol in these regression models.

In a recent meta-analysis of metabolic studies of alcohol and HDL-C, Rimm et al. (1999) estimated that a 30 g/day alcohol would increase HDL-C by 39.9 mg/l. If this increase in HDL-C was projected to rates of CHD from the Framingham Heart Study, the overall effect of 30 g/day of alcohol would lower the risk of CHD by 13.5%. If this estimate was adjusted for within-person variability in HDL-C levels, the overall reduction due to 30 g/day of alcohol would be ca. 16.5%. Since most prospective analyses of moderate alcohol use and risk of CHD report a 30–40% reduction in risk, the projected 16.5% reduction in risk due solely to changes in HDL-C is similar to the reduction suggested by the studies of Criqui and Langer discussed above (Criqui et al. 1987, Langer et al. 1992).

The above results suggest that about half of the protective effect of moderate alcohol use appears to be mediated by an HDL-C pathway and that other possible mechanisms are likely to play an important role. Decreased coagulation has been attributed to moderate alcohol use. Alcohol can lower fibrinogen (Meade et al. 1979) and inhibit platelet aggregation (Mikhailidis et al. 1983, Renaud et al. 1992a, b, Renaud et al. 1979). Thus, it is tempting to speculate that moderate drinking can inhibit CHD incidence both by inhibiting atherosclerosis (the HDL-C pathway) and by thrombotic occlusion of the coronary arteries (the coagulation pathway). Recent evidence also suggests that, independent of other known predictors of insulin, moderate drinking is associated with lowered fasting insulin levels (Kiechl et al. 1996, Vitelli et al. 1996, Lazarus et al. 1997).

Alcohol and Haemostasis

Platelet Function

It is now accepted that coronary thrombosis initiated by platelet aggregation is the primary trigger for MI. Anti-platelet drugs such as aspirin reduce coronary events by about half in unstable angina (Fuster et al. 1989) and in primary prevention (Steering Report, Physicians' Health Study 1989). The main effect of aspirin on platelets is to decrease secondary platelet aggregation to ADP (Zucker 1968) as evaluated by the *ex vivo* classical tests of platelet aggregation.

In man, platelet aggregation tests have been shown to predict coronary events (Thaulow et al. 1991) and to be significantly correlated with prevalent cases of MI (Elwood et al. 1991), independent of serum lipids.

Haut et al. (1974) demonstrated that alcohol added *in vitro* at a physiological dosage to human platelets markedly reduces the aggregation to thrombin, adrenaline and ADP (mostly secondary wave). Following this demonstration, several studies have confirmed that ethanol inhibits platelet aggregation and secretion (Fenn et al. 1982, Benistant et al. 1990, Mikhailidis et al. 1990, Rubin 1989).

Acute Effects Ex Vivo in Man

Collagen-induced platelet aggregation, *ex vivo*, was inhibited 30 min after the ingestion in man of 1 ml alcohol per kg body weight (Mikhaildis et al. 1983). This effect was lost at 60 min. In preliminary studies (Renaud et al. 1984), similar results were obtained for collagen and ADP aggregation, with rebound effects in some subjects.

These studies indicate that the acute effect of alcohol on platelets is transient in man, as is also observed in rats (Renaud et al. 1984, Renaud et al. 1996). Thus, it can be expected that any acute study failing to take a blood sample within 30 min of alcohol ingestion will not observe any inhibitory effects on platelets as was the case in the studies by Dunn et al. (1981) and Veenstra et al. (1990b). In the study of Hillbom et al. (1985), blood samples were obtained 4 h later. As a result, they observed a significant increase in the response of platelets to ADP-induced aggregation after the ingestion of 1.5 g alcohol per kg body weight, which lasted for an additional 8 h. This rebound effect, observed in alcoholics after alcohol withdrawal (Fink et al. 1983), could be the explanation for sudden CHD deaths after drunken episodes (Kozarevic et al. 1988). By contrast (Jackson et al. 1992), the risks of non-fatal MI and coronary death were consistently lower in people who had drunk alcohol in the previous 24 h.

Long-Term Effects Ex Vivo in Man

More important for the usual relationship with CHD is the effect of long-term alcohol use on platelet reactivity. Pikaar et al. (1987) studied, over a period of 5 weeks, the effect of consumption of a standard dose of wine. A significant decrease in collagen-induced platelet aggregation was observed, even when alcohol was not present in the circulation. After 2 weeks of alcoholic beverage administration, others (Seigneur et al. 1990) found that red wine, but not diluted alcohol or white wine, would decrease platelet aggregability to ADP. In contrast, Pellegrini (1996) found that red wine or alcohol (30 g/day) for 3 weeks had similar effects on reducing collagen-induced platelet aggregation. De-alcoholized wine had no effect on platelet aggregation. Results from several short-term feeding studies and large cross-sectional studies (Veenstra et al. 1990b, Renaud et al. 1981, 1992a, b, 1996, Meade et al. 1986, Pelligrini et al. 1996) suggest that the acute effect of alcohol on platelets may result in a permanent decrease of aggregation tendency.

Does the Effect of Alcohol on Haemostasis Explain the Effect of Alcohol on Coronary Heart Disease?

There is a consensus that part of the effect of alcohol on CHD is through an effect on haemostasis. There is also a consensus that, *in vitro*, alcohol inhibits platelet aggregation induced by several agonists, especially secondary aggregation to ADP. Although there are only a few long-term studies, these indicate that the acute inhibitory effects of moderate alcohol use may extend to longer-term benefits.

Although *ex vivo* tests of platelet aggregation have been criticized as not necessarily reflecting what occurs *in vivo*, there is increasing evidence that these tests are good indicators of CHD risk. Nevertheless, further studies are certainly required to definitely prove the role of platelet reactivity in CHD in relation to alcohol.

Alcohol and Fibrinolysis

In several epidemiological studies (Meade et al. 1986, Ernst et al. 1993) the level of fibrinogen has been found to be independently and significantly associated with the risk of CHD. Many, but not all, studies have found an inverse association between fibrinogen level and alcohol use (Kluft et al. 1992). In feeding studies, the association has not been consistent, with some (Burr et al. 1986, Pelligrini et al. 1996), but not all (Elmer et al. 1984, Kluft et al. 1992), reporting reduced fibrinogen levels among participants provided with alcohol for several weeks (Rimm et al. 1999).

The relationship between alcohol use and fibrinolytic activity has been previously reviewed (Veenstra 1990, Kluft et al. 1992). Recent results show large effects of moderate alcohol use on the specific fibrinolytic factors t-PA (tissue-type plasminogen activator) and PA1 (plasminogen activator 1), which play a crucial role in the ability to prevent and dissolve clots (Veenstra 1992, Hendriks et al. 1994). In a randomized cross-over study of a single dose of 40 g of beer, red wine or spirits, PA1 was increased up to 9 h after a test meal given with alcohol (compared to the placebo meal with no ethanol). t-PA was also increased, but t-PA activity decreased up to 5 h after the meal, and was significantly higher the following morning. The changes in fibrinolytic activity were not different by beverage type. After feeding periods of 4 weeks and 6 weeks, Pelligrini et al. (1996) and McConnell et al. (1997) both found increases in t-PA levels and McConnell et al. also reported an increase in PA1 activity.

Since both t-PA and PA1 display a strong circadian pattern, the effect of alcohol will strongly depend on the time of drinking. Further, the effects of alcohol on thrombolytic factors may depend on the extent of any pre-existing disease, since circulating levels of some of these markers have been associated with preclinical atherosclerosis.

Alcohol and Blood Pressure

A relationship between alcohol use and blood pressure elevation was first suggested by Lian in 1915, who noted that French service men drinking 2.5 litres of wine or more per day had an increased prevalence of hypertension (Lian 1915). Since 1967, attention has shifted to the question whether an association exists between alcohol use and blood pressure in populations not selected on the basis of alcohol intake. A large number of cross-sectional studies, a smaller number of prospective cohort studies and a few experimental studies have addressed this question. Most studies reported a positive association between alcohol use and blood pressure (Keil et al. 1993a, b).

Cross-Sectional Studies

The relation between alcohol and blood pressure has been investigated worldwide in at least 33 cross-sectional studies: 10 in Europe (Gyntelberg et al. 1974, Kozarevic et al. 1982, Milon et al. 1982, Salonen et al. 1983, Cairns et al. 1984, Kornhuber et al. 1985, Kromhout et al. 1985, Keil et al. 1989, 1991, Bulpitt et al. 1987), 12 in North America (Clark et al. 1967, Dyer et al. 1977, Klatsky et al. 1977, 1986, Harburg et al. 1980, Criqui et al. 1981, Kagan et al. 1981, Fortmann et al. 1983, Gordon et al.1983b,

1986, Coates et al. 1985, Gruchow et al. 1985), 6 in Australia (Mitchell et al. 1980, Baghurst et al. 1981, Cooke et al. 1982, Arkwright et al. 1982, Savdie et al. 1984, MacMahon et al. 1984), 2 in New Zealand (Paulin et al. 1985, Jackson et al. 1985) and 2 in Japan (Ueshima et al. 1984, Kondo and Ebihara 1984) and the Intersalt Study comprising 50 centres worldwide (Marmot et al. 1994).

In all the European studies evidence was obtained for an association between alcohol and blood pressure that was independent of a number of putative confounding factors such as age, body mass index (BMI), physical activity, smoking, coffee use, educational attainment and Type A/B behaviour. Intake of specific nutrients was not assessed in most of the studies.

In the Munich Blood Pressure Study (MBS) (Cairns et al. 1984) and in the Lübeck Blood Pressure Study (LBS) (Keil et al. 1989) the blood pressure of non-drinkers was in general either higher than or similar to those consuming 10–20 g of alcohol per day. In the LBS, blood pressure was higher in drinkers than it was in non-drinkers at consumption levels of 40 g of alcohol or more per day. In the MBS the respective drinking level was ≥60 g/day for men and ≥40 g/day for women.

The MONICA Augsburg Survey 1984/85 (Keil et al. 1991) confirmed the MBS results in that blood pressure was clearly higher in drinkers than in non-drinkers at drinking levels of ≥60 g/day for men and ≥40 g/day for women. Among the three studies performed in Germany with the same methodology, a clear J-shaped curve for the relation between alcohol and systolic blood pressure was found in LBS men (Keil et al. 1989) and in men and women aged 55–64 in Augsburg (Keil et al. 1991).

With the exception of the Canada Health Study (Coates et al. 1985), all of the 12 North American studies currently available have reported a significant positive association between alcohol and blood pressure. In the first Kaiser Permanente Study (Klatsky et al. 1977), only a small difference in systolic or diastolic blood pressure was found between non-drinking men and those drinking 10–20 g/day. In women, systolic and diastolic blood pressures were higher in non-drinkers than in those drinking 10–20 g/day, suggesting a J-shaped relationship. The findings of this study appear to indicate the presence of a threshold effect at 30 g of alcohol per day for blood pressure elevation in men and women. Several subsequent North American studies have confirmed these findings (Criqui et al. 1981).

In the 6 Australian and the 2 New Zealand studies linear, J-shaped and U-shaped associations between alcohol and blood pressure were observed, with the exception of one study (Baghurst et al. 1981). In the National Heart Foundation of Australia Risk Factor Prevalence Study (MacMahon et al. 1984) and in the Auckland Study (Jackson et al. 1985) there was evidence of elevated blood pressure levels in drinkers compared to non-drinkers at drinking levels of 30 g/day and above. Both Japanese studies (Ueshima et al. 1984, Kondo et al.1984) reported independent linear associations of alcohol with blood pressure. The Intersalt study revealed a significant relation of drinking $\geq$36 g/day to blood pressure in both men and women, and in both younger and older men. This relation was independent of BMI or urinary excretion of sodium and potassium (Marmot el al. 1994).

Cohort Studies

There are at least 7 prospective cohort studies that have addressed the association between alcohol and blood pressure (Kromhout et al. 1985, Dyer et al. 1977, Gordon et al.1983, 1986, Dyer et al. 1981, Reed et al. 1982, Witteman et al. 1989). The results of all but the Honolulu Heart Study (Reed et al. 1982) are consistent with those of the cross-sectional studies and indicate a positive relation between alcohol intake and blood pressure level. The effects of changing alcohol intake on blood pressure levels have been investigated prospectively over a 4-year period in the Framingham Heart Study (Gordon et al. 1983b). In both men and women an increase in alcohol consumption over 4 years was associated with a significant increase in blood pressure, whereas a decrease in alcohol use was associated with a significant decrease in blood pressure. In the Nurses' Health Study (Witteman et al. 1989), in a cohort of 58,000 US nurses not diagnosed as hyper-tensive, 3275 participants reported an initial diagnosis of elevated blood pressure during a four-year follow-up period. Women drinking 20-34 g/day alcohol had an approximate 1.4-fold higher risk of hypertension during follow-up than non-drinkers. In those drinking 35 g or more per day the relative risk was 1.9.

Table 2
Overview of observational studies on the association between alcohol and blood pressure

Differences in blood pressure between categories with the highest and the lowest alcohol intake. In general, the lowest category refers to abstainers, but in some cases light drinkers were also included. Studies are categorized by the unit of measurement.

Reference	Sex	Age	Highest drinking level	Difference in BP (mmHg) SBP	DBP
Reporting in "units"/day*					
Gyntelberg et al. 1974	M		6–10	8.1	4.8
Kozarevic et al. 1982	M		≥1	7.7	4.3
Coates et al. 1985	M	20–34	≥2.14	1.9	0.4
	M	35–49	≥2.14	2.9	4.0
	M	≥60	≥2.14	–3.4	–0.5
	F	20–34	≥2.14	1.8	–0.1
	F	35–49	≥2.14	–2.4	–5.4
	F	≥60	≥2.14	–5.7	–2.1
Bulpitt et al. 1987	M		>10	20.0	7.3
	F		>10	5.5	3.4
Lang et al. 1987	M		>5	8.9	5.3
	F		>5	14.3	6.1
Weissfeld et al. 1988	M	18–39	>2	3.3	3.7
	M	40–59	>2	0.7	1.9
	M	≥60	>2	2.4	4.5
	F	18–39	>2	8.4	6.9
	F	40–59	>2	6.1	2.8
	F	≥60	>2	9.7	3.3
Wannamethee 1991	M		>6	6.5	4.0
Reporting in ml/day*					
Klatsky et al. 1977	M		≥72	5.4	2.1
	F		≥72	10.9	4.5
Arkwright et al. 1981	M		>50	5.1	n.s.
Milon et al. 1982	M	<40	≥12	n.s.	n.s.
	M	40–49	≥12	10.6	n.s.
	M	>50	≥12	11.9	n.s.
Fortmann et al. 1983	M	20–34	≥30	2.6	-1.6
	M	35–49	≥30	3.0	1.2
	M	50–74	≥30	15.4	6.6
	F	20–34	≥30	2.3	1.5
	F	35–49	≥30	-0.4	-0.2
	F	50–74	≥30	12.8	6.5
Gordon et al. 1983b	M		≥74.7	7.3	n.s.
	F		≥74.7	8.4	n.s
Elliott et al. 1987	M		>42.8	13.2	5.4
Trevisan et al. 1987	M		>114	3.0	1.0
	F		>114	6.7	0.4
Dyer et al. 1990	M white		>30	2.4	2.0
	M black		>30	2.8	0.9
	F white		>30	1.5	1.5
	F black		>30	-0.3	2.4

Table 2 (continued)

Reference	Sex	Age	Highest drinking level	Difference in BP (mmHg) SBP	DBP
Klag et al. 1990	M Japan.		>58	14.1	8.9
	M white		>30	5.6	3.6
Yamada et al. 1991	M		>58	4.9	3.9
Marmot et al. 1994	M		>71	4.6	3.0
	F		>43	3.9	3.1
Reporting in g/day					
Myrhed 1974	M+F		>27.4	9.6	6.7
Dyer et al. 1977	M alcoholics		4.7	n.s.	
	M		≥25	9.7	5.9
Marmot et al. 1981	M		>34	2.8	2.3
Cooke et al. 1983	M		>30	7.7	4.7
	F		>30	5.0	3.8
Ueshima et al. 1984	M urban		>83	17.4	10.3
	M rural		>83	16.9	8.5
Cairns et al. 1984	M		≥60	2.4	1.2
	F		≥40	n.s	2.4
Jackson et al. 1985	M	>50	>34	4.8	1.7
	F	>50	>34	10.2	4.5
Paulin et al. 1985	M		≥42.8	9.8	8.9
	F		≥42.8	−6.0	1.0
Simon et al. 1988	M		>50	n.s.	n.s.
Keil et al. 1989	M	30–69	≥40	5.5	4.5
	F	45–69	≥20	_**	_**
Keil et al. 1991	M	25–34	≥80	5	5
	M	25–34	≥80	5	5
	M	35–44	≥80	8	5
	M	45–54	≥80	11	6
	M	55–64	≥80	3	2
	F	25–34	≥40	3	3
	F	35–44	≥40	6	5
	F	45–54	≥40	6	3
	F	55–64	≥40	2	1
Reporting in oz/day*					
Harburg et al. 1980	M		≥2.27	5.8	3.8
	F		≥1.98	2.0	5.5
Kagan et al. 1981	M		≥1.97	6.1	3.4
Gordon et al. 1986	M		≥2.96	7.3	5.6
Miscellaneous measures					
Clark et al. 1967	M		"yes"	1.9	1.6
Schnall et al. 1992	M		"regular use"	3.6	2.8

* 1 unit = 10–20 g alcohol; 1 ml = 0.9 g alcohol; 1 oz (ounce) = 28 g alcohol.
** Association only in smokers.
BP, blood pressure; SBP, systolic blood pressure; DBP, diastolic blood pressure.

Table 3

Change in alcohol intake (categorical, in g/day) in men (*n* = 1818) and women (*n* = 1832) between 1984/85 and 1987/1988. MONICA Augsburg Cohort Study 1984-199

Men		Women	
change in alcohol intake	***n* (%)**	**change in alcohol intake**	***n* (%)**
reduction >30 g	231 (12.7)	reduction >10 g	349 (19.0)
reduction 10–30 g	384 (21.1)	reduction 2–10 g	315 (17.2)
from reduction by 10 g to increase by 10 g	755 (41.5)	from reduction by 2 g to increase by 2 g	694 (37.9)
increase 10–30 g	303 (16.7)	increase by 2–10 g	229 (12.5)
increase >30 g	145 (8.0)	increase >10 g	

Source: Keil et al. (1998).

Table 2 provides an overview of observational studies on the association between alcohol and blood pressure. In this table the studies are categorized by the unit of measurement of alcohol intake.

The MONICA Augsburg cohort study similarly provides data on changes in alcohol intake and changes in blood pressure in 1818 men and 1832 women aged 25-64 over a 3-year period from 1984/85 to 1987/88 (Keil et al. 1998). Table 3 shows changes in alcohol intake categories for men and women over this 3-year period. Obviously, the net absolute effects for each sex are more persons changing their status from drinker to non-drinker than in the other direction. Table 4 depicts the changes in systolic and diastolic blood pressure with changes in alcohol use in men. Men who lower their alcohol intake show, on average, a decrease in systolic and diastolic blood pressure whereas men who increase their drinking level exhibit an increase in blood pressure values. This applies both to the crude changes (differences) and to changes adjusted for age, baseline blood pressure,antihypertensive medication and smoking. Table 5 shows the respective changes for women with findings similar to those in men. As women drink much less alcohol than men the changes in alcohol intake over the 3 years are much smaller as are the changes in blood pressure.

Table 4
Change in systolic (SBP) and diastolic blood pressure (DBP) by changes in alcohol intake among men 25–64 years old. MONICA Augsburg Cohort Study, 1984–1988

Change in alcohol use (g/day)	n	Crude differences		Adjusted differences[a]	
		SBP (mmHg)	DBP (mmHg)	SBP (mmHg)	DBP (mmHg)
reduction >30 g	231	−3.9	−2.2*	−3.2	−1.4
reduction 10–30 g	384	−1.8	−0.9	−1.1	−0.6
from reduction by 10 g to increase by 10 g	755	−1.1	−0.5	−1.5	−0.7
increase 10–30 g	303	1.1*	1.6*	0.6*	1.1*
increase >30 g	145	2.4*	1.8*	2.4*	1.5

* Significant difference (*P*<0.05) relative to the central change category (from 10 g/day reduction to 10 g/day increase).
[a] Adjusted in analysis of covariance for age, baseline blood pressure, antihyper-tensive medication and smoking.
Source: Keil et al. (1998).

Table 5
Change in systolic (SBP) and diastolic blood pressure (DBP) by changes in alcohol intake among women aged 25–64

Change in alcohol use (g/day)	n	Crude differences		Adjusted differences[1]	
		SBP (mmHg)	DBP (mmHg)	SBP (mmHg)	DBP (mmHg)
reduction >10 g	349	−1.8	−1.1	−1.7	−1.0
reduction 2–10 g	315	−1.1	−0.3	−1.0	−0.3
from reduction by 2 g to increase by 2 g	694	−0.7	−0.3	−0.5	−0.2
increase 2–10 g	229	0.2	−0.4	−0.2	−0.4
increase >10 g	245	0.6	0.6	0.2	0.2

[1] Adjusted in analysis of covariance for age, baseline blood pressure, antihyper-tensive medication and smoking.
Source: Keil et al. (1998).

Table 6
Randomized trials of changes in alcohol intake and their impact on blood pressure[1]

Design	Initial alcohol intake	Final alcohol intake	Duration	Initial BP	Change in BP[a]	*P*
Potter et al. (1984), 16 hypertensives, mean drinking level 80 ml/day						
crossover	80 ml/d	0 ml/d	3 days	174/104	−19/−5	<0.05
	0 ml/d	80 ml/d	4 days	156/100	+12/+5	<0.01
Puddey et al. (1985b), 46 normotensives, mean drinking level 366 ml/week						
crossover	426 ml/wk	85 ml/wk	6 weeks	130/73	−3.7/−1.4	<0.001
Howes et al. (1986), 10 normotensives, mean drinking level 40 ml/day						
crossover	55 ml/d	0 ml/d	7 days	116/60	−3.0/−3.1	<0.05/ <0.01
Puddey et al. (1987), 44 hypertensives, mean drinking level 472 ml/week						
crossover	452 ml/wk	64 ml/wk	6 weeks	142/84	−5/−3	<0.001
Parker et al. (1990), 59 hypertensives, mean drinking level 480 ml/week						
parallel group	537 ml/wk	57 ml/wk	4 weeks	138/85	−5.4/−3.2	<0.01
Maheswaran et al. (1992), 41 hypertensives, mean drinking level 480 ml/week						
parallel group	480 ml/wk	240 ml/wk	8 weeks	149/101	−/5.2	n.s./ <0.05

[a] Blood pressure (BP), in mmHg (systolic/diastolic BP).

Trials: Acute Withdrawal

Blood pressure rises when alcohol is acutely withdrawn in very heavy drinkers. This response is associated with clinical evidence of sympathetic nervous system activation (tachycardia and sweating) and raised plasma catecholamines, renin activity, aldosterone and cortisol (Bannan et al. 1984, Eisenhofer et al. 1985). Withdrawal of alcohol in hypertensives may also give rise to postural hypotension. In some but not all patients who show this effect the catecholamine response to standing is inhibited, suggesting impaired cardiovascular reflexes (Eisenhofer et al. 1985).

Trials: Chronic Withdrawal

Few studies have examined the effect of withdrawing for several days or weeks in moderate to heavy drinkers. To detect blood pressure lowering effects, such studies have to be carefully designed. To control for potential confounders and placebo effects, randomized controlled trials are to be preferred. Table 6 provides an overview of a number of randomized trials addressing changes in alcohol intake and their impact on the blood pressure of hypertensive and normotensive subjects.

Using a crossover design, Potter et al. (1984) admitted a group of heavy-drinking hypertensive patients to the hospital and withdrew alcohol from half of the group for three days and maintained the other half on normal alcohol intake. Then alcohol was withdrawn from the latter group and given to the former group for the next four days. The period of alcohol withdrawal in both groups was associated with significant lowering of blood pressure. Puddey et al. (1985b, 1987) also performed a crossover trial but employed an intervention period of six weeks. Subjects were also "blinded" to the level of alcohol intake by being given a low-alcohol lager with or without alcohol added. The aims of "blinding" are to exclude placebo intervention effects and to remove observer bias. Both groups showed a significant lowering of blood pressure on reduction of alcohol intake in heavy drinkers both in normotensive and hypertensive subjects. Other reports have confirmed the blood pressure-lowering effect of alcohol withdrawal using both crossover and parallel group designs (Howes et al. 1986, Parker et al. 1990, Maheswaran et al. 1992).

The intervention trials show a remarkable consistency in demonstrating a potentially valuable decrease in blood pressure when heavy drinkers abstain or restrict their alcohol intake (Table 6). The decrease in blood pressure induced in these studies is as large as would be predicted from associations found in populations. Taken together, the observational and intervention studies provide strong support for the view that alcohol use is an important life-style factor in the aetiology of elevated blood pressure.

From observational and intervention studies it appears that above a daily alcohol intake of 30 g a further increment of 10 g/day, on average, increases systolic blood pressure by 1 to 2 mmHg and diastolic blood pressure by 1 mmHg.

Interpretation of Findings on the Relation between Alcohol and Blood Pressure

MEASUREMENT PROBLEMS

Measurement of alcohol intake is a critical issue in research into the relation between alcohol and blood pressure. In many population-based studies, alcohol intake was estimated on the basis of oral or written information provided by the subject. Self-reporting may be obtained by having participants keep daily diaries on their alcohol use. Alternatively, consumption over periods ranging from the most recent week to lifetime may be recalled. One issue relates to problems in recalling the exact amount of alcohol consumed over a period such as one day, week, month or longer periods. Another issue is the heterogeneity of the group that claims to drink no alcohol at all (Colsher at al. 1989).

A retrospective recall method has been compared to a 3-day or 7-day prospective record method in men aged 45–64 participating in the MONICA Augsburg survey of 1984/85. Both methods produced very similar results for mean reported daily alcohol intake (Pearson correlation coefficient 0.75) (Schaeffer et al. 1991, Döring et al. 1993).

The blood alcohol concentration (BAC) provides a "gold standard" for the quantity of alcohol consumed recently (Puddey et al. 1985a). However, determination of BACs becomes impractical when alcohol consumption in large numbers of people and over longer time periods need to be assessed. Moreover, BACs may not be elevated in moderate drinkers several hours after their last drink. Several biochemical determinations are recommended to estimate regular alcohol use: GGT, mean corpuscular volume (MCV) and HDL-cholesterol (Chick et al. 1981). In general, studies relating biomarkers for alcohol intake to blood pressure levels have obtained results similar to studies relying on reported intake. However, none of these biochemical parameters appears to be sufficiently sensitive or specific to replace or substantiate interview or questionnaire data.

The "non-alcohol group" is a problem group comprising lifelong abstainers, drinkers who deny their drinking, those who already suffer from health problems and those who are too sick to drink alcohol (Midanek et al. 1990). The effects of misclassification in the non-alcohol group on the relation between alcohol and blood pressure may be diverse. In this respect, it is important to note that the positive association between alcohol consumption and blood pressure is particularly pronounced among those with a higher than average alcohol intake.

The findings for moderate and light drinking are less clear-cut. Some have described a "threshold phenomenon" where the mean blood pressure was only elevated if alcohol intake exceeded about three glasses (30 g) per day (Klatsky 1977, Dyer 1977). Others have reported a J-shaped relation between alcohol and blood pressure with moderate drinkers having a lower blood pressure than teetotallers (Gyntelberg et al. 1974, Harburg et al. 1980). There is inadequate information on light drinkers or non-drinkers, as the group of teetotallers may be "contaminated" by subjects who do not admit their heavy drinking, and this may explain some of the inconsistency in such findings. Such misclassification could theoretically cause an inverse relationship at the beginning of the curve although the general view is that this phenomenon, if present, may not completely account for the absence of an association between light to moderate alcohol use and blood pressure.

Another problem is that people might underreport their alcohol intake. Relative to the true distribution of intake the observed distribution will be shifted to the left. Such general, non-differential under-reporting will probably result in an overestimate of the association at any specific level of actual alcohol intake, although the overall strength of the association will not be affected. Moreover, if a threshold really exists the estimated threshold level might be higher if there is a systematic underreporting of alcohol use (MacMahon 1987).

CONFOUNDERS

Valid interpretation of the association between alcohol intake and blood pressure is affected not only by the quantification and potential misclassification of alcohol use, but also by various putative confounding factors. This applies in particular to age, gender and body weight, and in most of the investigations adjustments have been made for these factors. Several other variables have, however, often not been included in the analyses because relevant information was not available or assessment was too difficult. This applies, for example, to dietary factors such as electrolyte intake (notably sodium, potassium and magnesium), medication and physical activity. As it has also repeatedly been found that drinkers smoke more cigarettes (Gordon et al. 1983b), it is not inconceivable that alcohol use is related to a life-style that could have an effect on blood pressure independent of alcohol use (Calahan 1981). In addition, a poor nutritional condition could play a role, especially for heavy drinkers. Perhaps even more difficult to assess is the potentially confounding effect of psychosocial stress. It is generally accepted that alcohol may reduce tension under stressful circumstances. In view of the potential stress-buffering capacity of alcohol at a cognitive level, the blood pressure of subjects who do not drink may be more responsive to stressful conditions and life events. However, the debate about putative confounders can be closed on two grounds. First, analyses in which variables such as age, gender, BMI, smoking, coffee consumption, physical activity, Type A/B behaviour and educational attainment were controlled have confirmed the unadjusted associations between alcohol and blood pressure, i.e. have not changed the estimates of the associations (Keil et al. 1991). Second, randomized trials have confirmed the results from observational studies. As randomized trials have the advantage of controlling for both known and unknown confounders, the argument that the observed effect of alcohol on blood pressure might be due to uncontrolled confounding such as nutrition or psychosocial factors or unknown confounders can be refuted. The extent to which some of these factors modify the individual response of blood pressure to alcohol intake remains to be established (van Leer et al. 1994).

MECHANISMS

Alcohol is widely distributed in body fluids and exerts important actions on the physico-chemical properties and biological function of cell membranes. Different dose-dependent effects and divergence between acute and chronic actions make the interaction between alcohol and blood pressure a complex one, and it is extremely unlikely that a single mechanism accounts for the association between blood pressure and alcohol described in population studies. It is likely that chronic alcohol administration exerts a direct or indirect pressor effect on the cardiovascular system, which is not evident in acute studies, where the predominant effect is blood pressure-lowering. The pressor effect could be mediated by a neurogenic mechanism, a humoral mechanism or directly through actions on the vessels which maintain peripheral resistance. In summary, the acute and chronic physiological effects of alcohol on the cardiovascular system are quite distinct. The pressor effect of chronic ingestion is still poorly understood. At present neural, humoral and direct vascular mechanisms are thought to be possible mediators of the association between alcohol and blood pressure, but the role of each of these factors, if any, is still unclear.

IMPLICATIONS FOR PREVENTION AND TREATMENT

In most epidemiological studies, blood pressure levels were elevated at drinking levels ≥40 g/day relative to 10–20 g/day (MacMahon 1987, Keil et al. 1989). About 25% of studies reported blood pressure elevations at drinking levels <30 g/day compared with the blood pressure of non-drinkers. About 40% of studies reported the blood pressure of non-drinkers to be higher than of those drinking 10–20 g/day. It is doubtful whether these findings actually reflect a blood pressure-lowering effect of small amounts of alcohol. Thus, it is still unclear whether the relationship between alcohol and blood pressure is linear or curvilinear. One possible explanation for the J-shaped relationship is that "non-drinkers" are a heterogeneous group. More research is needed to better understand that group and its influence on the shape of the relationship between alcohol and blood pressure.

If a threshold dose for hypertension risk exists, it is probably ca. 30–60 g alcohol per day and likely lower for women than for men.

From a public health perspective it is important to estimate what proportion of hypertension in the community might be caused by alcohol use and, more importantly, how much hypertension in the community could be eliminated if drinking more than, for example, 40 g alcohol daily was avoided. Focusing on the population attributable-risk percentage, it was calculated from Lübeck Blood Pressure Study data that about 7% of hypertension in men in the community is drinking more than 40 g alcohol per day (Keil et al. 1989). The respective calculations from US and Australian population studies suggest that alcohol use could account for as much as 11% of hypertension in men but much less in women because of their much lower alcohol intake (MacMahon et al. 1984, Friedman et al. 1982). Chronic alcohol intake ≥30–60 g/day can be viewed as the second-most important risk factor for hypertension, closely behind obesity.

In spite of many unanswered questions (such as the threshold level and the shape of the association) concerning the relationship between alcohol and blood pressure, it seems clear that a causal association exists between consumption of ≥30–60 g alcohol per day and blood pressure elevation in men and women. The presence of a causal relationship is justified because chance, and to a large degree bias and confounding, have been ruled out as plausible explanations of the association in most observational studies. More importantly, intervention studies support the observational studies and show a similar quantitative relationship thus emphasizing that confounding factors are not responsible for the observed relationship.

Furthermore, the consistency in observations across cross-sectional, prospective cohort and intervention studies is high. In addition, a clear time sequence between cause and effect seems to be present. However, the underlying mechanisms must be clarified further. Recent techniques for studying vascular physiological and molecular mechanisms may shed more light on the mechanisms underlying the relationship between alcohol and blood pressure.

It is conceivable that a major improvement in the assessment of the exposure to alcohol will contribute to a more precise delineation of the association between alcohol and blood pressure and will transform the frequently found J-shaped curves to a more linear or curvilinear relationship with a more precise estimate of the threshold level in the range of a chronic intake of 30–60 g alcohol per day for hypertension.

Alcohol and Insulin Sensitivity

In addition to the effects of alcohol on atherosclerosis and thrombosis, recent evidence suggests that moderate drinking may be associated with increased insulin sensitivity. Several previous studies have suggested that heavy drinking may inhibit secretion of insulin and lead to pancreatitis and overt diabetes. However, recent evidence from experimental, cross-sectional and prospective studies suggests that moderate drinking may increase insulin sensitivity and decrease the risk of diabetes (Facchini et al. 1994, Kiechl 1996, Vitelli 1996, Rimm 1995). Some have suggested that the effect of alcohol on insulin sensitivity could mediate some of the reported beneficial effects of alcohol on HDL-C (Kiechl 1996). In a prospective analysis from the Bruneck Study (Kiechl 1996), 9–35% of changes in HDL-C and apolipoprotein A1 among drinkers were due to changes in insulin sensitivity. More research is needed to determine if the reported associations between alcohol and insulin sensitivity directly lower the risk of CHD independent of lipid and haemostatic factors.

Alcohol and Stroke

The relationship between stroke and alcohol consumption has been extensively reviewed (van Gijn et al. 1993) for studies reported up to 1992. The extent to which conclusions in the report by van Gijn et al. need to be updated or revised in view of recent research findings is considered here.

Stroke can be briefly defined as a focal neurological deficit of sudden onset, caused by a vascular lesion of the brain. Three subtypes of stroke can be distinguished: (1) cerebral infarction (75% to 85% of all strokes) or ischaemic necrosis of a part of the brain due to the occlusion by an embolus or a thrombus in a cerebral artery; (2) cerebral haemorrhage (10% of all strokes) or extravasation of blood into the brain parenchyma caused by a rupture of a small perforating artery or, in young adults, of an arteriovenous malformation; (3) subarachnoid haemorrhage (5% of all strokes) or extravasation of blood primarily in the subarachnoid space caused by a ruptured aneurysm. These three types of stroke, which can be diagnosed by computerized tomography (CT) scan, all have different causes, and it is unlikely that the effect of alcohol would be the same for all types. Unfortunately, studies reported in the period 1993-1998 are still generally based on total stroke without separating out the different types.

Total Stroke

Van Gijn et al. (1993) concluded that there is no convincing evidence for an association between habitual drinking and overall risk of total stroke except for a modest increase in risk at high drinking levels. Recent results from the Physicians' Health Study (Robbins et al. 1994) corroborate this conclusion. In this study 22,071 men, 40 to 84 years of age, were followed for 9.7 years; 312 non-fatal and 28 fatal strokes occurred. Although the main purpose of the study was not to evaluate the effect of alcohol, the relative risk for total stroke with consuming alcohol monthly, weekly and daily was 0.95 (CI 0.56–1.61), 0.75 (CI 0.47–1.22) and 1.14 (CI 0.63–2.05), respectively, compared to abstainers. In a prospective study in Shanghai on 18,244 middle-aged men with 6 to 9 years of follow-up (Ross et al. 1997, Yuan et al. 1997) moderate drinking (1–28 drinks/week) was not associated with an increased risk of death from stroke. By contrast, heavy drinking (29 drinks/week on average) over a sustained period was associated with a 65% increase in overall stroke mortality. In the huge study on half a million US adults with a 9-year follow-up (Thum et al. 1997), 1307 men and 1072 women died from stroke. Compared to abstainers, a 10 to 30% lower mortality from stroke was found with no increase in risk at whatever level of alcohol use (after adjustment for 4 (men) or 5 (women) variables). The Copenhagen City Heart Study analysis (Gronbæk et al. 1995) comprised 13,285 subjects with 10–12 years of follow-up. The risk of death from cardiovascular and cerebrovascular disease was 60% lower for drinkers of 3–5 glasses of wine per day than for abstainers. For beer drinkers, the reduction was 28% with 3–5 drinks/day compared to not drinking beer. However with a daily use of 3–5 drinks of spirits risk increased by 34%.

The potential risk associated with spirits is in contrast to other findings on the relative benefits and risks of various alcoholic beverages (Rimm et al. 1996) and requires further research. A recent study in eastern France which included 34,000 predominantly wine-drinking men (with 82% of the alcohol drunk as wine) was followed up for 12 years (Renaud et al. 1998). In this large cohort, mortality from cardiovascular (including cerebrovascular) disease was significantly lower, by 33%, even with 10 drinks per day, after adjustment for several confounding factors. These results agree with those of Gronbæk et al. (1995) concerning the effect of wine on overall cardiovascular death. As the consumption of spirits was rare in the French cohort, beverage-specific effects could not be evaluated. In a prospective study in the UK of 6369 treated hypertensive subjects (Palmer et al. 1995), a 66% lower risk of overall stroke death was found in men and a 48% lower risk in women after adjusting for age, smoking and blood pressure after drinking. In this study most participants drank wine, but a lower risk was also found for men who drank both wine and beer. Again, the small number of users of spirits prevented a separate analysis. In conclusion, recent results in prospective studies performed in the USA, China, Denmark, France and the UK confirm that habitual moderate drinking (up to 3 to 4 drinks per day) is not associated with an increased risk of overall stroke. At a higher intake, a modest increase in stroke mortality has been observed in some studies. The possible beverage-specific risks and benefits for total stroke require further study.

Haemorrhagic Stroke

According to van Gijn et al. (1993), substantial evidence suggests an association between habitual drinking and the risk of haemorrhagic stroke at high levels of intake. The dose range for this adverse effect was unclear, as were the differential effects of habitual versus short-term (binge) drinking. In a recent report from the state of Washington, 149 cases of subarachnoid haemorrhage were compared to 298 matched controls (Longstreth et al. 1992). In light drinkers (<1 drink/day) the relative risk of haemorrhage was 0.7 (95% CI 0.4–1.1) compared to non-drinkers. In moderate drinkers (1–2 drinks/day) the relative risk was 1.5 (95% CI 0.7–3.0) and in heavy drinkers (>2 drinks/day) 3.8 (95% CI 1.7–8.4). In the latter group risks were reduced to 2.2 (95% CI 0.9–5.1) after adjustment for smoking. After adjustment for smoking, the relative risk for habitual drinkers was 0.6 (95% CI 0.3–1.0) but reached 4.3 (95% CI 1.5–12.3) in those binging at least once a week. The Hisayama study in Japan is a prospective study on 1621 subjects with a follow-up of 26 years (Kiyohara et al. 1995); during that period 244 subjects developed a cerebral infarction and 60 a cerebral haemorrhage. The relative risk of haemorrhage was non-significantly higher in normotensive light drinkers (up to 33 g alcohol per day; RR 1.35, 95% CI 0.57–3.32)) or heavy drinkers (>34 g/day; RR 1.69, 95% CI 0.58–4.91) compared to non-drinkers. However, risks were significantly higher in hypertensive heavy drinkers (RR 3.13, 95% CI 1.08–9.10). The results appear to apply to regular heavy drinking. In a study from the Helsinki University Hospital (Juvela et al. 1993), 278 consecutive patients with aneurysmal subarachnoid haemorrhage were compared to 314 hospitalized matched controls. After adjusting for age, hypertension and smoking status, men who consumed 1 to 40 g alcohol within the 24 h preceding the onset of illness had a relative risk of haemorrhage of 0.3 (95% CI 0.1–0.8). However, relative risks were 4.5 (95% CI 1.5–12.9) for those consuming >120 g/day. Women who had drunk 1–40 g alcohol in the past 24 h had a relative risk of haemorrhage of 0.4 (95% CI 0.2–0.8) but of 6.4 (95% CI 2.3–17.9) when their alcohol intake was higher than 40 g. In that study, both recent heavy drinking (more than 40 g/day) and current smoking were strong independent risk factors for aneurysmal subarachnoid haemorrhage. From the same hospital, a subsequent case-control study included 156 consecutive patients with a first intracerebral haemorrhage and 332 matched controls (Juvela et al. 1995). The adjusted relative risk (RR) of haemorrhage was 0.33 (95% CI

0.16–0.72, *P*<0.01) compared to abstainers for up to 40 g alcohol consumed within 24 h of the onset of illness. The relative risk increased to 4.56 (95% CI 2.20–9.42, *P*<0.001) for 41–120 g/day and 11.34 (95% CI 3.00–42.79, *P*<0.001) for an intake above 120 g. For alcohol use in the week before the onset of symptoms, excluding the last 24 h, the adjusted relative risks was 2.0 (95% CI 1–3.5) for 1–150 g, 4.3 (95% CI 1.6–11.7) for 151–300 g and 6.5 (95% CI 2.4–17.7) for >300 g per week. The authors concluded that moderate to heavy recent alcohol use is, with hypertension, the most important risk factor for intracerebral haemorrhage. In a Swedish population-based register including 15,077 middle-aged and older men and women followed up for 20 years (Hansagi et al. 1995), 769 deaths from stroke were recorded, 195 of which were haemorrhagic. After adjustment for age and smoking, mortality was not significantly related to the intake of alcohol. A possible explanation for these Swedish results could be the low level of alcohol intake in the population. Only 25% of the men and 7% of the women used alcohol on a daily basis, and only 1% of the men and 0.08% of the women drank more than 40 g/day. An increased risk was only observed for ischaemic stroke, predominantly in men reporting intoxication or binge drinking a few times a year.

In summary, results from research (one cohort and three case-control studies) reported in the past six years confirm that heavy drinking, both regular and short-term, is an independent risk factor for haemorrhagic stroke. In one additional prospective study with most of the subjects drinking less than 40 g alcohol per day, there was no relationship between the intake of alcohol and haemorrhagic stroke (Hangasi et al. 1995). These collective findings suggest that the use of more than 40 g alcohol per day, and in particular irregular or binge drinking, increases the risk of haemorrhagic stroke. At present, little can be said about beverage-specific risk of haemorrhagic stroke over and beyond the effects of alcohol.

Ischaemic Stroke

Van Gijn et al. (1993) concluded that substantial evidence suggests that there is no association between habitual drinking and the risk of ischaemic stroke, even at high drinking levels. In a small case-control study in England (Shinton et al. 1993) on 81 ischaemic stroke cases and 198 matched controls, a protective effect of light or moderate alcohol use was found which was attenuated after adjustment for potential confounders. Excessive drinking had little effect on the risk of stroke (adjusted RR 0.83, 95% CI 0.33–1.35). In a case-control study in 156 hospitalized patients with acute ischaemic stroke and 153 hospitalized matched male controls in Helsinki University Hospital (Palomäki et al. 1993), the risk was assessed using stepwise multiple logistic regression adjusted for 7 covariables one of which was hypertension. In regular light drinkers (up to 150 g alcohol evenly distributed over the week) the risk of ischemic stroke was significantly reduced (OR 0.12, 95% CI 0.02–0.65), as it was in moderate drinkers (150–300 g/week; OR 0.55, 95% CI 0.14–2.08), but it was markedly increased in heavy drinkers (>300 g/week; OR 4.45, 95% CI 1.09–18.1), especially in those with an irregular pattern of drinking.

The prospective study of Kiyohara et al. (1995) in Japan on 1621 subjects followed for 26 years found a slight reduction in ischaemic strokes for a moderate drinking level (<34 g/day for both men and women). Among heavy drinkers (>34 g/day) a modestly increased risk (RR 1.96, 95% CI 1.08–3.57) was reported for hypertensive men. In the Swedish cohort of 15,077 middle-aged men and women (Hansagi et al. 1995) with a follow-up of 20 years (574 ischaemic strokes) alcohol was not associated with the risk of stroke in men. In women, the lowest risk was with 0–5 g/day (RR 0.6, 95% CI 0.5–0.8). Interesting results were obtained after adjustment for age and smoking in that men who drank infrequently ran twice the risk of dying of ischaemic stroke than lifelong abstainers (RR 2.0, 95% CI 1.3–3.2). Those who reported binge drinking had an elevated risk (RR 1.6, 95% CI 1.1–2.5 if they were intoxicated occasionally; RR 1.8, 95% CI 1.1–2.8 if they were intoxicated frequently). By contrast, women reporting infrequent drinking had a 40% reduction in ischaemic stroke risk (RR 0.6, 95% CI 0.4–0.9), those reporting drinking once a month to once a week a 30% reduction (RR 0.7, 95% CI 0.5–0.9), and those drinking almost daily a 20% reduction (RR 0.8, 95% CI 0.5–1.4). Binge-drinking women and those who felt occasionally intoxicated had no increased risk (RR 0.9, 95% CI 0.4–2.4). The highest risk in women for ischaemic stroke in relation to alcohol was found for former drinkers (RR 3.3, 95% CI 1.5–7.2). However, in the cohort average intake of alcohol was >40 g/day for only 1% of men and 0.08% of women.

In summary, findings in the few case-control and prospective studies reported since 1992 on alcohol use and ischaemic stroke suggest that light and moderate habitual drinkers have a slightly lower risk of ischaemic stroke than teetotallers, most clearly seen in women, although this may reflect their generally lower alcohol use. In heavy drinkers, especially binge drinkers, a 2- to 4-fold increased risk of ischaemic stroke was reported in 3 out of the 4 recent studies confirming that heavy drinking is associated with an increased rate of ischaemic stroke. Methodological problems in some studies include over-adjustment. In particular, both blood pressure and serum cholesterol could play an intermediary role by being increased by large intakes of alcohol.

Ischaemic Stroke and Light Drinking

At the time of the report by van Gijn et al. (1993), no consensus appeared to exist regarding a possible decreased risk of ischaemic stroke with low to moderate drinking levels. The subsequent few reports that addressed this issue in some detail seem to suggest that light drinking is associated with a reduced risk of ischaemic stroke, most clearly among women. This protective effect in women may reflect their low intake (0–5 g/day) as it was associated with a 40% reduction in risk in the prospective study by Hansagi et al. (1995). This is consistent with previous prospective studies (Stampfer et al. 1988; Klatsky et al. 1990) reporting a borderline significant protective effect for an alcohol use of less than one drink daily.

Since a protective effect of alcohol on CHD is reasonably well established (Rimm et al. 1996), a modest level of protection against ischaemic stroke is plausible, the two diseases sharing common aetiologies. Nevertheless, large prospective studies are still needed to definitely settle the possible protective effect of light drinking on ischaemic stroke in both men and women. Still, as 75 to 85% of all strokes in Western societies are ischaemic, one may expect that the protective effects on overall stroke in large prospective studies predominantly reflect an effect on ischaemic stroke. For example, the large American Cancer Society cohort (Thun et al. 1997), including 1307 deaths from stroke in men and 1072 in women, showed that one drink or less per day was associated with a 30% lower risk for both men and women. In this cohort, even at an intake of >4 drinks/day a lower risk of ischaemic stroke in men (RR 0.7, 95% CI 0.6–0.9) and women (RR 0.9, 95% CI 0.7–1.2) was found. However, in that study binge drinkers and very heavy drinkers were excluded or under-represented.

When collectively considering previous and recent results on ischaemic stroke and overall stroke, it seems clear that light to moderate regular drinking is associated with a protective effect on ischaemic stroke. Further research is needed to determine whether wine drinking may have a stronger protective effect on ischaemic stroke than other alcoholic beverages, as suggested by Palmer et al. (1995) and Grønbæk et al. (1995).

Binge Drinking and Stroke

Recent studies on overall stroke considered very few binge drinkers or heavy drinkers. However, for stroke subtypes (ischaemic or haemorrhagic), several case-control and prospective studies have addressed this issue. In a case-control study of Palomäki et al. (1993) in Finland, a significant reduction in the risk of ischaemic stroke for regular alcohol use did not hold true for irregular drinking despite similar weekly alcohol consumption (up to 300 g). Above 300 g/week, alcohol consumption increased the risk of stroke by more than four-fold after adjustment for several confounders. In the Kiyohara et al. (1995) prospective study on 1621 middle-aged subjects in Japan, heavy drinking (probably regular) associated with hypertension increased the risk of ischaemic stroke close to two-fold and the risk of haemorrhagic stroke more than three-fold. In a case-control study in the USA (Longstreth et al. 1992) on subarachnoid haemorrhage, the relative risk for heavy drinking was 2.2 (95% CI 0.9–5.1) after adjustment for smoking but increased to 4.3 (95% CI 2.2–8.4) for those binging at least once a week. In carefully selected patients for a case-control study on risk factors for intracerebral haemorrhage in Finland (Juvela et al. 1995), the use of alcohol within the 24 h preceding the onset of illness was evaluated. The relative risk for subarachnoid haemorrhage (adjusted for 10 confounders) was 0.3 (95% CI 0.2–0.7) when alcohol intake was 1–40g/day. The relative risk, however, increased to 4.6 (95% CI 2.2–9.4) when the intake was 41–120 g and 11.3 (95% CI 3.0–42.8) for an intake of >120 g/day. In contrast, in the Hansagi et al. (1995) prospective study in Sweden, men reporting binge drinking (and sometimes or often intoxication) had only an 80% increased risk (RR 1.8, 95% CI 1.1–2.8, adjusted for age and smoking) of ischaemic stroke and no increased risk of haemorrhagic stroke. However, the overall level of alcohol intake in that cohort was generally low.

In summary, results from Finland (two studies), Japan, the USA and Sweden confirm the results previously reported (van Gijn et al. 1993) that consumption in a few hours of a large quantity of alcohol (binge drinking) for intoxication is associated with an increased risk of mainly haemorrhagic but also ischaemic stroke. Again, most recent results stem from case-control studies (3 out of 5) as they appear the most appropriate to evaluate intake of alcohol just before the event. Two prospective studies also report a significant increased risk of stroke after binge drinking, although the risk was not as spectacular (2- to 3-fold) as in case-control studies. A recent prospective study of 2682 men from Finland (Kauhanen et al. 1997) suggested that the pattern of drinking might have independent effects on risk not explained by total quantity of alcohol drunk. In that study (69% beer drinkers) the pattern of heavy acute beer drinking was associated with a 3-fold increased risk of all-cause mortality, and a 6.5-fold increase in fatal myocardial infarction independently of the total average quantity consumed. Taken together, convincing evidence exists that acute alcohol intoxication is associated with a sizeable increased risk of stroke and of additional health problems, especially violent death.

Future Research

In most aspects of the research areas mentioned, a better understanding of the relation between alcohol and CHD and stroke is needed.

There are now a large number of both case-control and prospective cohort studies addressing the question of alcohol and CHD, and these reveal quite consistent findings. In the past few years, prospective studies with data from more than 1,000,000 subjects have been reported. Additional observational studies may help to refine certain questions if more detail is collected on beverage choice, drinking patterns, and other correlated drinking behaviours. The latter is particularly relevant to the effect of alcohol use on subtypes of stroke.

Re-analysis of Existing Studies

Meta-analysis of the association between alcohol and CHD and stroke is needed and feasible.

A few studies suggest that wine could have stronger beneficial effects than other alcoholic beverages. A recent review of prospective studies suggests that alcohol from all beverage sources has similar benefits (Rimm 1996) and that changes in lipids and haemostatic factors are dependent on alcohol content rather than beverage type (Rimm 1999). However, the cause of differences in results by beverage between studies has not been fully elucidated. The following influences of drinking patterns should be explored: (1) drinking with meals; (2) episodic drinking (weekend vs. daily); (3) substances other than alcohol present in red wine or other alcoholic beverages altering the antioxidant profile.

Pearson (1994) calculated that similar numbers of lives are lost due to alcohol-related mortality as are saved thanks to reduced CHD mortality in the USA. However, a more detailed cost-benefit analysis could be conducted taking into account alcohol-related (or prevented) morbidity and mortality. Such an analysis is clearly needed to substantiate public health policy on the sensible use of alcohol.

Some studies have suggested that alcohol may alter levels of circulating carotenoids and, in a recent study of folate and CHD (Rimm 1998), moderate drinking was found to complement the reduced risk of CHD associated with folate. A clearer understanding of the effect of alcohol on other dietary factors is needed.

Randomized Controlled Trials

The dose-response U-shape of the alcohol-CHD curve needs further evaluation. Where data are available, cohort studies should evaluate the timing of alcohol use during the course of the day, the association for ex-drinkers and the possible differences in dietary factors as potential confounding variables, and should utilize measures of changes in drinking pattern over time. Prospective observational studies with repeated assessments of alcohol and non-invasive vascular measures, or invasive measures such as angiography, would be helpful.

A randomized double-blind trial of alcohol use and CHD events could give a definitive answer, but it seems unlikely that such a trial will ever be done. Methodological problems include the difficulty of maintaining controls on a zero-alcohol regimen over several years, and the obvious difficulty with providing an appropriate placebo for the control group and maintaining "blinding". Other approaches will be required.

Large intervention trials of alcohol use and CHD morbidity and mortality cannot be undertaken. Therefore, limited intervention studies in healthy human volunteers to evaluate the specificity of alcohol's effects on CVD risk factors would be useful, since risk factors such as blood pressure, lipids and lipoproteins as well as fibrinogen, platelets, fibrinolysis and other coagulation factors are likely mediating variables for alcohol's effect. Experimental studies to date reveal some inconsistency concerning platelets and fibrinolysis (Veenstra 1991, Rimm et al. 1999). If we could determine dose-response relationships, including some probable non-linear relationships between alcohol and such mediating variables, we could begin to investigate whether such effects could be produced or modified by specific dietary or other behavioural regimens.

Conclusions

The epidemiological and clinical literature is replete with studies which show that light to moderate drinking is associated with a reduced risk of CHD, total and ischaemic stroke and total mortality in middle-aged and elderly men and women. A number of alternative explanations for the findings have been suggested but do not appear to explain the observed inverse association. These findings are supported by evidence from animal, clinical and biochemical studies. Despite the absence of a randomized intervention trial, it is highly likely that the association is causal.

From a public health point of view, the fear of stimulating alcohol overuse prevents us from advising individuals to start drinking if they have previously abstained. However, guidelines for moderation which have been adopted in the USA, the UK and elsewhere suggest that individuals who do consume alcohol responsibly may achieve some benefit if daily consumption is limited to 2 to 3 drinks.

References

Arkwright PD, Beilin LJ, Rouse I, et al. (1981) Alcohol: effect on blood pressure and predisposition to hypertension. Clin Sci 61: 373s–75s

Arkwright PD, Beilin LJ, Rouse I, et al. (1982) Effects of alcohol use and other aspects of lifestyle on blood pressure levels and the prevalence of hypertension in a working population. Circulation 66: 60–66

Baghurst K, Dwyer T (1981) Alcohol consumption and blood pressure in a group of youngAustralian males. J Human Nutr 35: 257–64

Bannan LT, Potter JF, Beevers DG, et al. (1984) Effect of alcohol withdrawal on blood pressure, plasma renin activity, aldosterone, cortisol and dopamine beta-hydroxylase. Clin Sci 66: 659–63

Barboriak JJ, Anderson AJ, Hoffmann RG (1979) Interrelationship between coronary artery occlusion, high-density lipoprotein cholesterol, and alcohol intake. J Lab Clin Med 94: 348–53

Barboriak JJ, Anderson AJ, Hoffmann RG (1982) Smoking, alcohol and coronary artery occlusion. Atherosclerosis 43: 277–82

Benistant C, Rubin R (1990) Ethanol inhibits thrombin-induced secretion by human platelets at a site distinct from phospholipase C or protein kinase C. Biochem J 269: 489

Brummer P (1969) Coronary mortality and living standard II. Coffee, tea, cacao, alcohol and tobacco. Acta Med Scand 186: 61–63

Bulpitt CJ, Shipley MJ, Semmence A (1987) The contribution of a moderate intake of alcohol to the presence of hypertension. J Hypertens 5: 85–91

Burr ML, Fehily AM, Butland BK, et al. (1986) Alcohol and high-density-lipoprotein cholesterol: a randomized controlled trial. Br J Nutr 56: 81–86

Cairns V, Keil U, Kleinbaum D, et al. (1984) Alcohol consumption as a risk factor for high blood pressure: Munich Blood Pressure Study. Hypertension 6: 124–31

Calahan D (1981) Quantifying alcohol consumption: patterns and problems. Circulation 64: 7–14

Camargo CA, Stampfer MJ, Glynn RJ, et al. (1997) Moderate alcohol consumption and risk for angina pectoris or myocardial infarction in U.S. male physicians. Ann Intern Med 126: 364–71

Chick J, Plant M, Kretiman N (1981) Mean cell-volume and gamma-glutamyltranspeptidase as markers of drinking in working man. Lancet i: 1249–51

Clark VA, Chapman JM, Coulson AH (1967) Effects of various factors on systolic and diastolic blood pressure in the Los Angeles Heart Study. J Chronic Dis 20: 571–81

Clevidence BA, Reichman ME, Judd JT, et al. (1995) Effects of alcohol consumption on lipoproteins of premenopausal women: a controlled diet study. Arterioscler Thromb Vasc Biol 15: 179–84

Coates RA, Corey PN, Ashley MJ, et al. (1985) Alcohol consumption and blood pressure: analysis of data from the Canada Health Survey. Prev Med 14: 1–14

Colsher PL, Wallace RB (1989) Is modest alcohol consumption better than none at all? An epidemiologic assessment. Annu Rev Public Health 10: 203–19

Cooke KM, Frost GW, Stokes GS (1983) Blood pressure and its relationship to low levels of alcohol consumption. Clin Exp Pharmacol Physiol 10: 229–33

Cooke KM, Frost GW, Thornell IR, et al. (1982) Alcohol consumption and blood pressure: survey of the relationship in a health screening clinic. Med J Aust 1: 65–69

Criqui MH, Wallace RB, Mishkel M, et al. (1981) Alcohol consumption and blood pressure: the Lipid Research Clinics Prevalence Study. Hypertension 3: 557–65

Criqui MH, Cowan LD, Tyroler HA, et al. (1987) Lipoproteins as mediators for the effects of alcohol consumption and cigarette smoking on cardiovascular mortality. Results from the Lipid Research Clinics Follow-up Study. Am J Epidemiol 126: 629–37

Criqui MH et al. (1990) The reduction of coronary heart disease with light to moderate alcohol consumption: effect or artifact? Br J Addict 85: 854–57

Criqui MH, Ringel BL (1994) Does diet or alcohol explain the French paradox? Lancet 344: 1719–23

Demirovic J, Nabulsi A, Folsom AR, et al. (1993) Alcohol consumption and ultrasonographically assessed carotid artery wall thickness and distensibility. Circulation 88:2787–93

Doll R, Peto R, Hall E, et al. (1994) Mortality in relation to consumption of alcohol: 13 years' observations on male British doctors. Br Med J 309: 911–18

Döring A, Filipiak B, Stieber J, et al. (1993) Trends in alcohol intake in a Southern German population from 1984-1985 to 1989-1990: results of the MONICA Project Augsburg. J Stud Alcohol 54: 745–49

Dunn EL, Cohen RG, Moore EE, et al. (1981) Acute alcohol ingestion and platelet function. Arch Surg 116: 1082–83

Dyer AR, Stamler J, Paul O, et al. (1977) Alcohol consumption, cardiovascular risk factors, and mortality in two Chicago epidemiologic studies. Circulation 56: 1067–74

Dyer AR, Stamler J, Paul O (1981) Alcohol, cardiovascular risk factors and mortality: the Chicago experience. Circulation (suppl 3) 64: 20–27

Dyer AR, Cutter GR, Liu KQ, et al. (1990) Alcohol intake and blood pressure in young adults: the Cardia Study. J Clin Epidemiol 43: 1–13

Eisenhofer G, Whiteside EA, Johnson RH (1985) Plasma catecholamine responses to changes of posture in alcoholics during withdrawal and after continued absence from alcohol. Clin Sci 68: 71–78

Elliott P, Fehily AM, Sweetnam PM, et al. (1987) Diet, alcohol, body mass, and social factors in relation to blood pressure: the Caerphilly Heart Study. J Epidemiol Comm Health 41: 37–43

Elmer O, Goransson G, Zoucas E (1984) Impairment of primary hemostasis and platelet function after alcohol ingestion in man. Haemostasis 14: 223–28

Elwood PC, Renaud S, Sharp DS, et al. (1991) Ischaemic heart disease and platelet aggregation. The Caerphilly collaborative heart disease study. Circulation 83: 38–44

Ernst E, Resch KL (1993) Fibrinogen as a cardiovascular risk factor: a meta-analysis and review of the literature. Ann Intern Med 118: 956–63

Facchini F, Chen YD, Reaven GM (1994) Light-to-moderate alcohol intake is associated with enhanced insulin sensitivity. Diabetes Care 17: 115–19

Fenn CG, Littleton JM (1982) Inhibition of platelet aggregation by ethanol in vitro shows specificity for aggregating agent used and is influenced by platelet lipid composition. Thromb Haemost 48: 49–53

Fink R, Hutton RA (1983) Changes in the blood platelets of alcoholics during alcohol withdrawal. J Clin Pathol 36: 337–40

Food and Nutrition Board (1989) Recommended Dietary Allowances, 10th revised edition. National Academy of Sciences, Washington, DC.

Fortmann SP, Haskell WL, Vranizan K, et al. (1983) The association of blood pressure and dietary alcohol: Differences by age, sex and estrogen use. Am J Epidemiol 118: 497–507

Frankel EN, Kanner J, German JB, et al. (1993) Inhibition of oxidation of human low-density lipoprotein by phenolic substances in red wine. Lancet 341: 454–57

Friedman LA, Kimball AW (1986) Coronary heart disease mortality and alcohol consumption in Framingham. Am J Epidemiol 124: 481–89

Friedman GD, Klatsky AL, Siegelaub AB (1982) Alcohol, tobacco and hypertension. Hypertension (suppl 3) 4: 143–50

Fuchs CS, Stampfer MJ, Colditz GA, et al. (1995) Alcohol consumption and mortality among women. N Eng J Med 332: 1245–50

Fuster V, Cohen M, Halpern J (1989) Aspirin in the prevention of coronary disease (editorial). N Engl J Med 321: 183–85

Gaziano JM, Buring JE, Breslow JL, et al. (1993) Moderate alcohol intake, increased levels of high-density lipoprotein and its subfractions and decreased risk of myocardial infarction. N Eng J Med 329: 1829–34

Goldberg DM, Hahn SE, Parkes JG (1995) Beyond alcohol: beverage consumption and cardiovascular mortality. Clin Chim Acta 237: 155–87

Gordon T, Doyle JT (1986) Alcohol consumption and its relationship to smoking, weight, blood pressure, and blood lipids: the Albany Study. Arch Intern Med 146: 262–65

Gordon T, Kannel WB (1983a) Drinking habits and cardiovascular disease. The Framingham Study. Am Heart J 105: 667–73

Gordon T, Kannel WB (1983b) Drinking and its relation to smoking, blood pressure, blood lipids and uric acid. Arch Intern Med 143: 1366–1374

Gronbæk M, Deis A, Sorensen TIA, et al. (1995) Mortality associated with moderate intakes of wine, beer or spirits. Br Med J 310: 1165–69

Gruchow HW, Hoffmann RG, Anderson AJ, et al. (1982) Effects of drinking patterns on the relationship between alcohol and coronary occlusion. Atherosclerosis 43: 393–404

Gruchow HW, Sobocinski KA, Barboriak JJ (1985) Alcohol, nutrient intake, and hypertension in US adults. JAMA 253: 1567–70

Gyntelberg F, Meyer J (1974) Relationship between blood pressure and physical fitness, smoking and alcohol consumption in Copenhagen males aged 40-59. Acta Med Scand 195: 375–80

Hansagi H, Romelsjö A, Gerhardson de Verdier M, et al. (1995) Alcohol consumption and stroke mortality. 20 year follow-up of 15,077 men and women. Stroke 26: 1768–73

Harburg E, Ozgoren F, Hawthorne VM, et al. (1980) Community norms of alcohol usage and blood pressure. Am J Public Health 70: 813–20

Haut MJ, Cowan DH (1974) The effect of ethanol on hemostatic properties of human blood platelets. Am J Med 56: 22–33

Hegsted DM, Ausman LM (1988) Diet, alcohol and coronary heart disease in men. J Nutr 118: 1184–89

Hendriks HFJ, Veenstra J, Velthuis-te Wierik EJM, Schaafsma G, Kluft C (1994) Effect of a moderate dose of alcohol with evening meal on fibrynolytic factors. Br Med J 308: 1003–06.

Hillbom M, Kangasaho M, Kaste M, et al. (1985) Acute ethanol ingestion increases platelet reactivity: is there a relationship to stroke? Stroke 16: 19–23.

Hirst AE, Hadley GG, Gore I (1965) The effect of chronic alcoholism and cirrhosis of the liver on atherosclerosis. Am J Med Sci 46: 143–49

Howes LG, Reid JL (1986) Changes in blood pressure and autonomy reflexes following regular moderate alcohol consumption. J Hypertension 4: 421–25

Jackson R, Stewart A, Beaglehole R, et al. (1985) Alcohol consumption and blood pressure. Am J Epidemiol 122: 1034–44

Jackson R, Scragg R, Beaglehole R (1991) Alcohol consumption and risk of coronary heart disease. Br Med J 303: 211–16

Jackson R, Scragg R, Beaglehole R (1992) Does recent alcohol consumption reduce the risk of acute myocardial infarction and coronary death in regular drinkers? Am J Epidemiol 136: 819–24

Jackson R, Beaglehole R (1993) The relationship between alcohol and coronary heart disease: is there a protective effect? Curr Opin Lipidol 4: 21–26

Juvela S, Hillbom M, Numminen H, et al. (1993) Cigarette smoking and alcohol consumption as risk factors for aneurysmal subarachnoid hemorrhage. Stroke 24: 639–46

Juvela S, Hillbom M, Palomäki H (1995) Risk factors for spontaneous intracerebral hemorrhage. Stroke 26: 1558–64

Kagan A, Katsuhiko Y, Rhoads GG, et al. (1981) Alcohol and cardiovascular disease: the Hawaiian experience. Circulation 64 (suppl 3): 27–31

Kannel WB (1988) Alcohol and cardiovascular disease. Proc Nutr Soc 47: 99–110

Kaufman DW, Rosenberg L, Helmrich SP, et al. (1985) Alcoholic beverages and myocardial infarction in young men. Am J Epidemiol 121: 548–54

Kauhanen J, Kaplan GA, Goldberg DE, et al. (1997) Beer binging and mortality: results from the Kuopio ischemic heart disease risk factor study, a prospective population based study. Br Med J 315: 846–51

Keil U, Chambless L, Remmers A (1989) Alcohol and blood pressure: results from the Lübeck Blood Pressure Study. Prev Med 18: 1–10

Keil U, Chambless L, Filipiak B, et al. (1991) Alcohol and blood pressure and its interaction with smoking and other behavioural variables: results from the MONICA Augsburg Survey 1984/85. J Hypertension 9: 491–98

Keil U, Swales JD, Grobbee DE (1993a) Alcohol intake and its relation to hypertension. Cardiovascular Risk Factors 3: 189–200

Keil U, Swales JD, Grobbee DE (1993b) Alcohol intake and its relation to hypertension. In: Verschuren PM (eds) Health issues related to alcohol consumption. International Life Sciences Institute Europe (ILSI Europe), Brussels, pp. 17–42

Keil U, Chambless LE, Doring A, et al. (1997) The relation of alcohol intake to coronary heart disease and all cause mortality in a beer-drinking population. Epidemiology 8: 150–56.

Keil U, Liese A, Filipiak B, et al. (1998) Alcohol, blood pressure and hypertension. In: Alcohol and cardiovascular diseases. Wiley, Chichester, UK, pp. 125–51.

Kiechl S, Willet J, Poewe W, et al. (1996) Insulin sensitivity and regular alcohol consumption: large, prospective, cross sectional population study (Bruneck study). Br Med J 313: 1040–44

Kitamura A, Iso H, Snakai T, et al. (1998) Alcohol intake and premature coronary heart disease in urban Japanese men. Am J Epidemiol 147: 59–65

Kiyohara Y, Kato I, Iwamoto H, et al. (1995) The impact of alcohol and hypertension on stroke incidence in a general Japanese population. The Hisayama Study. Stroke. 26: 368–72

Klag MJ, Moore RD, Whelton PK, et al. (1990) Alcohol consumption and blood pressure: a comparison of native Japanese to American men. J Clin Epidemiol 43: 1407–14

Klatsky AL (1996) Alcohol, coronary disease, and hypertension (review). Annu Rev Med 47: 149–60

Klatsky AL, Friedman GD, Siegeland AB, et al. (1977) Alcohol consumption and blood pressure. N Engl J Med 296: 1194–1200

Klatsky AL, Friedman GD, Siegelaub AB (1981a) Alcohol use and cardiovascular disease: the Kaiser-Permanente experience. Circulation 64 (suppl III): 32–41

Klatsky AL, Friedman GD, Siegelaub MS (1981b) Alcohol and mortality. A ten year Kaiser-Permanente experience. Ann Intern Med 95: 139–45

Klatsky AL, Friedman GD, Armstrong MA (1986) The relationships between alcoholic beverage use and other traits to blood pressure: a new Kaiser Permanente Study. Circulation 73: 628–36

Klatsky AL, Armstrong MA, Friedman GD (1990) Risk of cardiovascular mortality in alcohol drinkers, ex drinkers and non-drinkers. Am J Cardiol 66: 1237–42

Klatsky AL, Armstrong MA, Friedman GD (1997) Red wine, white wine, liquor, beer, and risk of coronary heart disease hospitalization. Am J Cardiol 80: 416–20

Kluft C, Jie AFH, Kooistra T, et al. (1992) Alcohol and fibrinolysis. In: Veenstra J, van der Heij DG (eds) Alcohol and cardiovascular disease. Pudoc, Wageningen, Netherlands, pp. 45–63

Kondo K, Ebihara A (1984) Alcohol consumption and blood pressure in a rural community of Japan. In: Lovenberg W, Yamori Y (eds) Nutritional prevention of cardiovascular disease. Academic Press, Orlando, FL, pp. 217–24

Kono S, Handa K, Kawano J, et al. (1991) Alcohol intake and nonfatal acute myocardial infarction in Japan. Am J Cardiol 68: 1011–14

Kono S, Ikeda M, Tokudome S, et al. (1986) Alcohol and mortality: a cohort study of male Japanese physicians. Int J Epidemiol 15: 527–31

Kornhuber HH, Lisson G, Suschka-Sauermann L (1985) Alcohol and obesity: a new look at high blood pressure and stroke; an epidemiological study in preventive neurology. Eur Arch Psychiatry Neurol Sci 234: 357–62

Kozarevic D, Racic Z, Gordon T, et al. (1982) Drinking habits and other characteristics: the Yugoslavia Cardiovascular Disease Study. Am J Epidemiol 116: 287–301

Kozarevic DJ, McGee D, Vojvodic N, et al. (1980) Frequency of alcohol consumption and morbidity and mortality: the Yugoslavia Cardiovascular Disease Study. Lancet 1: 613–16

Kozarevic DJ, Vojvodic N, Gordon T, et al. (1988) Drinking habits and death. The Yugoslavia cardiovascular disease study. In J Epidemiol 12: 145–50

Kromhout D, Bosschieter EB, de Lezenne Coulander C (1985) Potassium, calcium, alcohol intake and blood pressure: the Zutphen Study. Am J Clin Nutr 41: 1299–1304

La Porte RE, Cresanta JL, Kuller LH (1980) The relationship of alcohol consumption to atherosclerotic heart disease. Prev Med 9: 22–40

Lang T, Degoulet P, Aime F (1987) Relationship between alcohol consumption and hypertension prevalence and control in a French population. J Chron Dis 40: 713–20

Langer RD, Criqui MH, Reed DM (1992) Lipoproteins and blood pressure as biologic pathways for the effect of moderate alcohol consumption on coronary heart disease. Circulation 85: 910–15

Lazarus NB, Kaplan GA, Cohen RD, et al. (1991) Change in alcohol consumption and risk of death from all causes and ischaemic heart disease. Br Med J 303: 553–56

Lazarus R, Sparrow D, Weiss ST (1997) Alcohol intake and insulin levels. The Normative Aging Study. Am J Epidemiol 145: 909–16

Lian C (1915) L'alcoholisme, cause d'hypertension artérielle. Bull Acad Natl Méd Paris 74: 525–28

Longstreth Jr WT, Nelson LM, Koepsell TD, et al. (1992) Cigarette smoking, alcohol use and subarachnoid hemorrhage. Stroke 23: 1242–49

Maclure M (1993) Demonstration of deductive meta-analysis: ethanol intake and risk of myocardial infarction. Epidemiol Rev 15: 328–51

MacMahon S (1987) Alcohol consumption and hypertension. Hypertension 9: 111–21

MacMahon SW, Blacket RB, MacDonald GJ et al. (1984) Obesity, alcohol consumption and blood pressure in Australian men and women. The National Heart Foundation of Australia Risk Factor Prevalence Study. J Hypertension 2: 85–91

Maheswaran R, Beevers M, Beevers DG (1992) Effectiveness of advice to reduce alcohol consumption in hypertensive patients. Hypertension 19: 79–84

Marmot MG, Shipley MJ, Rose G, et al. (1981) Alcohol and mortality: a U-shaped curve. Lancet ii: 580–83

Marmot M, Brummer E (1991) Alcohol and cardiovascular disease: the status of the U-shaped curve. Bt Med J 303: 565–68

Marmot MG, Elliott P, Shipley MJ, et al. (1994) Alcohol and blood pressure: the Intersalt study. Br Med J 308: 1263–67

Marques-Vidal P, Ducimetiere P, Evans A, et al. (1996) Alcohol consumption and myocardial infarction: a case-control study in France and Northern Ireland. Am J Epidemiol 143: 1089–93

McConnell MV, Vavouranakis I, Wu LL, et al. (1997) Effects of a single, daily alcoholic beverage on lipid and hemostatic markers of cardiovascular risk. Am J Cardiol 80: 1226–28

McElduff P, Dobson AJ (1997) How much alcohol and how often? Population based case-control study of alcohol consumption and risk of a major coronary event. Br Med J 314: 1159–64

Meade TW, Chakrabarti R, Haines A, et al. (1979) Characteristics effecting fibrinolytic activity and plasma fibrinogen concentrations. Br Med J 1: 153–56

Meade TW, Mellows S, Brozovic M, et al. (1986) Haemostatic function and ischaemic heart disease: principal results of the Northwick Park Heart Study. Lancet ii: 533–37

Midanek LT, Klatsky AL, Armstrong MA (1990) Changes in drinking behaviour: demographic, psychosocial and biochemical factors. Int J Addict 25: 599–619

Mikhailidis DP, Jeremy JY, Barradas A, et al. (1983) Effect of ethanol on vascular prostacyclin (prostaglan oodin I_2) synthesis, platelet aggregation, and platelet thromboxane release. Br Med J 287: 1495–98

Mikhailidis DP, Barradas MA, Jeremy JY (1990) The effect of ethanol on platelet function and vascular prostanoids. Alcohol 7: 171–80

Miller NE, Bolton CH, Hayes TM, et al. (1988) Associations of alcohol consumption with plasma high-density lipoprotein cholesterol and its major subfractions: the Caerphilly and Speedwell Collaborative Heart Disease studies. J Epidemiol Commun Health 42: 220–25

Milon H, Froment A, Gaspard P, et al. (1982) Alcohol consumption and blood pressure in a French epidemiological study. Eur Heart J 3: 59–64

Mitchell PI, Morgan MJ, Boadle DJ, et al. (1980) Role of alcohol in the etiology of hypertension. Med J Aust 2: 198–200

Moore RD, Pearson TA (1986) Moderate alcohol consumption and coronary artery disease: a review. Medicine 65: 242–67

Myrhed M (1974) Alcohol consumption in relation to factors associated with ischemic heart disease. Act Med Scand (suppl I) 195: 567

Palmer AJ, Fletcher AE, Bulpitt CJ, et al. (1995) Alcohol intake and cardiovascular mortality in hypertensive patients: report from the department of health hypertension care computing project. J Hypertension 12: 957–64

Palomäki H, Kaste M (1993) Regular light-to-moderate intake of alcohol and the risk of ischemic stroke. Is there a beneficial effect? Stroke 24: 1828–32

Parker M, Puddey IB, Beilin LJ, et al. (1990) A 2-way factorial study of alcohol and salt restriction in treated hypertensive men. Hypertension 16: 398–406

Parrish HM, Eberly Jr AL (1961) Negative association of coronary atherosclerosis with liver cirrhosis and chronic alcoholism. a statistical fallacy. J Indiana Med Ass 54: 341–47

Paulin JM, Simpson FO, Waal-Manning HJ (1985) Alcohol consumption and blood pressure in a New Zealand community study. NZ Med J 98: 425–28

Pearson TA, Terry P (1994) What to advise patients about drinking alcohol. The clinician's conundrum (editorial). JAMA 272: 967–68

Pellegrini N, Pareti FI, Stabile F, et al. (1996) Effects of moderate consumption of red wine on platelet aggregation and haemostatic variables in healthy volunteers. Eur J Clin Nutr 50: 209–213

Pikaar NA, Wedel M, van der Beek E, et al. (1987) Effects of moderate alcohol consumption on platelet aggregation, fibrinolysis, and blood lipids. Metabolism 36: 538–47

Pohorecky L (1991) Stress and alcohol interaction: an update on human research. Alcohol Clin Exp Res 15: 438–59

Poikolainen K (1991) Epidemiologic assessment of population risks and benefits of alcohol use. Alcohol Alcoholism 1 (suppl): 27–34

Potter JF, Beevers DG (1984) Pressor effect of alcohol in hypertension. Lancet i: 119–22

Puddey IB, Vandongen R, Beilin LJ, et al. (1985a) Alcohol stimulation of renin release in man: its relation to the hemodynamic, electrolyte and sympatho-adrenal responses to drinking. J Clin Endocrinol Metabol 61: 37–42

Puddey IB, Beilin LJ, Vandongen R, et al. (1985b) Evidence for a direct effect of alcohol consumption on blood pressure in normotensive men: a randomized controlled trial. Hypertension 7: 707–13

Puddey IB, Beilin LJ, Vandongen R (1987) Regular alcohol use raises blood pressure in treated hypertensive subjects: a randomized controlled trial. Lancet i: 647–51

Reed D, McGee D, Yano K (1982) Biological and social correlates of blood pressure among Japanese men in Hawaii. Hypertension 4: 406–14

Rehm JT, Bondy SJ, Sempos CT, et al. (1997) Alcohol consumption and coronary heart disease morbidity and mortality. Am J Epidemiol 146: 495–501

Renaud SC, Morazain R, McGregor L, et al. (1979) Dietary fats and platelet functions in relation to atherosclerosis and coronary heart disease. Hemostasis 8: 234–51

Renaud SC, Morazain R, Godsey F, et al. (1981) Platelet function in relation to diet and serum lipids in British farmers. Br Heart J 46: 562–70

Renaud SC, McGregor L, Martin JL (1984) Influence of alcohol on platelet functions in relation to atherosclerosis. In: Pozza G, et al. (eds), Diet, diabetes and atherosclerosis. Raven Press, New York, pp. 177–87

Renaud SC, Beswick AD, Fehily AM, et al. (1992a) Alcohol and platelet aggregation: the Caerphilly prospective heart disease study. Am J Clin Nutr 55: 1012–17

Renaud SC, de Lorgeril M (1992b) Wine, alcohol, platelets and the French paradox for coronary heart disease. Lancet 339: 1523–26

Renaud SC, Ruf JC. (1996) Effects of alcohol on platelet functions (review). Clin Chim Acta 246: 77–89

Renaud SC, Gueguen R, Schenker J, et al. (1998) Alcohol and mortality in middle-aged men from eastern France. Epidemiology 9: 184–88

Rhoads GG, Blackwelder WC, Stemmermann GN, et al. (1978) Coronary risk factors and autopsy findings in Japanese-American men. Lab Invest 38: 304–11

Rimm EB, Giovannucci E, Willet WC, et al. (1991a) Alcohol and mortality. Lancet 338: 1073–74

Rimm EB, Giovannucci EL, Willet WC, et al. (1991b) Prospective study of alcohol consumption and risk of coronary disease in men. Lancet 338: 464–68

Rimm EB, Chan J, Stampfer MJ, et al. (1995) Prospective study of cigarette smoking, alcohol use and the risk of diabetes in men. Br Med J 310: 55–59

Rimm EB, Klatsky A, Grobbee D, et al. (1996) Review of moderate alcohol consumption and reduced risk of coronary heart disease: is the effect due to beer, wine or spirits? Br Med J 312: 731–36

Rimm EB, Williams P, Fosher K, et al. (1999) A biologic basis for moderate alcohol consumption and lower coronary heart disease risk: a meta-analysis of effects on lipids and hemostatic factors. Br Med J (in press).

Rissanen V (1974) Coronary and aortic atherosclerosis in chronic alcoholics. Z Rechtsmed 75: 183–89

Robbins AS, Manson JE, Lee IM, et al. (1994) Cigarette smoking and stroke in a cohort of US male physicians. Ann Intern Med. 120: 458–62

Rosenberg L, Slone D, Shapiro S, et al. (1981) Alcoholic beverages and myocardial infarction in young women. Am J Public Health 71: 82–85

Ross RK, Yuan JM, Henderson BE, et al. (1997) Prospective evaluation of dietary and other predictors of fatal stroke in Shangaï, China. Circulation 96: 50–55

Rubin R (1989) Ethanol interferes with collagen-induced platelet activation by inhibition of arachidonic acid mobilization. Arch Biochem Biophys 270: 99

Sackett L, Gibson RW, Bross IDJ, et al. (1968) Relation between aortic atherosclerosis and the use of cigarettes and alcohol: an autopsy study. N Engl J Med 279: 1413–20

Salonen JT, Tuomilehto J, Tanskanen A (1983) Relation of blood pressure to reported intake of salt, saturated fats, and alcohol in a healthy middle aged population. J Epidemiol Commun Health 37: 32–37

Savdie E, Grosslight GM, Adena MA (1984) Relation of alcohol and cigarette consumption to blood pressure and serum creatinine levels. J Chronic Dis 37: 617–23

Schaeffer V, Döring A, Winkler G, et al. (1991) Erhebung der Alkoholaufnahme: Vergleich verschiedener Methoden. Ernährungs-Umschau 38: 490–94

Schnall PL, Schwartz JP, Landsbergis PA, et al. (1992) Relation between job strain, alcohol, and ambulatory blood pressure. Hypertension 19: 488–94

Seigneur M, Bonnet J, Dorian B, et al. (1990) Effect of the consumption of alcohol, white wine and red wine on platelet function and serum lipids. J Applied Cardiol 5: 215–22

Shaper AG, Wannamethee G, Walter M (1988) Alcohol and mortality in British men: explaining the U-shaped curve. Lancet ii: 267–73

Shinton R, Sagar G, Beevers G (1993) The relation of alcohol consumption to cardiovascular risk factors and stroke. The West Birmingham stroke project. J Neurol Neurosurg Psychiatry 56: 458–62

Simon J, Filipovsky J, Rosolova H, et al. (1988) Cross-sectional study of beer consumption and blood pressure in middle-aged men. J Human Hypertension 2: 1–6

St Leger AS, Cochrane AL, Moore F (1979) Factors associated with cardiac mortality in developed countries with particular reference to the consumption of wine. Lancet i: 1017–20

Stampfer MJ, Colditz GC, Willett WC, et al. (1988) A prospective study of moderate alcohol consumption and the risk of coronary disease and stroke in women. N Engl J Med 319: 267–73

Stampfer MJ, Sacks FM, Salvini S, et al. (1991) A prospective study of cholesterol, apolipoproteins, and risk of myocardial infarction. N Engl J Med 325: 373–81

Steering Committee of the Physicians' Health Study Research Group (1989) Final report on the aspirin component of the ongoing Physicians' Health Study. N Engl J Med 321: 129–35

Suh I, Shaten BJ, Cutler JA, et al. (1992) Alcohol use and mortality from coronary heart disease: the role of high density lipoprotein cholesterol. Ann Intern Med 116: 881–87

Suhonen O, Aromas A, Reunanen A, et al. (1987) Alcohol consumption and sudden coronary death in middle-aged Finnish men. Acta Med Scand 221: 335–41

Thaulow E, Erikssen J, Sandvik L, et al. (1991) Blood platelet count and function are related to total and cardiovascular death in apparently healthy men. Circulation 84: 613–17

Thum MJ, Peto R, Lopez AD, et al (1997) Alcohol consumption and mortality among middle-aged and elderly US adults. N Engl J Med 337: 1705–14

Trevisan M, Krogh V, Farinaro E, et al. (1987) Alcohol consumption, drinking pattern and blood pressure: analysis of data from the Italian National Research Council Study. Int J Epidemiol 16: 520–27

Ueshima H, Shimamoto T, Iida, et al. (1984) Alcohol intake and hypertension among urban and rural Japanese populations. J Chronic Dis 37: 585–92

Valimaki M, Taskinen MR, Ylikahri R, et al. (1988) Comparison of the effect of two different doses of alcohol on serum lipoproteins, HDL-subfractions and apolipoproteins A-I and A-II: a controlled study. Eur J Clin Invest 18: 472–80

van Gijn J, Stampfer MJ, Wolfe C, et al. (1993). The association between alcohol and stroke. In: Verschuren PM (ed.) Health issues related to alcohol consumption. ILSI Europe, Brussels, pp. 43–79

van Leer EM, Seidell JC, Kromhout D (1994) Differences in the association between alcohol consumption and blood pressure by age, gender, and smoking. Epidemiology 5: 576–82

Veenstra J (1990) Alcohol and fibrinolysis. Fibrinolysis 4 (suppl 2): 64–68

Veenstra J (1991) Moderate alcohol use and coronary heart disease: a U-shaped curve? In: Simopoulos AP (ed), Impacts on nutrition and health. World Reviews on Nutrition and Diet 65. Karger, Basel, pp. 38–71

Veenstra J (1992) Effects of alcohol on the cardiovascular system. In: Veenstra J, van der Heij G (eds), Alcohol and Cardiovascular Disease. Pudoc, Wageningen, Netherlands, pp. 87–113

Veenstra J, Ockhuizen Th, van de Pol H, et al. (1990a) Effects of a moderate dose of alcohol on blood lipids and lipoproteins postprandially and in the fasting state. Alcohol Alcoholism 25: 371–77

Veenstra J, van de Pol H, Schaafsma G (1990b) Moderate alcohol consumption and platelet aggregation in healthy middle-aged men. Alcohol 7: 547–49

Viel B, Donoso S, Salcedo D, et al. (1966) Alcoholism and socioeconomic status, hepatic damage and arteriosclerosis. Arch Intern Med 117: 84–91

Vitelli LL, Folsom AR, Shahar E, et al. (1996) Association of dietary composition with fasting serum insulin level: the ARIC study. Nutr Metab Cardiovasc Dis 6: 194–202

Wannamethee G, Shaper AG (1991) Alcohol intake and variations in blood pressure by day of examination. J Human Hypertension 5: 59–67

Weissfeld JL, Johnson EH, Brock BM, et al. (1988) Sex and age interactions in the association between alcohol and blood pressure. Am J Epidemiol 128: 559–69

Witteman JCM, Willett WC, Stampfer MJ, et al. (1989) A prospective study of nutritional factors and hypertension among US women. Circulation 80: 1320–27

Yamada Y, Ishizaki M, Kido T, et al. (1991) Alcohol, high blood pressure, and serum γ-glutamyl transpeptidase level. Hypertension 18: 819–26

Yano K, Rhoads GG, Kagan A (1977) Coffee, alcohol and risk of coronary heart disease among Japanese men living in Hawaii. N Engl J Med 297: 405–09

Yuan J, Ross RK, Gao Y, et al. (1997) Follow up study of moderate alcohol intake and mortality among middle aged men in Shanghai, China. Br Med J 314: 18–23

Yuan JM, Ross RK, Gao YT, et al. (1997). Follow-up of moderate alcohol intake and mortality among middle-aged men in Shanghaï, China. Br Med J 314: 18–23

Zucker MB, Peterson J (1968) Inhibition of adenosine diphosphate-induced secondary aggregation and other platelet functions by acetylsalicylic acid ingestion. Proc Soc Exp Biol Med 127: 547–51

Chapter **6**

Alcohol and Pregnancy

M. L. Plant
Alcohol & Health Research Centre, Edinburgh, UK

E. L. Abel
C.S. Mott Center, Detroit, MI, USA

C. Guerri
Valencia Foundation of Biomedical Investigations, Spain

Abstract

This chapter reviews the large and growing evidence on the effects of parental levels and patterns of alcohol consumption on the offspring. This information is assessed in the light of new developments in both diagnostic paradigms and nomenclature. Furthermore, given that it is now over thirty-five years since the first scientific reports were published, evidence of possible alcohol-related harm in older children and adults is also reconsidered.

Evidence is also reviewed on the possible adverse effects of maternal and paternal alcohol consumption on pregnancy and on the development of the foetus and the child. Clinical studies support the conclusion that chronic heavy maternal drinking, consistent with a diagnosis of "alcohol dependence" or "alcoholism", is an aetiological factor giving rise to foetal alcohol syndrome (FAS). Recent follow-up studies of adolescent and adult patients diagnosed with FAS revealed that while both physical features of FAS and growth deficits are less distinctive after puberty, cognitive and neurobehavioural problems continue and are the most deleterious outcome. The control of confounding factors in epidemiological studies (e.g. low socioeconomic status, poor maternal health, and use of tobacco and illicit drugs) is essential for determining the real influence of high and low levels of alcohol on children's neurobehavioural outcome. Animal studies have provided evidence that the effects of alcohol on the foetus are dose-related. These studies have also demonstrated that the brain is the most sensitive organ and many of the neurobehavioural effects observed in humans have been reproduced in animals. Although the causes of the apparent vulnerability are not fully understood, studies suggest that various biological and environmental factors, along with the amount and timing of alcohol intake may, at least in part govern the adverse effects of alcohol. Individual differences in maternal metabolism and genetic factors may explain why the infants of some problem-drinking mothers are more affected than are others. Current evidence is not consistent in showing a clear-cut relationship between adverse effects in pregnancy or individual pathognomonic effects on the foetus or child and lower levels of maternal alcohol consumption. There is some evidence of a threshold of drinking below which adverse effects cannot be detected. Current information is still insufficient to define exactly where this threshold lies, but it may be around 30–40 g per day (i.e. 4–5 UK drinks or 2½–3½ US drinks per day; Abel

1998b). It should be noted that this is well above the levels defined as moderate drinking for non-pregnant women.

Glossary

Atrial septal defect: defect in the upper chamber of the heart

Autism: failure to develop relationships with others involving non-responsiveness and delay in language development

Cerebellum: the largest part of the hind brain

Cognitive disabilities: problems in the processes of thinking, understanding and reasoning

Hippocampus: area of the brain

Hydronephrosis: an obstruction causing atrophy of the kidney structure

Hyperactivity disorder: disorder involving constant movement, restlessness, sometimes increased speed of speech and irritability

Morphogenesis: the stimulated growth of structure and form

Myopia: short sight

Neocortex: the outer layer of part of the brain

Learning deficits: problems in the area of learning; severe learning difficulties were originally known as mental handicap

Spontaneous abortion: miscarriage

Strabismus: squint in the eye

Ventricular septal defect: defect in the larger chambers of the heart

Introduction

Considerable advances in our understanding of foetal alcohol syndrome (FAS) and related individual abnormalities resulting from prenatal exposure to alcohol have occurred since the previous review (Plant et al. 1993). Changes in nomenclature and a new diagnostic paradigm have been proposed. New estimated incidence data have been published and risk factors contributing to the syndrome have been clarified. Furthermore, new models describing the mechanism of action underlying FAS have been formulated. The present overview reassesses our knowledge of the syndrome in the light of these new developments. Over the past few years a number of studies on the longer-term effects of alcohol consumption during pregnancy have been published; these too have been included in this update. Researchers have attempted in recent years to identify biological, genetic and environmental factors contributing to FAS and to answer questions such as: which of the alterations observed in FAS are permanent and which are transitory? Can low levels of maternal alcohol consumption during pregnancy also be detrimental to the developing foetus? Are some different patterns or styles of drinking (e.g. chronic or binge drinking) more dangerous for the foetus than others? At what periods during gestation is the foetus particularly vulnerable to the effects of alcohol?

Human Studies

In the late 1950s and early 1960s, reports started to emerge from Europe, mainly France, on the possible consequences of maternal and paternal alcohol consumption on the foetus (Lecomte 1950, Christiaens et al. 1960). In 1968, Lemoine et al. published a report of 127 cases of alcohol-related birth damage. These findings were followed in the early 1970s by work from the United States (Ulleland 1972) and, by 1973, Jones and Smith's group identified a cluster of anomalies occurring in the children of alcohol-dependent mothers. As noted by the latter authors: "A pattern of altered growth and morphogenesis has lately been described in eight offspring of chronic alcoholic mothers. We call this disorder the 'foetal alcohol syndrome' " (Jones et al. 1973).

The pattern of anomalies in FAS consists of defects in the following categories (Rosett 1980):

(1) pre- and/or postnatal growth deficiency, including intrauterine growth retardation, small-for-dates, failure to thrive, and continuing growth below the l0th percentile for gestational age;

(2) morphological anomalies, including a distinctive facial appearance;

(3) central nervous system dysfunction, including cognitive disabilities, the most serious of which are severe learning disorders.

There is a further consideration related to the mothers of these children. The mothers were noted to have an "identifiable" drinking problem. This latter category was important, first of all because it highlighted the often highly chaotic and atypical drinking patterns of these women. (Note also that the drinking problem was described as identifiable, not necessarily identified). It is one of the puzzles of FAS that this fourth category was often ignored in the climate of the work of the 1970s and early 1980s.

Over the years several screening tests have been designed specifically related to the second category. A recent addition in relation to the facial phenotype has been designed and successfully tested by Astley and Clarren (1996).

In addition to the pattern of anomalies defining FAS, a number of individual features have also been associated with drinking during pregnancy. These include intrauterine and postnatal growth retardation, limb anomalies, cardiac anomalies (ventricular and atrial septal defects), urogenital anomalies (labial hypoplasia, hydronephrosis) and ophthalmological problems (external eye lesions, myopia, optic nerve hypoplasia, strabismus) (Chan et al. 1991). Further reported anomalies include otological problems (hearing deficits, serious infections), neurophysiological anomalies and neuroanatomical anomalies (Plant et al. 1993).

Finally, a number of behavioural problems have been associated with FAS such as fine and gross motor dysfunction, attention deficit disorder/hyperactivity, autism, sleep disorders and poor sucking reflex.

It is important to note the wide range of anomalies, many of which can also be found in children of mothers who have no history of drinking problems. A major issue is the problem of attributing a causal relationship to alcohol at lower consumption levels where the influence of confounders is high. Consensus as to FAS, in contrast to individual alcohol-related birth defects, is based on the fact that FAS has specific criteria and is present only in women who have a clearly identifiable drinking problem (Sokol and Abel 1992).

Concern still persists about the consistency of information pregnant women are receiving. Some countries state that even small amounts of alcohol can cause irreparable damage to the foetus. Other countries take a less extreme view. FAS and "alcohol-related birth defects" (ARBDs) are not confined to any one country. However, a recent comparison of incidence data from around the world, based on prospective studies, indicates that the USA has the highest incidence of FAS (2 cases per 1000) relative to Europe and other industrialized countries (0.4 per 1000) (Abel 1995). This shows up another of the confusions in this confusing picture: the USA has the highest incidence of this disorder, yet has a national per capita alcohol consumption level that is not particularly high. Abel has named this the "American Paradox" (Abel 1998a). However, the debate still continues with a recent US report by Sampson et al. (1997) re-analysing European data suggesting that the incidence of FAS in some European countries is similar to that in the USA.

Diagnostic Paradigms

Until 1996 two main paradigms were used to make a diagnosis of FAS. One was that proposed by the Foetal Alcohol Study Group of the Research Society on Alcoholism and basically comprises the criteria described earlier in this chapter. This group also defined the terms "foetal alcohol effects" (FAE) and "alcohol-related birth defects" (ARBD) which were coined to define those individuals with only some features of FAS. Majewski (1981) formed the other paradigm in the 1980s. This was a numerical measure, which listed specific individual components of the syndrome and assigned a numerical score to them, which was then tallied to give a diagnosis. The severity of the diagnosis related to the total point score.

In 1996, the US Institute of Medicine developed a diagnostic paradigm that departed markedly from its two predecessors by including maternal alcohol exposure as part of the diagnosis. This measure also included several anomalies not previously specified, such as hearing loss. Another innovation was the division of FAS into three categories, namely:

1) FAS with confirmed maternal alcohol exposure
2) FAS without confirmed maternal alcohol exposure
3) Partial FAS with confirmed maternal alcohol exposure.

Category 2 is similar to the earlier FAS Study Group definition, as is category 1, except for the inclusion of a confirmed maternal drinking history.

One problem in this categorization is the inclusion of issues such as patient care and research into the formulation of the category 2 grouping. The stated rationale was a wish to make it easier for patients to receive the benefits of a clinical diagnosis of FAS despite a lack of information about their mothers. Identification of "problem drinking" is certainly not a skill in which many midwives and obstetricians in Europe would feel adequately trained. The US Institute of Medicine also clearly indicated issues of services and reimbursement had influenced its formulation of category 3, which it described as "partial FAS with confirmed maternal alcohol exposure". Since uncertainty might make it more difficult to obtain insurance coverage for "appropriate services and reimbursement for these services" (Institute of Medicine 1996: 75), the Institute of Medicine felt the end justified the means. However, while this was well intentioned, it introduced social and political issues into what had previously been an objective standard for medical diagnosis.

A fourth category included alcohol-related birth defects (ARBD) and an innovative feature introduced by the Institute of Medicine was the creation of a distinct category called "alcohol-related neuro-developmental disorders" (ARND) which includes "neurological hard or soft signs" (Institute of Medicine 1996: 76–77) as well as behavioural problems. Apart from category 1, the other categories can include a number of groupings found in more than one of the above diagnostic criteria.

Level and Pattern of Maternal Drinking

An important question not yet completely clarified is whether social drinking during pregnancy can also be detrimental to the developing brain. The reactivity and capability of developing compensatory mechanisms seem to differ in the developing brain and in the adult brain and the toxic effects of alcohol generally appears more direct and less reversible for the developing brain than for the developed brain. The fact that the brain passes through some developmental stages at which it is particularly vulnerable to teratogenic agents (Coles, 1994), including alcohol, means that the threshold dose of alcohol capable of producing detrimental effects is likely to vary with the age of development. Therefore, proper attention must be given to factors such as the timing and pattern of alcohol drinking, which are potentially very important in determining the magnitude and nature of the developmental damage. A recently published study from Mexico noted a strong relationship between low birth weight and the pattern of drinking in that country. This pattern was an extreme one of "infrequent binge drinking with episodic drunkenness of high amounts of alcohol consumption" (Borges et al. 1993:363).

A prospective study carried out in Detroit, USA, found that prenatal alcohol exposure is associated with deficient cognitive processing speed, longer visual fixation on infant recognition memory and a slower reaction time at 12 months of age (Jacobson et al., 1992, 1994a). The lowest level of alcohol at which these deficits have been detected is "an average" of 14 g per day during gestation. However, Jacobson and colleagues make the point that none of the mothers drank this "average" amount of alcohol. Commonly the pattern was of the drinking being concentrated in two days in the week. These findings suggest that, in their study, this pattern of drinking produces a specific effect on speed of information processing rather than a general delay, and are consistent with Streissguth's suggestion of an alcohol-related deficit in "speed of central processing" in older children (Streissguth et al. 1995). In other prospective studies on children exposed prenatally to varying amounts of alcohol, the results are not as clear. In the cohort from Ottawa, decreased language comprehension was found in two- and three-year-old children exposed to relatively low maternal alcohol intake (mean 4.3 g alcohol per day) (Fried et al. 1988, 1990). However no deficits in language comprehension or in attention were found at 5 or 6 years of age (Fried et al. 1992a, b). A three-year follow-up study in a Cleveland (USA) cohort (Greene et al. 1990) found no significant relationship between alcohol exposure at the level of 28 g alcohol per day during gestation and language indices.

Studies carried out by the Seattle team indicate that drinking >19 g alcohol a day prior to pregnancy recognition and binge drinking (defined as 70 g alcohol on one occasion per week) during pregnancy have the greatest impact on developmental outcomes (Streissguth et al., 1990, 1994b). These findings are consistent with the Detroit study, in which functionally significant deficits were seen primarily in infants born to mothers who averaged at least 70 g alcohol (6 US standard drinks) per occasion on an average of one occasion per week during pregnancy. A recent study has also shown an association between binge drinking (42 g alcohol per occasion) or continuous drinking (ca. 98 g per week) during pregnancy and perinatal brain injury in premature infants (Holzman et al. 1995). These reports indicate that a single binge, at a critical period during gestation, could have a significant impact on behavioural outcome.

The methodology of studies in this area is constantly being questioned (Ernhart et al. 1988, Day et al. 1989, Verkerk 1992). One possible reason why so little thought has been given to including "alcohol abuse" or "problem drinking" in the ARBD nomenclature is that several epidemiological studies have been interpreted as suggesting that individual anomalies can occur in conjunction with relatively low levels of maternal drinking in pregnancy. This point of view would suggest that the low drinking levels might be seen to be a statistical artefact. Instead of focusing on the actual drinking occasion, some researchers have calculated "average" drinking levels for a week, a month etc. This means that the level of alcohol consumption, which occurs over a relatively discreet period, such as a Saturday night, is treated statistically as if it were the cumulative result of drinking every day of the week. In other words, consumption of seven drinks on one evening is analysed as an "average" of one drink a day. Although the "average" is clearly stated in the methods, it is often ignored in the discussion of an article or when it is discussed in reviews (Abel 1998b).

A number of researchers have noted that drinking pattern may have an important influence on the possible consequences of alcohol use (Plant et al. 1997, Grant et al. 1997).

Clearly related to this is the issue of the accuracy of recall in pregnant problem drinkers (Jacobson et al. 1991, Russell et al. 1991, da Costa Pereira et al. 1993).

In summary, although some consistent results emerge from these studies, research will still need to monitor the impact, if any, of low-level maternal drinking on children's behavioural and cognitive development. The possible long-term consequences of moderate prenatal alcohol exposure demonstrated in several studies continues to justify attention and rigorous examination of individuals exposed to alcohol *in utero*.

Threshold Doses

In human neurobehavioural studies, the threshold for observing effects is usually defined in terms of the level of exposure to a toxin below which average group performance is not adversely affected. However, there are marked individual differences in vulnerability to any given exposure. Because the threshold values derived from human studies are based on group averages, it is not appropriate to infer that exposure just below a threshold level is necessarily "safe", because some individuals could be markedly more sensitive than others. Taking this under consideration and on the basis of the results obtained in the Seattle study, Streissguth et al. (1993) suggest that there is no statistical evidence of any "risk-free" level of drinking or any "threshold" level of prenatal alcohol exposure in the context of dose-response analysis. However, Jacobson et al. (1994b), using the results obtained by the Detroit cohort, estimated a lower threshold of ca. 14 g alcohol per day for producing intellectual deficits in offspring.

These authors emphasize that this threshold represents a sample average and should not be taken to imply that drinking below that level is "safe" (Jacobson et al. 1994a). They suggest that even if no functional deficits are associated with a given level of exposure in infancy and childhood, there is the potential for unobservable neurostructural damage, which could lead to functional deficits at older age (Streissguth et al. 1994a, b).

Critical Periods of Exposure

Although the complex nature of human behavioural development makes it difficult to find a relationship between particular behavioural outcomes and alcohol exposure during different stages of pregnancy, some conclusions can be drawn. Early heavy exposure leads to the most severe consequences and is associated with morphological anomalies, severe learning difficulties and sensory deficits. For example, Ernhart et al. (1987) report a dose-response relationship between craniofacial anomalies in children and maternal alcohol intake (28–85 g alcohol per day) around the time of conception. The anomalies were also related to later intellectual development, and the greater dysmorphia was associated with lower IQ. However, more subtle behavioural effects, such as learning disabilities and attention deficits, can result from lower levels of alcohol exposure. For example, Streissguth et al. (1989, 1990, 1994a, b) found moderate drinking (17 g alcohol per day) either before pregnancy recognition (which included the first month of gestation) or at mid-pregnancy to be associated with relatively mild late deficits on neuropsychological tasks. Larsson et al. (1985) found that pre-school children who had been exposed to alcohol throughout gestation (28–85 g alcohol per day) were more likely to show hyperactivity, language problems and motor deficits than the offspring of mothers who stopped drinking by the second trimester. This implies that these effects result from later exposure. Similar results were obtained by Coles et al. (1997) in a follow-up on school-age children who had been exposed to alcohol (44 g alcohol per day) during part or all of pregnancy. These results suggest that each abnormal outcome in brain function has its own dose-response relation and gestational timing and that stopping drinking is likely to have a beneficial outcome on behavioural functions.

Parental Characteristics

As noted in the previous review (Plant et al. 1993), features of FAS may result from a variety of adverse influences. These influences can be summarized in relation to (1) parental characteristics and (2) developmental stages of the foetus, the infant, the child, the adolescent and the adult.

MATERNAL FACTORS

The previous review on this topic listed some maternal factors associated to a greater or lesser degree with FAS (Plant et al. 1993). Amongst the most powerful is socio-economic status. In nearly every case where FAS has been found, the mother has been of low socioeconomic status (Sokol et al. 1986, Abel and Sokol 1987). In many societies this variable is closely linked with ethnicity, which of itself can be a risk factor for alcohol-related adverse pregnancy outcome (Abel and Sokol 1987). In the USA, for example, the incidence of FAS among poor women is about 2.29 cases per 1000 compared to 0.2 cases among middle-class women (Abel 1995).

Other maternal factors include poor nutritional status. Heavy drinking leads to an imbalance and/or deficiency in micronutrients and vitamins, which are essential for maintenance of a healthy pregnancy. Access and use of prenatal care has also been highlighted. In most prospective studies the proportion of women giving birth to babies with FAS who obtain prenatal care is relatively low. One of the causes of this may be the lifestyle of many problem drinkers, which makes them less likely to attend regular prenatal checks (Abel et al. 1991). Therefore, many of the "at-risk" women are not included in these studies. Obstetric history is also a factor: if a female problem drinker has given birth to one child with FAS, there is a greatly increased risk of subsequent children also being affected if the problem drinking continues (Abel 1988). Other risk factors identified in relation to obstetric status are a history of spontaneous abortion and previous obstetric problems (Cavallo et al. 1995). Maternal age may be a risk factor simply because the older the woman, the greater the likelihood of a longer drinking history. The studies of Jacobson et al. (1993) indicate that maternal age affects the risk and severity of the neurobehavioural deficits associated with moderate-to-heavy prenatal alcohol exposure. It was shown that exposure to an average of ca. 14 g absolute alcohol per day doubled the risk of functional deficits observed with the Bayley Mental Development Index (BMDI). In this study, the risk increased by a factor of five if the mother was above the age of 30 years.

Further studies on the relevance of age have produced conflicting results in relation to the use of alcohol and other drugs. Waterson et al.

(1990) showed "risk" drinking to be more common in couples who were older and of higher socioeconomic status (SES). This study also noted that the expectant mothers were more likely to reduce their alcohol use and smoking if their partners also reduced their use of these substances. Abma and Mott (1991), in a US cohort study of young mothers, showed younger, less educated women to be more likely than older, well-educated women to smoke cigarettes or marijuana during pregnancy. However, Cornelius et al. (1994), again in the USA, found white adolescent pregnant women drinking in a way which put their unborn children at greater risk due to "intermittent high-peak alcohol exposure". This study also showed an increase in smoking later in pregnancy, a finding again not shown in the older age group.

There is a strong association between heavy drinking, heavy smoking and heavy caffeine use (Meyer et al. 1994). All of these factors affect birth weight. The effects of the use of drugs other than alcohol or their use in combination with alcohol have always been a complicated aspect of the drinking in pregnancy debate. For example, the use of illegal substances such as cocaine (Streissguth et al. 1991a, O'Connor et al. 1993) and legal substances such as tobacco (Cassano et al. 1990, Davis 1992, Floyd et al. 1993) are highly correlated.

Furthermore, research into the effects of a wide range of substances on both the foetus and the child have continued to be published. Studies on illegal substances include opiates (Lindenberg et al. 1993), methadone (DePetrillo et al. 1995), cocaine (Strickland et al. 1993), cocaine and heroin (Glantz et al. 1993) and marijuana (Day et al. 1991, 1994, Chandler et al. 1996). Clearly, there is cross-over between the use of legal and illegal substances, such as tobacco and marijuana (Fried 1993, 1995). Various authors have noted that, in several cultures, people who are heavy drinkers may also use other forms of psychoactive drugs heavily and may also engage in a variety of "risky" behaviours (Plant et al. 1992). Other studies have concentrated on more commonly used substances such as caffeine and tobacco (Meyer et al. 1994) and tobacco itself (Cliver et al. 1992, Floyd et al. 1993, Orlebeke et al. 1994, McGee et al. 1994). These studies have produced mixed results with some showing a clear relationship between foetal harm and maternal drinking and others showing no such link.

In certain areas, particularly in the UK and the USA, use of illicit drugs such as marijuana, cocaine and heroin is also high, especially amongst teenagers and young adults (Hibell et al. 1997). The concomitant use of alcohol with tobacco and illicit or prescribed drugs raises the possibility of additive or synergistic effects on the embryo/foetus.

Metabolic factors have also been noted. There has been much controversy about the role of acetaldehyde in the aetiology of FAS. Even so, the precise role of acetaldehyde in FAS is still uncertain (Schenker et al. 1990). Indeed, animal studies from the 1970s raised the issue of alcohol withdrawal being of importance (Himwich et al. 1977) but this has not been followed up.

Finally, the general health of alcohol-dependent women or other problem drinkers is often poor. Immune deficiency is commonplace among alcohol-dependent people (Plant 1992, 1997). Liver damage is commonly associated with heavy drinking and it is now clear that alcohol exacerbates the progress of viral infections such as hepatitis B and hepatitis C, leading to the possibility of hepatocellular carcinoma (Nalpas et al. 1998). Clearly, if any of these factors are present there will be an increased risk of poor pregnancy outcome.

PATERNAL FACTORS

Available evidence on paternal drinking in cases of FAS suggests that heavy alcohol consumption is common (Abel 1991). In relation to the outcome of pregnancy, factors include small, but significant decreases in birth weight (Sokol et al. 1993, Little et al. 1987, Windham et al. 1995), cardiac anomalies, particularly ventricular septal defect (Savitz et al. 1991) and immune system problems (Gottesfeld et al. 1991). Perhaps more powerful aspects of paternal alcohol use relate to social factors. The risks and concerns of having a male partner who drinks in a problematic way, the inconsistent behaviour which is often a hallmark of problem drinking (Plant 1997) and the increase in stress and fear both for herself and her unborn child should not be underestimated. Women with drinking problems not uncommonly move from one traumatic relationship to another, feeling more and more helpless and powerless as each relationship collapses (Lammers et al. 1995, Plant 1997). Any pregnancy at these times is vulnerable to harm.

Foetal Development

As noted earlier, in addition to the cluster of anomalies characterizing the syndrome, a large array of individual anomalies from within FAS's core symptoms, referred to interchangeably as foetal alcohol effects (FAEs) or alcohol-related birth defects (ARBDs), have been associated with prenatal alcohol exposure. However, in human studies no single anomaly is specific to or is reliably associated with drinking during pregnancy. As a result of the difficulties in unambiguously attributing individual effects to alcohol use, there has been a tendency, particularly in the USA, to over-diagnose anomalies with uncertain aetiologies as FAEs. Some dysmorphologists have recently urged that these terms be dropped from the diagnostic lexicon (Aase et al. 1995). This recommendation only applies to clinical situations, to clinical diagnosis only, rather than to the concept itself.

Indeed, in 1994, two of the original workers in this field, Lemoine from France and Jones from the USA, both suggested discontinuing the use of the term FAE (Kaskutas 1995). Jones noted:

"[I] recommended that physicians document alcohol exposure *in utero*, low birth weight, and behavioural difficulties, when they occur, but to avoid the FAE diagnosis which carries an implication of causation.

… Citing inappropriate use over the years, they argue that such overdiagnosis impedes the search for other causes of children's problems, frustrates any accurate assessment of the true magnitude of the problem caused by maternal consumption, stigmatises mothers whose drinking may in fact not have damaged their children, and affects misdiagnosed children by lowering others' expectations of them" (Kaskutas 1995:1540).

Another reason why a number of dysmorphologists have recommended abandonment of the term FAE is a confusion as to whether these individual effects are the result of a lesser exposure to alcohol and are therefore not as serious as if they occurred in the context of the syndrome. It has been suggested that the damage is the same whether it occurs in isolation or as part of the full-blown syndrome, because the levels of consumption are the same. It may be that the difference is in the pattern of consumption, with prolonged heavy drinking at one end of the spectrum and periodic heavy drinking at the other. Changes in nomenclature both for the syndrome and individual effects have also been proposed to reflect their aetiologies more accurately (Abel 1998b). For instance, many clinicians and researchers acknowledge that the syndrome only occurs in the context of maternal alcohol abuse as stated by Jones et al. (1973) in their original work. It has been suggested that the syndrome would be more accurately named foetal alcohol abuse syndrome (FAAS) (Abel 1998b). This would give a more accurate picture of the abuse of alcohol than alcohol per se. Changes in the nomenclature for both the syndrome and these individual effects have also been proposed to reflect their aetiologies more accurately (Abel 1998b).

However, yet again, the debate continues with some workers such as Mattson et al. (1997) noting that central nervous system (CNS) abnormalities are the most dramatic and permanent consequences of "*in utero*" alcohol exposure and can occur in the absence of other gross morphological defects associated with FAS. Recent follow-up studies from different countries revealed that although many of the physical characteristics of FAS become less prominent with maturity, cognitive behavioural deficits appear to endure with age (Aronson 1997, Spohr et al. 1994, Steinhausen 1996, Lemoine et al. 1992, Streissguth et al. 1994a, b). Recently, new technology such as positron emission tomography (PET) and magnetic resonance imaging (MRI) has made it possible to examine the brains of living children with FAS and FAE and to examine the relation between the pattern of malformation seen in the brain and behavioural profiles. The studies revealed brain damage in these adolescents in areas involving balance, co-ordination and some aspects of cognition (Mattson et al. 1996, Sowell et al. 1996). Other anomalies have also been shown such as midline brain anomalies (Riley et al. 1995, Swayze et al. 1997) and areas involved in transferring messages from one part of the brain to another (Mattson et al. 1996). Some of these alterations in the structure of the brain in children with FAS were related to mental impairment and behavioural problems (Knight et al. 1993). In addition, a high proportion of children with FAS present hearing, language, visual and dentofacial disorders (Church et al. 1998). Most of these findings have been replicated in animal studies (Church et al. 1984, Driscoll et al. 1990, Pinazo-Durán 1997).

Growth Deficits and Physical Anomalies

A number of prospective longitudinal studies conducted in the USA and Canada (NIAAA 1993) have examined the relationship between the full range of drinking patterns during pregnancy and childhood development. These studies confirm that chronic alcohol intake or heavy drinking (defined as an average of more than 30–40 g alcohol per day) during pregnancy induced growth deficits and dysmorphology in some of the most severely affected children. These outcomes have not been clearly observed when the level of alcohol consumption during pregnancy is lower (<40 g alcohol per day). Even so, some recent epidemiological data show a discrete decrease in birth weight (150 g) with a daily consumption of 14 g alcohol or more during gestation (Windham et al. 1995, Shu et al. 1995, Passaro et al. 1996).

In consonance with these findings, it has been found that, when alcohol use is discontinued by the beginning of the second trimester, the children of drinkers may approach the growth rate of children of non-drinkers. In addition, third-trimester exposure has been associated with growth retardation and neurobehavioural disturbances (Coles 1994). These findings indicate either that the growth deficit associated with alcohol occurs in the third trimester, when the foetus is growing rapidly, or that being alcohol-free during this time allows the previously exposed foetus to catch up in growth.

With respect to physical abnormalities, animal and epidemiological studies strongly suggest that the facial malformations characteristic of FAS result from exposure to high levels of ethanol during the first trimester, more specifically, during the first two months of gestation (Ernhart et al. 1987, Graham et al. 1988, Day et al. 1989). Indeed, Ernhard et al. (1987) report a dose-response relation between craniofacial anomalies in children and maternal alcohol intake (28–85 g per day) around the time of conception, and found that greater dysmorphia was associated with lower intellectual development (lower IQ).

Child Development

During the past twenty years a number of prospective studies have allowed researchers to measure maternal drinking during pregnancy as well as other factors that may influence both prenatal and postnatal development in the offspring (NIAAA 1993). Among them, the Detroit longitudinal study examined 382 children of moderate-to-heavy drinkers during pregnancy. In this study, Jacobson et al. (1993) reported a dose-dependent relation between the Bayley Mental Developmental Index (BMDI) of 13-month-old children and maternal drinking during pregnancy (7–56 g/day). This relationship was less significant when the mother only drank around the period of conception. In contrast, these results found that the effects of alcohol exposure on the Psychomotor Development Index (PDI) were not dose-related, and the PDI scores were reduced only at the highest levels of exposure (56 g alcohol per day) (Jacobson et al. 1993). Schandler et al. (1995) showed spatial learning deficit in pre-school children of problem drinkers. They also noted these were more supportive of a cognitive model than one of personal development.

The large multi-centre European study carried out in the early 1990s showed an adverse effect on growth in babies born to women drinking the equivalent of 120 g per week. Yet no lasting impairment, either mental or physical, was noted when the children were examined at 18 months (Florey et al. 1992). Except for facial anomalies, a similar result was reported for children up to 4 years and 10 months of age (Greene et al. 1991). Chandler et al. (1996) found children (aged 3 years) of mothers who were described as "light to moderate users" of alcohol and marijuana not to show negative effects on gross motor performance.

Similarly, Russel et al. (1991) noted a decrease in verbal IQ of 7.1 points in children (aged 6 years) born to mothers having more than one indicator of problem drinking. The follow-up of the Seattle study of 500 children whose mothers consumed different amounts of alcohol showed daily exposure to 26 g alcohol during mid pregnancy to be associated with a 6.7 point decrement in full-scale IQ at the age of 7 (Streissguth et al. 1990). However, other studies of prenatal exposure to lower levels of alcohol (<26 g/day) did not detect variations in intellectual performance at 4 years (Greene et al. 1991) or 6 years of age (Fried et al. 1992a, b).

The most serious problems of all are severe learning difficulties (IQ below 70), which occur in about 50% of the children with FAS (Abel 1982). The remaining 50% of children have IQs ranging from 70 to normal. A study in which maternal IQ rather than educational level or occupation was taken into account showed that alcohol consumption no longer significantly affected IQ in alcohol-exposed children who do not have FAS (Greene et al. 1991). The contribution of parental IQ has not received adequate attention in many studies. A failure to consider attention deficits and hyperactivity in the parents may likewise lead to false attribution of effects in the children to maternal alcohol intake.

Attention deficits, learning problems and language processing disorders were also found to be associated with moderate alcohol consumption during pregnancy in the Seattle study. Among the most salient sequelae are: reduced speed of information processing at the age of 4, poor academic performance as measured by the second-grade teacher ratings and low scores on arithmetic at the age of 7 (Streissguth et al. 1990).

However, a study by Coles et al. (1997) questioned the view that the most commonly mentioned behavioural effects associated with

FAS/ARBD are attention deficit disorder (ADD) and hyperactivity disorder (HD). It has been widely assumed that these conditions are invariably associated. Although ADD and HD are considered synonymous, they are clinically distinct disorders (American Psychiatric Association 1994). Coles et al. compared four groups of children to determine if indeed ADD/HD were related to FAS/ARBD. One group was prenatally exposed to alcohol and exhibited physical signs of such exposure. Another group was exposed to alcohol but did not bear any physical signs of exposure, a third group was clinically diagnosed as ADD/HD and a fourth was a control group whose mothers did not drink during pregnancy and did not have any signs of ADD/HD. Whereas 85% of the children previously identified as ADD/HD were reclassified as such, only 44% of the dysmorphic children with FAS/ARBD received this diagnosis. Children with ADD/HD and FAS/ARBD also differed on several other cognitive and attention measures, leading to the conclusion that whereas HD may in fact be related to FAS/ARBD, ADD was not. This conclusion has important implications for treatment particularly in relation to pharmacological treatment.

Longer-term follow-up examination of infants diagnosed at birth as FAS or FAE showed that growth retardation in these infants tends to persist throughout the neonatal period (Spohr et al. 1996, Aronson 1997, Lemoine et al. 1992). Some of these individuals experience a catch-up growth during adolescence (14 years) (Sampson et al. 1994).

Regarding the dysmorphic features of FAS, it seems that they also become less prominent in adolescents, although certain features, such as long philtrum and microcephaly as well as distinct mental and cognitive impairments, tend to persist (Streissguth et al. 1991b, Spohr et al. 1994). These studies suggest that alcohol-induced growth deficiency and dysmorphology are not useful indicators of the adverse effects of prenatal ethanol exposure in adolescents, whereas cognitive and behavioural deficits seem to persist into adulthood (Sampson et al. 1994, Aronson 1997, Spohr et al. 1994, Steinhausen, 1996). At 14 years of age there is a continued dose relationship between maternal drinking during pregnancy and alcohol-related attention/memory and spatial/learning deficits in offspring (Streissguth et al. 1994b, 1995) and low scores on arithmetic (Streissguth et al. 1994a).

Health Education and Intervention/Prevention Programmes

As in many areas, the results in these programmes are mixed (Waterson et al. 1990, Schorling 1993, Greenfield 1997, Plant 1997) with many interventions not adequately evaluated. However, recent attempts such as May's "multiple-level, comprehensive approach" to prevention (1995) suggest a broader view is now being taken. Large-scale programmes such as the introduction of warning labels on alcoholic beverages in the USA have not shown promising results in relation to drinking in pregnancy. There appears to have been little effect on antenatal drinking in general and, sadly, no impact on the heaviest drinkers (Hankin et al. 1996a, b, Kaskutas 1995). Although countries differ in their assessment or recommendations for drinking during pregnancy it is heartening to note some consistency in the recommendation of never drinking to the point of intoxication.

The Role of Animal Models

In animal research, it is possible to eliminate many confounding factors that are commonly associated with chronic alcohol use (e.g. malnutrition, disease, socioeconomic status, smoking, other drug use). This work has not only confirmed that alcohol is a teratogen (Guerri, 1995), but has also shown that the foetal brain is the organ most vulnerable to the effects of alcohol, and that the severity of the damage is dose- and time-dependent (West et al. 1994). A variety of neurobehavioural effects observed in children with FAS and FAE have also been detected in animals upon prenatal alcohol exposure (Driscoll et al. 1990). Optic nerve hypoplasia observed in animals exposed to alcohol has been associated with impaired vision in children with FAS and FAE (Pinazo-Durán et al. 1997). Moreover, this research has provided insight into the structure-function relationship underlying the abnormal behavioural development that results from prenatal alcohol exposure. For example, learning and memory deficits have been demonstrated in animals and are related to alcohol-induced damage in the hippocampus, a part of the brain that plays an important role in mediating these mental activities. Motor co-ordination problems have also been linked to structural defects in the cerebellum (Guerri 1998). Such structure-function associations observed in animal models have recently been observed with brain imaging techniques (e.g. MRI), as indicated above. However, care should be taken in extrapolating the results of animal studies to humans because there are species differences in alcohol metabolism, the timing of brain development and the complexity of the CNS.

Critical Periods for Prenatal Alcohol Exposure

There are problems involved in using animals as models for studying the effects of alcohol on man however; for example, aspects such as social behaviour and higher cognitive functions cannot be examined in experimental animals. Research on the timing of alcohol exposure in animals has yielded valuable information on physical anomalies in man. Experimental data have demonstrated that ethanol interferes with all brain developmental stages, and that the extent and type of neurotoxic effects are dose-dependent (higher alcohol levels produce greater damage) (Bonthius et al. 1990) and time-dependent (some periods in brain development are particularly susceptible to the toxic effects of alcohol). For example, as mentioned above, it is clear that exposure to high levels of alcohol during the gastrulation phase of embryogenesis (gestation days 7–8 in rodents and to the third week of gestation in women) produces significant dysmorphia and neurological damage (Ernhart et al. 1987).

Levels of Alcohol Intake

Although blood alcohol concentrations (BACs) are generally not available in human studies, animal studies have found that it is precisely the BAC, rather than the absolute dose of alcohol, that provides a meaningful estimate of alcohol bioavailability, given the differences in alcohol metabolism among species. For example, the ethanol intake of a rat on a 5% ethanol liquid diet is ca. 12 g per kg per day (e.g. Sanchis et al. 1986). This is considerably more than the dose a woman can be reasonably expected to consume on a body weight basis. However, the BAC with the 5% alcohol liquid diet is about 10 mg/dl (e.g. Sanchis et al. 1986), which is similar to the levels found in pregnant chronic drinkers (Halmesmäki 1988) or when a 60 kg woman has 3–5 drinks within an hour. Even the BAC of 20 mg/dl that can be obtained in animals by the intubation method is in line with the BACs found in women who give birth to infants with FAS (Abel 1984). The alcohol levels to which the foetal brain is exposed are similar to the BACs achieved by the pregnant rat (Guerri et al. 1985).

Brain Developmental Stages

Although all mammals pass through the same stages of brain development, the timing of these stages relative to birth varies considerably from one species to another. For example, in the human embryo the major brain regions are recognisable at five weeks of gestation. Brain cells undergo two periods of rapid growth: from week 15 to week 20 of gestation and again from week 25 of gestation to a year after birth. However, in the rat, the full gestation is equivalent to the first two trimesters in women, and the first 10 days of postnatal life are considered equivalent to the third trimester of human gestation (Dobbing et al. 1979).

In summary, from the experimental data it is clear that alcohol interferes in all the stages of brain development and that the amount, duration and timing are important factors influencing the type and severity of the damage. At the same time, although in some of the studies mentioned above the foetus was exposed to relatively high BACs to demonstrate the time-dependent effects of alcohol, binge drinking at any of the different stages of pregnancy may occur. This could induce deficits in CNS functions, as reported in several clinical studies.

Alcohol-Induced Specific Damage in Different Brain Regions

There is also experimental evidence that the effects of alcohol on the developing brain are not uniform. Some regions are more affected than others, and even within a given region some cell populations are more vulnerable to the effects of alcohol than others. Collectively, clinical and experimental data support the idea that the regions in which the toxic effects of alcohol are felt most strongly are the neocortex, hippocampus and cerebellum (Guerri 1998).

Experimental data also support the conclusion that binge drinking and perhaps moderate drinking during the period of "brain growth spurt" (corresponding to the third trimester in human gestation) can induce structural and functional deficits in the hippocampus and cerebellum which may explain the long-lasting cognitive and motor deficits observed in the children and animals exposed to relatively low alcohol doses.

Neurochemical Effects

It has been established that the developing nervous system is influenced by a number of neurotransmitters as well as by intracellular factors (cyclic AMP, Ca^{2+}), the levels of which are modulated by transmembrane signalling. The results of a number of studies lead to the conclusion that "*in utero*" or postnatal exposure to alcohol markedly impaired several neurotransmitter systems. However, exposure to low BACs (<10 mg/dl) produces little effect on whole-brain neurotransmitter levels (e.g. dopamine, serotonin, norepinephrine), while exposure to BACs of 11–13 mg/dl results in a significant CNS deficiency of norepinephrine, dopamine and serotonin in different brain areas (Druse 1992).

Finally, an abnormal neurotransmitter system may be consistent with the alcohol-induced cell depletion in some brain regions, leading to fewer neurons that can send projections to target areas. Since these effects have been identified in animals that exhibit no external physical abnormalities, they may represent the neurobiological basis of some of the behavioural deficits induced by *in utero* alcohol exposure.

Neuroendocrine Influence

Hormones also influence the development of the nervous system. The receptors for steroid and thyroid hormones and retinoic acid are members of a family of nuclear receptors that regulate DNA transcription and cell growth and differentiation (Tsai et al. 1994). Prenatal alcohol exposure in the rat (all of gestation or end of gestation and first week of postnatal life) has been shown to induce several hormonal alterations including changes in thyroxine concentrations (e.g. Portoles et al. 1988). Defects in both pituitary and central regulation of the hypothalamic-pituitary-gonadal axis (Weinberg 1994) have also been shown. As a result of the latter alteration, sexual maturation is delayed, sexual behaviour is disrupted, hormone levels are abnormal and reproductive function is altered in both males and females (e.g. McGivern et al. 1984, Esquifino et al. 1986). Animal studies have also shown that *in utero* alcohol exposure can have major effects on development and function of the hypothalamic-pituitary-adrenal (HPA) axis. Alcohol increases plasma and brain levels of corticosterone at birth (Weinberg 1994). In addition, adrenocortical hyper-responsiveness to stressors has also been observed after early postnatal ethanol exposure. Since glucocorticoids are known to have modulatory effects on behavioural responses to stressful situations, it is possible that this elevation results in the increased response to stress and suppression of immune responsiveness that have also been seen in animals (Abel 1998b). Finally, most of these findings in animals have been observed in the offspring of mothers fed with alcohol-containing liquid diets, which produced BACs of 10–15 mg/dl.

Mechanisms of Foetal Alcohol Damage

Given the multitude of different types of defects, the involvement of all the major organ systems, and the involvement of many dysfunctional neurochemical and biochemical processes, the search for the underlying mechanism(s) is a difficult task. Research on the pathogenesis of foetal alcohol damage has traditionally focused on the toxicity of acetaldehyde, placenta dysfunction and impaired foetal nutrition, foetal hypoxia and abnormal prostaglandin metabolism (Schenker et al. 1990). More recently, other potential molecular mechanisms have also been proposed such as free radical damage (e.g. Kotch et al. 1992, 1995, Guerri et al. 1994), disruption of retinoic acid metabolism (Deltour et al. 1996), suppression of *msx2* gene expression (Rifas et al. 1997) and alteration of foetal DNA methylation of specific genes (Garro et al. 1991, Vallés et al. 1997). Since any of these proposed mechanisms can explain the overall alterations observed in FAS, it is quite possible that several different mechanisms are responsible for the various deleterious effects of prenatal alcohol exposure.

Conclusions and Discussion

Available evidence supports the conclusion that alcohol-dependent women who drink heavily during pregnancy may produce offspring exhibiting features of FAS. Such women also have an increased risk of experiencing spontaneous abortion. FAS, as noted above, is based on a pattern of defects rather than on one or two features unique to the offspring of alcohol-dependent women. The aetiology of FAS is complex and, in addition to alcohol, is related to maternal life-style and health. Whereas chronic heavy drinking is a necessary component in the aetiology of alcohol-related birth defects, other factors are also present. Even though most alcohol-dependent women do not give birth to FAS babies, this does not mean that heavy drinking does not pose a danger to the embryo/foetus. Heavy drinking is invariably associated with a variety of causal factors related to poor pregnancy outcome, including low socioeconomic status, poor diet and general health, heavy use of tobacco, illicit drug use and a previous poor obstetric history. The contribution of these factors to FAS needs to be clarified.

Adequate definitions of alcohol use are a prerequisite to any future epidemiological studies if the results are to be meaningful to the public. For instance, one drink in the UK contains 8 g alcohol, while in the USA it contains 12 g. Epidemiological studies on the effects of maternal alcohol use at lower levels need to cover a broad range of confounding variables; concentrating solely on alcohol to the exclusion of other factors will not clarify the issue. A wider spectrum of postnatal development must also be considered. One area that has yet to be examined is the risk of psychopathological behaviour resulting from prenatal alcohol exposure.

The research focus should also encompass paternal drinking as well as other risk factors that may affect pregnancy outcome.

Recent follow-up studies of adolescents and adults patients, in whom FAS was diagnosed at birth or during childhood, revealed that while physical features of FAS are less distinctive after puberty and the weight-to-height age ratio changes from low to high, cognitive and neurobehavioral problems continue and are the most debilitating outcomes. In addition, evidence emerging from some prospective longitudinal studies suggests the impact of a low or moderate level of maternal drinking on children's behavioural and cognitive development. Even so, not all the studies have replicated these findings. Underestimation of prenatal alcohol exposure has been considered a potential problem in these studies. However, the importance of such findings justifies continued attention and rigorous examination of individuals exposed *in utero* to alcohol and suggests that further longitudinal studies should be undertaken and follow-up should extend into school age to identify which effects are permanent and which are transient. The control of confounding factors in these studies (Plant et al. 1993) is essential for determining the real influence of low levels of alcohol exposure on children's neurobehavioural outcomes. Finally, efforts should be made to incorporate BACs and quantitative assessment of alcohol exposure in future longitudinal studies. As noted earlier, the drinking pattern and the accuracy of recording this is of great importance. Animal models have provided evidence that foetal alcohol effects are dose-dependent. These studies have clearly demonstrated that the peak maternal blood alcohol level and the pattern of drinking (e.g. binging) are the most important determinants of the magnitude of FAE or ARBD in the offspring. However, different aspects of development may be sensitive to different levels of alcohol, although a threshold for the different outcome remains to be determined. Future investigations should attempt to clarify specific aspects of alcohol-related behavioural dysfunction and relate them with alcohol-induced alterations in neurochemical, neurohormonal or cellular components during specific stages of the developing brain.

We must now accept that there have been times in the recent past when the "morality" of FAS has had a louder voice than the science. It appears that we are now entering a period where it is possible to question and even challenge extreme positions without being judged uncaring. This can only be to the good for a group of severely damaged babies and their mothers, both of whom need help and compassion.

References

Aase MM, Jones KL, Clarren SK (1995) Do we need the term "FAE"? Pediatrics 95: 428–30

Abel EL (1982) Consumption of alcohol during pregnancy: a review of effects on growth and development of offspring. Human Biol 54: 421–53

Abel EL (1984) Fetal alcohol syndrome and fetal alcohol effects. Plenum Press, New York

Abel EL (1988) Fetal alcohol syndrome in families. Neurotoxicol Teratol 10: 1–2

Abel EL (1991) Fetal alcohol syndrome. Medical Economics Books, Oradell, NJ

Abel EL (1995) An update on the incidence of FAS: FAS is not an equal opportunity birth defect. Neurotoxicol Teratol 17: 437–43

Abel EL (1998a) Fetal alcohol syndrome: the American paradox. Alcohol Alcoholism 33: 195–201

Abel EL (1998b) Fetal alcohol syndrome revisited. Plenum Press, New York

Abel EL, Sokol RJ (1987) Incidence of fetal alcohol syndrome and the economic impact of FAS-related anomalies. Drug Alcohol Depend 19: 51–70

Abel EL, Sokol RJ (1991) A revised conservative estimate of the incidence of FAS and its economic impact. Alcohol Clin Exp Res 15: 514–24

Abma JC, Mott FL (1991) Substance use and prenatal care during pregnancy among young women. Family Planning Persp 23(3): 117–22

American Psychiatric Association (1994) Diagnostic and Statistical Manual of Mental Disorders, 4th ed. American Psychiatric Association, Washington, DC.

Aronson M. (1997) Attention deficits and autistic spectrum problems in children exposed to alcohol during gestation: a follow-up study. Dev Med Child Neurol 39: 583–87

Astley SJ, Clarren SK (1996) A case definition and photographic screening tool for the facial phenotype of fetal alcohol syndrome. J Pediatr 129: 33–41

Bonthius DJ, West JR (1990) Alcohol-induced neural loss in developing rats: increased brain damage with binge exposure. Alcohol Clin Exp Res 14: 107–18

Borges G, Lopez-Cervantes M, Medina-Mora ME, et al (1993) Alcohol consumption, low birth weight and preterm delivery in the National Addiction Survey (Mexico). Int J Addict 28: 355–68

Cassano PA, Koepsell TD, Farwell JR (1990) Risk of febrile seizure in childhood in relation to prenatal cigarette smoking and alcohol intake. Am J Epidem 132: 462–73

Cavallo F, Russo R, Zotti C (1995) Moderate alcohol consumption and spontaneous abortion. Alcohol Alcoholism 30: 195–201

Chan T, Bowell R, O'Keefe M et al (1991) Ocular manifestations in fetal alcohol syndrome. Br J Opthalmol 75: 524–26

Chandler LS, Richardson GA, Gallagher JD et al (1996) Prenatal exposure to alcohol and marijuana: effects on motor development of pre-school children. Alcohol Clin Exp Res 20: 455–461

Christiaens L, Mizon JP, Delmarle G (1960) Sur la descendance des alcooliques [On the offspring of alcoholics]. Am Pediatr 36: 37.

Church MW, Holloway JA (1984) Effects of parental exposure on the postnatal development of the brainstem auditory evoked potential in the rat. Alcohol Clin Exp Res 14: 674–83

Church MW, Abel EL (1998) Fetal alcohol syndrome. Hearing, speech, language and vestibular disorders. Obstet Gynecol Clin North Am 25: 85–97

Cliver SP, Goldenberg RL, Cutter GR et al (1992) The relationships among psychosocial profile, maternal size and smoking in predicting fetal growth retardation. Obstet Gynecol 80: 262–67

Coles C (1994) Critical periods for prenatal alcohol exposure. Alcohol Health Res World 18: 22–29

Coles CD, Platzman KA, Raskin-Hood CL, et al (1997) A comparison of children affected by prenatal alcohol exposure and attention deficit hyperactivity disorder (ADHD). Alcohol Clin Exp Res 21: 150–61

Cornelius MD, Geva,D (1994) Effects of prenatal marijuana exposure on the cognitive development of offspring at age three. Neurotoxicol Teratol 16: 169–75

da Costa Pereira A, Olsen J, Ogston S. (1993) Variability of self reported measures of alcohol consumption: implications for the association between drinking in pregnancy and birth weight. J Epidemiol Commun Health 47: 326–30

Davis RO (1992) The relationships among psychosocial profile, maternal size and smoking in predicting fetal growth retardation. Obstet Gynecol 80: 262–67

Day NL, Robles N (1989) Methodological issues in the measurement of substance abuse. Ann NY Acad Sci 562: 8–13

Day NL, Jasper MS, Richardson GA et al (1989) Prenatal exposure to alcohol. Effect on infant growth and morphologic characteristics. Pediatrics 84: 536–41

Day NL, Sambamoorthi U, Taylor P, et al (1991) Pre-natal marijuana use and neonatal outcome. Neurotoxicol Teratol 13: 329–34

Day NL, Richardson GA, Goldschmidt L et al (1994) Effect of pre-natal marijuana exposure on the cognitive development of offspring at age three. Neurotoxicol Teratol 16: 169–75

Deltour L, Ang HL, Duester G, et al (1996) Ethanol inhibition of retinoic acid synthesis as a potential mechanism for fetal alcohol syndrome. FASEB Monogr 10: 1050–57

DePetrillo PB, Rice JM (1995) Methadone dosing and pregnancy: impact on program compliance. Int J Addict 30: 207-17

Dobbing J, Sands J (1979) Comparative aspects of the brain growth spurt. Early Hum Dev 3: 79–83

Driscoll CD, Streissguth AP, Riley EP (1990) Prenatal alcohol exposure: comparability of effects in human and animal models. Neurotoxicol Teratol 12: 231–37

Druse MJ (1992) Effects of in utero ethanol exposure on the development of neurotransmitter systems. In: Watson RR (Ed.), Development of the central nervous system: effects of alcohol and opiates. Wiley-Liss, New York

Ernhart CB, Sokol RJ, Martier S, et al (1987) Alcohol teratology in the human: a detailed assessment of specificity, critical period and threshold. Am J Obstetr Gynecol 156: 33–39

Ernhart CB, Morrow-Tlucak M, Sokol RJ, et al (1988) Under-reporting of alcohol use in pregnancy. Alcohol Clin Exp Res 12: 506–11

Esquifino AL, Sanchis R, Guerri C (1986) Effect of prenatal alcohol exposure on sexual maturation in female rat offspring. Neuroendocrinology 44: 483–87

Florey C, Taylor D, Bolumar F, et al (1992) A European concerted action: maternal alcohol consumption and its relation to the outcome of pregnancy and child development at 18 months. Int J Epidemiol 21 (Suppl 1): S40–S44

Floyd RL, Rimer BK, Giovino GA et al (1993) A review of smoking in pregnancy: effects on pregnancy outcomes and cessation efforts. Annu Rev Public Health 14: 379–411

Fried PA (1993) Prenatal exposure to tobacco and marijuana: effects during pregnancy, infancy and early childhood. Clin Obstetr Gynecol 36: 319–37

Fried PA (1995) Prenatal exposure to marijuana and tobacco during infancy, early and middle childhood: effects and an attempt at synthesis. Arch Toxicol Suppl. 17: 233–60

Fried PA, Watkinson B (1988) Twelve and 24 month neurobehavioral follow-up of children prenatally exposed to marijuana, cigarettes and alcohol. Neurotoxicol Teratol 10: 305–31

Fried PA, Watkinson B (1990) Thirty-six and 48 month neurobehavioral follow-up of children prenatally exposed to marijuana, cigarettes and alcohol. J Dev Behav Pediatr 11: 49–58

Fried A, O'Connell CM, Watkinson B (1992a) Sixty and 72 month follow-up of children prenatally exposed to marihuana, cigarettes and alcohol: cognitive and language assessment. J Dev Behav Pediatr 13: 383–91

Fried PA, Watkinson B, Gray R (1992b) A follow-up study of attentional behavior in 6-year-old children exposed prenatally to marihuana, cigarettes and alcohol. Neurotoxicol Teratol 14: 299–311

Garro AJ, Mc'Beth DL, Lima V, et al (1991) Ethanol consumption inhibits fetal DNA methylation in mice: implications for the fetal alcohol syndrome. Alcohol Clin Exp Res 15: 395–98

Glantz JC, Woods JR (1993) Cocaine, heroin and phencyclidine: obstetric perspectives. Clin Obstetr Gynecol 36: 279–301

Gottesfeld Z, Abel EL (1991) Maternal and paternal use: effects on the immune system of the offspring. Life Sci 48: 1–8

Graham JM, Hanson JW, Darby BL, et al (1988) Independent dysmorphology evaluation at birth and 4 years of age for children exposed to varying amounts of alcohol in utero. Pediatrics 81: 772–78

Grant M, Litvak J (Eds.) (1997) Drinking patterns and their consequences. Taylor and Francis, Washington, DC

Greene T, Ernhart CB, Martier S, et al (1990) Prenatal alcohol exposure and language development. Alcohol Clin Exp Res 14: 937–54

Greene T, Ernhart CB, Ager J, et al (1991) Prenatal alcohol exposure and cognitive development in the preschool years. Neurotoxicol Teratol 13: 57–68

Greenfield T (1997) Warning labels: evidence on harm reduction from long-term American surveys. In: Plant MA, Single E, Stockwell T (Eds.), Alcohol: minimising the harm. What works? London Free Association Books, London, pp. 105–25

Guerri C (1995) Teratogenic effects of alcohol: current status on animal research and in vitro models. Arch Toxicol 18: 71–80

Guerri C (1998) Neuroanatomical and neurophysiological mechanisms involved in central nervous system dysfunctions induced by prenatal alcohol exposure. Alcohol Clin Exp Res 22: 304–12

Guerri C, Sanchis R (1985) Acetaldehyde and alcohol levels in pregnant rats and their fetuses. Alcohol 2: 267–70

Guerri C, Montoliu C, Renau-Piqueras J (1994) Involvement of free radical mechanism in the toxic effects of alcohol: implications for fetal alcohol syndrome. In: Armstrong D (Ed.), Free radicals in diagnostic medicine. Plenum Press, New York, pp. 291–305

Halmesmäki E (1988) Alcohol counselling of 85 pregnant problem drinkers: effect on drinking and fetal outcome. Br J Obstetr Gynaecol 89: 892–95

Hankin JR, Firestone IJ, Sloan JJ, et al (1996a) Heeding the alcoholic beverage warning labels during pregnancy: multiparae versus nulliparae. J Stud Alcohol 57: 171–77

Hankin JR, Sloan JJ, Firestone IJ, et al (1996b) Has awareness of the alcohol warning label reached its upper limits? Alcohol Clin Exp Res 20: 440–44

Hibell B, Andersson B, Bjarnason T, et al (1997) The 1995 ESPAD Report: alcohol and other drugs among students in 26 European countries. Swedish Council for Information on Alcohol and Other Drugs, Stockholm/Council of Europe (Pompidou Group)

Himwich WA, Hall JS, MacArthur WF (1977) Maternal alcohol and neonatal health. Biol Psychiatry 12: 495–505

Holzman C, Paneth N, Little R, et al (1995) Perinatal brain injury in premature infants born to mothers using alcohol in pregnancy. Pediatrics 95: 66–73

Institute of Medicine (1996) Fetal alcohol syndrome. National Academy Press, Washington, DC

Jacobson SW, Jacobson JL, Sokol RJ, et al (1991) Maternal recall of alcohol, cocaine and marijuana use during pregnancy. Neurotoxicol Teratol 13: 535–40

Jacobson SW, Jacobson JL, O'Neill JM, et al (1992) Visual expectation and dimensions of infant information processing. Child Dev 63: 711–24

Jacobson JL, Jacobson SW, Sokol RJ, et al (1993) Teratogenic effects of alcohol on infant development. Alcohol Clin Exp Res 17: 174–83

Jacobson SW, Jacobson JL, Sokol RJ (1994a) Effects of fetal alcohol exposure on infant reaction time. Alcohol Clin Exp Res 18: 1125–32

Jacobson JL, Jacobson SW (1994b) Prenatal alcohol exposure and neurobehavioral development: where is the threshold? Alcohol Health Res World 18: 30–36

Jones KL, Smith DW (1973) Recognition of the fetal alcohol syndrome in early infancy. Lancet ii: 999–1001

Kaskutas LA (1995) Interpretations of risk: the use of scientific information in the development of the warning label policy. Int J Addict 30: 1519–48

Knight JE, Kodituwakku PW, Orrison WW Jr et al (1993) Magnetic resonance imaging in high-functioning children with fetal alcohol syndrome who exhibit specific neuropsychological deficits. Alcohol Clin Exp Res 17: 485–92

Kotch LE, Sulik KK (1992) Experimental fetal alcohol syndrome: proposed pathogenic basis for a variety of associated facial and brain anomalies. Am J Med Genet 44: 168–76

Kotch LE, Chen S-Y, Sulik KK (1995) Ethanol-induced teratogenesis: free radical damage as a possible mechanism. Teratology 52: 128–36

Larsson G, Bohlin A.-B, Tunell R (1985) Prospective study of children exposed to variable amounts of alcohol in utero. Arch Dis Child 60: 315–21

Lammers MS, Schippers GM, van der Staak CPF (1995) Submission and rebellion: excessive drinking of women in problematic heterosexual partner relationships. Int J Addict 30: 901–17

Lecomte M (1950) Eléments d'hérédopathologie. Scalp 103: 1133–45

Lemoine P, Lemoine P (1992) Avenir des enfants de mères alcooliques (Etude de 105 cas retrouvés à l'âge adulte) et quelques constatations d'intérêt prophylactique [Following the infants of alcoholic mothers: study of 105 cases through adulthood and some notes on prophylaxis]. Ann Pédiatr (Paris) 39: 226–35

Lindenberg CS, Keith AB (1993) Opiate abuse in pregnancy. Annu Rev Nurs Res 11: 249-79

Little RE, Sing CF (1987) Father's drinking and infant birth weight: report of an association. Teratology 36: 59–65

McGee R, Stanton WR (1994) Smoking in pregnancy and child development to age nine years. J Paediatr Child Health 30: 263–68

McGivern RF, Clancy AN, Hill MA, et al (1984) Prenatal exposure alters adult expression of sexually dimorphic behavior in rats. Science 224: 896–98

Majewski F (1981) Alcohol embryopathy: some facts and speculations about pathogenesis. Neurobehav Toxicol Teratol 3: 129–44

Mattson SN, Riley EP, Sowell ER, et al (1996) A decrease in the size of basal ganglia in children with fetal alcohol syndrome. Alcohol Clin Exp Res 20: 1088–93

Mattson SN, Riley EP, Gramling L, et al (1997) Heavy prenatal alcohol exposure with or without physical features of fetal alcohol syndrome leads to IQ deficits. J Pediatr 131: 718–21

May PA (1995) A multiple-level, comprehensive approach to the prevention of fetal alcohol syndrome (FAS) and other alcohol-related birth defects (ARBD). Int J Addict 30: 1549–1602

Meyer LC, Peacock JL, Bland JM, et al (1994) Symptoms and health problems in pregnancy: their association with social factors, smoking, alcohol, caffeine and attitude to pregnancy. Paediatr Perinatal Epidemiol: 145–55

Nalpas B, Pol V, Thépot H, et al (1998) Relationship between excessive alcohol drinking and viral infections. Alcohol Alcoholism 33: 202–06

NIAAA (National Institute on Alcohol Abuse and Alcoholism) (1993) Eighth report to the US Congress on alcohol and health. NIH publication 94-3699. Government Printing Office, Washington, DC

O'Connor TA, Kilbride HW, Hayden LK (1993) Incidence of fetal alcohol syndrome among infants with intrauterine cocaine exposure. J Maternal-Fetal Invest 3: 29–31

Orlebeke JF, Boomsma DI, van Baal GC, et al (1994) Effects of maternal smoking on birth weight of twins: a study from the Dutch twin register. Early Hum Dev 37: 161–66

Passaro KT, Little RE, Savitz DA, et al (1996) The effect of maternal drinking before conception and in early pregnancy on infant birth weight. Epidemiology 6: 377–83

Pinazo-Durán MD, Renau-Piqueras J, Guerri C, et al (1997) Optic nerve hypoplasia in fetal alcohol syndrome: an update. Eur J Ophthalmol 7: 262–70

Plant ML (1992) Women and alcohol: a review of the international literature on the use of alcohol by females. World Health Organization, Copenhagen

Plant ML (1997) Women and alcohol: contemporary and historical perspectives. Free Association Books, London

Plant MA, Plant ML (1992) Risk takers: alcohol, drugs, sex and youth. Tavistock/Routledge, London

Plant ML, Sullivan FM, Guerri C, et al (1993) Alcohol and pregnancy. In: Verschuren PM (Ed.), Health issues related to alcohol consumption. International Life Sciences Institute (ILSI) Europe, Brussels, pp. 245–62

Plant MA, Single E, Stockwell T (eds) (1997) Alcohol: minimising the harm. What works? Free Association Books, London

Portolés M, Sanchis R, Guerri C (1988) Thyroid hormone levels in rats exposed to alcohol during development. Hormone Metab Res 20: 267–70

Rifas L, Towler DA, Avioli LV (1997) Gestational exposure to ethanol suppresses msx2 expression in developing mouse embryos. Proc Natl Acad Sci USA 94: 7549–54

Riley EP, Mattson SN, Sowell ER, et al (1995) Abnormalities of the corpus callosum in children prenatally exposed to alcohol. Alcohol Clin Exp Res 19: 1198–1202

Rosett HL (1980) A clinical perspective of the fetal alcohol syndrome. Alcohol Clin Exp Res 4: 119–22

Russell M (1991) Clinical implications of recent research on the fetal alcohol syndrome. Bull NY Acad Med 67: 207–22

Russell M, Czarnecki DM, Cowan R, et al. (1991) Measures of maternal alcohol use as predictors of development in early childhood. Alcohol Clin Exp Res 15: 991–1000

Sampson PD, Bookstein FL, Barr HM, et al. (1994) Prenatal alcohol exposure, birthweight, and measures of child size from birth to age 14 years. Am J Public Health 84: 1421–28

Sampson PD, Streissguth AP, Bookstein FL, et al. (1997) Incidence of fetal alcohol syndrome and prevalence of alcohol-related neurodevelopmental disorder. Teratology 5: 317–26

Sanchis R, Sancho-Tello M, Guerri C (1986) The effects of chronic alcohol consumption on pregnant rats and their offspring. Alcohol Alcoholism 21: 295–305

Savitz DA, Schwingl PJ, Keele MA (1991) Influence of paternal age, smoking and alcohol consumption on congenital anomalies. Teratology 44: 429–40

Schandler SL, Thomas CS, Cohen MJ (1995) Spatial learning deficit in preschool children of alcoholics. Alcohol Clin Exp Res 19: 1067–72

Schenker S, Becker HC, Randall CL, et al. (1990) Fetal alcohol syndrome: current status of pathogenesis. Alcohol Clin Exp Res 14: 635–47

Schorling JB (1993) The prevention of prenatal alcohol use: a critical analysis of intervention studies. J Stud Alcohol 54: 261–67

Shu XO, Hatch MC, Mills J et al. (1995) Maternal smoking, alcohol drinking, caffeine consumption, and fetal growth: results from a prospective study. Epidemiology 6: 115–20

Sokol RJ, Abel EL (1992) Risk factors for alcohol related birth defects: threshold, susceptibility and prevention. In: Sonderegger TB (Ed.), Perinatal substance abuse. Johns Hopkins University Press, Baltimore, MD

Sokol RJ, Ager JW, Martier SS, et al. (1986) Significant determinants of susceptibility to alcohol teratogenicity. Ann NY Acad Sci 477: 87–102

Sokol RJ, Martier SS, Ager JW, et al (1993) Paternal drinking may affect intrauterine growth. Am J Obstretr Gynecol 168: 48

Sowell ER, Jernigan TL, Mattson SN, et al. (1996) Abnormal development of the cerebellar vermis in children prenatally exposed to alcohol: size reduction in lobules I-V. Alcohol Clin Exp Res 20: 31–34

Spohr H-L, Willms J, Steinhausen H-C (1994) The fetal alcohol syndrome in adolescence. Acta Pediatr 83 (404):19–26

Spohr H-L, Steinhausen H-C (Eds) (1996) Alcohol, pregnancy, and the developing child. Cambridge University Press, New York

Steinhausen H-C (1996) Psychopathology and cognitive functioning in children with fetal alcohol syndrome. In: Spohr H-L, Steinhausen HC (Eds.), Alcohol, pregnancy and the developing child. Cambridge University Press, New York, pp. 227–46

Stockwell T, Single E (1997) Standard unit labelling of alcoholic containers. In: Plant MA, Single E, Stockwell T (Eds.) Alcohol: minimising the harm. What works? Free Association Books, London, pp. 85–104

Streissguth AP, Bookstein FL, Sampson PD, et al. (1989) Neurobehavioral effects of prenatal alcohol. Part III. PLS analyses of neuropsychologic test. Neurotoxicol Teratol 11: 493–507

Streissguth AP, Barr HM Sampson PD (1990) Moderate prenatal alcohol exposure: effects on child IQ and learning problems at 7½ years. Alcohol Clin Exp Res 14: 662–69

Streissguth AP, Grant TM, Barr HM, et al. (1991a) Cocaine and the use of alcohol and other drugs during pregnancy. Am J Obstetr Gynecol 164: 1239–43

Streissguth AP, Aase JM, Clarren SK, et al. (1991b) Fetal alcohol syndrome in adolescents and adults. J Am Med Ass 265: 1961–67

Streissguth AP, Bookstein FL, Sampson PD (1993) The enduring effects of prenatal alcohol exposure on child development, birth through 7 years: a partial least squares solution. University of Michigan Press, Ann Arbor, MI

Streissguth AP, Barr HM, Olson HC, et al. (1994a) Drinking during pregnancy decreases word attack and arithmetic scores on standardized tests: adolescent data from a population-based prospective study. Alcohol Clin Exp Res 18: 248–54

Streissguth AP, Sampson PD, Olson HC, et al (1994b) Maternal drinking during pregnancy: attention and short-term memory in 14 year old offspring. A longitudinal study. Alcohol Clin Exp Res 18: 202–18

Streissguth AP, Bookstein FL, Sampson PD, et al (1995) Attention: prenatal alcohol and continuities of vigilance and attentional problems from 4 through 14 years. Dev Psychopathol 7: 419–46

Strickland TL, James R, Myers H, et al. (1993) Psychological characteristics related to cocaine use during pregnancy: a postpartum assessment. J Natl Med Ass 85: 758–60

Swayze VW, Johnson VP, Hanson JW, et al. (1997) Magnetic resonance imaging of brain anomalies in fetal alcohol syndrome. Pediatrics 99: 232–40

Tsai MJ, O'Malley BW (1994) Molecular mechanisms of action of steroid/thyroid receptor superfamily members. Annu Rev Biochem 63: 451–86

Ulleland CN (1972) The offspring of alcoholic mothers. Ann NY Acad Sci 197: 167–69

Vallés S, Pitarch J, Renau-Piqueras J, et al. (1997) Ethanol exposure affects glial fibrillary acidic protein gene expression and transcription during rat brain development. J Neurochem 69: 2484–93

Verkerk PH (1992) The impact of alcohol misclassification on the relationship between alcohol and pregnancy outcome. Int J Epidemiol Suppl 21: 33–37

Waterson EJ, Evans C, Murray-Lyon IM (1990) Is pregnancy a time of changing drinking and smoking patterns for fathers as well as mothers? An initial investigation. Br J Addict 85: 389–96

Weinberg J (1994) Recent studies on the effects of fetal alcohol exposure on the endocrine and immune systems. Alcohol Alcoholism Suppl 2: 401–09

West JR, Chen WJ, Pantazis NJ (1994) Fetal alcohol syndrome: the vulnerability of the developing brain and possible mechanisms of damage. Met Brain Dis 9: 291–332

Windham GC, Fenster L, Hopkins B, et al. (1995) The association of moderate maternal and paternal alcohol consumption with birthweight and gestational age. Epidemiology 6: 591–97

Chapter 7

Alcohol and Breast Cancer

K. McPherson
London School of Hygiene and Tropical Medicine, UK

F. Cavallo
Università Degli Studi di Torino, Italy

E. Rubin
Jefferson Medical College, Philadelphia, PA, USA

Abstract

Biological theories concerning putative mechanisms for the development of breast cancer have been invoked to explain a possible association between alcohol use and elevated breast cancer risk. However such theories are merely suggestive rather than unambiguous and compelling. In this report we present the consensus of the research by reviewing the epidemiological evidence of some 70 studies for a causative association between alcohol consumption and the risk of breast cancer.

The accumulated evidence suggests the possibility of a weak association between alcohol use and breast cancer. Some studies seem to show a relationship with increasing drinking level, but this is not necessarily linear. The most likely causative relationship, from the mixed evidence, exists for heavy drinking, since the ability to distinguish the inconsistent observational evidence concerning moderate drinking from confounding by unknown or unmeasured risk factors for breast cancer remains inadequate.

Since the evidence for an association between alcohol use and breast cancer is all non-experimental, and since the aetiology of this tumour remains largely unexplained, the definitive interpretation of the evidence is necessarily problematic. In other words, the opportunities for important unknown confounding are large. In particular, aspects of diet (mostly fat but also other dietary factors) as well as psychological stresses of various kinds have been shown to be associated with breast cancer risk, and both of these are likely to be associated independently with lifetime exposure to alcohol.

Determining relevant exposures to foods, psychological stress or other unknown factors that may be implicated in the risk of breast cancer is difficult. It is often past exposures, possibly decades previously, that are important, and recall or memory of such exposures may be unreliable and possibly epidemiologically biased. In such circumstances the patterns of epidemiological findings reviewed are consistent with no causative effect, but rather show varying amounts of residual, possibly unmeasured, confounding.

Since experimental studies in which such confounding could be minimized are unlikely, the resolution of this question must await the ability to better adjust for such dietary or other confounding by knowing more about their roles as primary risk factors for breast cancer. This will involve prospective studies in which the consequences of contemporary dietary patterns or other risk factors are observed in the future.

In the meantime, any recommendation that women should limit their alcohol use to reduce their risk of breast cancer can only be supported in terms of reduction from excessive drinking. The evidence implicating moderate drinking in breast cancer risk is weak, and yet the evidence for an overall benefit on the health of women is strong. The balance of the risk of dying from causes for which alcohol is protective tends to be eliminated by the known risks of excessive drinking at 2 or 3 drinks per day for women, whatever the actual effect on breast cancer risk may be.

Introduction

Alcohol (ethanol) is unlikely to be carcinogenic to the breast *per se* (Rubin 1996), but has been postulated by some to facilitate the process of carcinogenesis by a number of recognized mechanisms. It has been amply demonstrated that ethanol per se is not directly mutagenic in any of the commonly used assays (Brooks 1997). All so-called promoters stimulate cell proliferation, whereas ethanol inhibits cell proliferation both *in vitro* and *in vivo*. Hence, it is unlikely that ethanol acts as a direct carcinogen, and any such effect would have to be indirect, for example through hormonal or dietary mechanisms. Some biological plausibility might be provided by, for instance, evidence that the primary metabolite of ethanol, acetaldehyde, does induce DNA replication and is mutagenic in cultured mammalian cells (Ristow et al. 1978, Dellarco 1988). There is no evidence, however, that carcinogenic changes in mammary tissue have occurred as a consequence, particularly since circulating levels of acetaldehyde are, at most, in the very low micromolar range. Some studies have found positive associations between alcohol intake and plasma oestrogen levels (Hankinson et al. 1995), whereas others have not (Newcomb et al. 1995).

The time span between menarche and first full-term pregnancy is known to be positively related to breast cancer risk, mediated possibly by exposure of the ductal system to repeated cycles of oestrogen and progesterone without progression to lactation (Drife 1981). It is conceivable that the use of alcohol could increase the sensitivity of the breast to these exposures, either by delaying the metabolic degradation of these hormones by a hepatotoxic effect in heavy drinkers or by increasing the production of electrophilic compounds through the induction of microsomal oxidases (Rubin et al. 1968). There is no evidence to support either of these opposing mechanisms. Moreover, it is not likely that such an effect will be demonstrated since, if present, it is small.

A similar result might be expected if alcohol consumption resulted in suppression of prolactin secretion by direct inhibition or through the stimulation of, for example, dopamine release. There is experimental evidence to support the suppression of prolactin by prolonged alcohol administration (Schrauzer et al. 1979). In man (male volunteers), alcohol was found to slightly increase prolactin levels in response to thyrotropin-releasing hormone (TRH), but this was followed by a phase in which TRH was without effect (Ylikahri et al. 1976). It is thus conceivable that chronic alcohol consumption leads to prolonged repression of the prolactin response, but there is no evidence in support of this concept.

Since breast cancer clearly has, in part, a hormonal aetiology (Key et al. 1988), any effect that alcohol may have on a woman's endogenous hormonal milieu might indirectly affect risk. Such a postulate must remain imprecise, however, since the exact role of endogenous hormones remains poorly understood. In principle, such a mechanism could reduce, increase or have no aggregate effect on risk. However some studies do show an increased endogenous oestrogen level associated with moderate alcohol intake (Hunter et al. 1996).

Interest in any possible association between alcohol use and breast cancer was aroused empirically in 1977 in a report by Williams et al. In the population-based Third National Cancer Survey, 7518 incident cases were interviewed about their lifetime use of tobacco and alcohol, as well as their socioeconomic status (SES). Associations were found between breast cancer and alcohol use and between breast cancer and SES. Comparisons of breast cancer patients and patients with other cancers were made, acknowledging the reasonable suspicion that tobacco, alcohol and SES are sufficiently correlated to be powerful confounding variables in the observed association. Breast cancer exhibited only a weak association with alcohol use.

Since then, a large number of epidemiological studies have been published, many confirming this association, but a substantial number failing to find any association, significant or otherwise. We have reviewed 12 cohort studies and nearly 50 case-control studies, of which 7 cohort studies and 37 case-control studies supplied sufficient data to look for a dose-response relationship. Around 45 articles commenting on the association, and about 40 articles suggesting and discussing biological mechanisms to explain any possible causal association, have been reviewed.

Possible Specific Associations

From these studies a large number of detailed possible specific associations between the consumption of alcohol and breast cancer emerge. These consist of any plausible combination of the following factors:

(1) Nature of consumption:
 – type of alcohol (e.g. beer, spirits or wine);
 – quantity drunk per week or per day;
 – age at consumption, possibly relative to diagnosis of breast cancer;
 – age at onset of drinking and duration of drinking

(2) Nature of breast cancer:
 – premenopausal or
 – postmenopausal;
 – oestrogen receptor-positive or
 – oestrogen receptor-negative;
 – local disease or
 – with dissemination;

(3) Nature of the association:
 – causal or
 – associative only.

The dominant associations suggested by epidemiological research consist of a general but weak relationship between increasing daily alcohol use and breast cancer risk. Importantly, nothing in the literature predicts a strong association of alcohol use with breast cancer. Since the consumption of alcohol is common and the incidence of breast cancer is high, the public health consequences of a weak association could be important. The other clear implication is that if a particular causal effect does exist, say duration of consumption with premenopausal breast cancer, then it should be evident against a background of generally low risks. The examination of the possible combinations in the research literature is, of course, subject to the vagaries of multiple hypothesis testing, and in any event is inconclusive.

The various hypotheses are investigated by observational epidemiological studies (case-control studies or cohort studies), in which the consumption of alcohol is measured according to amounts, sometimes type and sometimes temporal relationships. The responses to questions on alcohol use are generally categorized according to daily amounts, without detailed reference to the type of alcohol, when it was consumed or the maximum amount taken at one time. Since any biological hypothesis is so poorly specified *a priori*, many of the above possible associations have been investigated and published. Clearly this association has been subjected to strong and widespread scrutiny which, of course, compromises the interpretation of positive findings. Dickersin et al. (1987), for example, have published an extensive study of published and unpublished clinical trials that show the existence of a publication bias for positive findings of importance both to meta-analysis and reviews of the epidemiological literature. The extent of publication bias is unknown. English et al. (1995) have shown some evidence for possible bias in studies of modest drinking, where small studies showing positive effects appear to be over-represented.

The Scientific Consensus Concerning Possible Specific Associations Between Alcohol and Breast Cancer Risk

We begin with the main hypothesis that alcohol consumption itself causes an increased breast cancer risk. A current scientific consensus probably does exist and is best argued by Steinberg et al. (1991), in which the epidemiological literature is well reviewed and summarized. More recently, Schatzkin et al. (1994) and Roth et al. (1994) have both reviewed the entire literature, 50 studies and 38 case-control studies respectively, and concluded that whether the observed association is causal is essentially unproved. Plant (1992) concludes that evidence for a causal link is lacking and is concerned that undue obsession with this association diverts attention from the real possibilities for preventing breast cancer.

In our view, the current consensus holds that there is insufficient evidence to support a general causal relationship between alcohol and breast cancer risk. The studies that do find an association find only a weak positive one (with a relative risk of up to about 1.5), and this is not consistently found. With such a weak association and a poor understanding of the aetiology of breast cancer, it is impossible to exclude systematic confounding with some known or unknown risk factor. No particular specific relationship stands out, except the possibility that the association is strongest for high reported drinking levels and premenopausal breast cancer. But the strength and consistency of even this particular subgroup analysis are not indicative of a strong relationship.

Confounding will be present when alcohol use is itself associated with exposure to some independent established or unknown risk factor. The most likely confounding factors are some aspects of diet, for which many well-established candidates exist (Henderson et al. 1997) and which are often perforce poorly measured. Stress may be an independent risk factor for breast cancer (Redd et al. 1991) and, needless to say, might well be associated with alcohol use. A review of the evidence for stress as a risk factor for breast cancer is, not surprisingly, inconclusive (Bryla 1996) but this may be a reflection of the intrinsic methodological difficulties that go with measuring and attributing stress as a risk factor for any chronic disease. Notwithstanding all these problems, the pattern of consumption empirically found to be associated with breast cancer risk is not sufficiently consistent.

Epidemiological Evidence

The epidemiological studies we have reviewed are not of an even methodological quality. A very important source of variation is the definition and measurement of the amount and timing of alcohol use. How difficult this is for the interpretation may be illustrated by the following definitions used in some of these studies: recent use, recent and past use, lifetime use, usual intake, frequency of drinking, current use, use 3 years ago, use in the preceding year, use in the preceding 5 years, use more or less than 4 days per week, use per week, moderate use, infrequent use, use per day, use per month, and use with meals.

For the dose-response relationship, we have translated the use into grams of pure alcohol per day whenever possible. One drink (wine, beer or spirits) is described as containing 9–13 g ethanol; we chose to regard "one drink" as containing 10 g. Moderate use usually means 5–10 g/day. The numbers of "heavy drinkers" (more than 30 g/day) are usually very low, and their estimated relative risks are correspondingly volatile.

Many studies worked with questionnaires that asked about current use or drinking in the past year. Some studies mentioned use before the age of 30 or 35 years or specified duration of use as less or more than 30 years. The ratio of non-drinkers to drinkers differs considerably in the studies (sometimes 84% non-drinkers, which is certainly not average). Non-drinkers are defined in several ways: using less than 10 g/week (Talamini et al. 1984), not having used alcohol in the past 5 years (Webster et al. 1983), or just "ex-drinkers" (Sneyd et al. 1991).

In some studies alcohol use is differentiated into wine, beer, spirits and total use. Some case-control studies have used hospital controls (cancer controls, non-cancer controls), but the more recent ones usually used population controls who were often matched on important confounding variables. Roth et al. (1994) report lower estimated odds ratios and significantly lower dose-response relationships in the 17 studies using community controls than in those using hospital controls. The use of screening programmes also has a possible weakness, because controls are possibly self-selected to volunteer in the programme (Harvey et al. 1987).

There are considerable differences in the extent and type of the questionnaires used to elicit alcohol histories. Some studies specify that the subjects were interviewed at their homes by trained interviewers. There is the ubiquitous problem (for alcohol use in particular) of possible underreporting, which if associated with disease status in case-control studies will result in bias. In cohort studies this information is collected before the diagnosis, but may have been gathered long ago, and not all studies have reported more recent interviews Sometimes information has been collected by telephone (Nasca et al. 1990).

Some studies were designed specifically for examining the question of an association between alcohol and breast cancer (Williams et al. 1977, Rosenberg et al. 1990), but many studies were started long ago and were re-analysed subsequently when the question of an association between alcohol and breast cancer was suggested. In one instance the questionnaires had been collected in 1959 (Garfinkel et al. 1988).

Well-known risk factors for breast cancer were usually, but not always, taken into account (age, age at menarche and age at menopause, marital status, age at first full-term pregnancy, family history of breast cancer, etc.), but there are more possible confounding variables. These include oestrogen use, socioeconomic status, different population groups, tobacco use, body mass index, dietary factors and psychological health. The published relative risks are not always corrected for the latter risk factors and not always adjusted for best known confounding factors. Clearly, it is not possible to adjust for unknown confounding factors, although they could be dominant.

One small study on male breast cancer and alcohol use (Casagrande et al. 1981) found no association with alcohol use, but an association with high body mass index at the age of 30 years. Rohan et al. (1989) reported no association between benign breast lesions and alcohol consumption. Lindegard (1987) found no association between the prevalence of breast cancer and alcohol-related diseases in a large homogeneous population study (commented upon by Graham 1987).

Overviews

Several papers have presented overviews or "meta-analyses" of a number of individual studies. Longnecker et al. (1989) calculated dose-response curves, using data extracted from 16 published studies. They fitted mathematical models to the pooled data from the available literature. Some of the analyses were weighted by the assessed quality of the studies. The authors concluded that a small relative risk (RR), which was dose-related in a linear fashion, was consistent with the overall data. For case-control studies, the estimated RR increased linearly to 1.5 for 36 g alcohol or more per day. The results of cohort studies indicated a slightly higher RR of about 2.0 and a steeper linear relationship. These authors interpreted their findings as no proof of causality, but strongly supportive of an association between alcohol use and breast cancer.

Howe et al. (1991) performed a formal meta-analysis with original data from six dietary case-control studies, including two published studies (Rohan et al. 1988, Toniolo et al. 1989). This study does represent stronger evidence for a causal association between alcohol and breast cancer, because it consists of the raw data from the majority of case control studies in which an attempt at obtaining detailed dietary histories was made. These authors conclude that the adjusted RR for 40 g/day or more of alcohol is 1.7 (see Table 1) and unity for any lower consumption. However, the estimates for this particular cut-off of drinking level are derived entirely from the data and not from any prior hypothesis suggested by other studies. Moreover, out of 3500 subjects with and without breast cancer, only 91 cases and 72 controls consumed 40 g ethanol or more daily in the whole study. This is a relatively high drinking level and is, therefore, likely to be found only in a unique group of women; in addition, since this dose relationship differs from the unadjusted analyses of Longnecker et al. (1988), it cannot be regarded as strong evidence for a causal relationship.

The authors conclude that the observed association is not due to confounding by a number of diet-related factors. This is justified, however, by their analysis that statistical adjustments of the RR associated with alcohol show little evidence of confounding with individual measured dietary components. What is unclear is the extent to which a complex of

Table 1

Relative risk of breast cancer for daily alcohol intake from Howe et al. (1991)

Alcohol (g/day)	Cases	Controls	Relative risk (RR)	95% Confidence interval (CI)
0	523	607	1.0	0.8–1.1
0–10	479	642	0.9	0.9–1.3
10–20	282	376	1.1	0.9–1.3
20–30	138	210	1.0	0.6–1.4
30–40	60	76	0.9	0.6–1.4
40+	91	72	1.7	1.2–2.4

dietary adjustment alters the strength of this association. From the tabulations, it appears that the RR associated with 40 g alcohol or more per day drops from around 1.74 to 1.69 after adjustment for all recorded dietary components, from which some evidence for confounding is apparent. The effect that dietary adjustments had on the estimated RR of around unity for consumption of less than 40 g/day remains unclear. This is an important unanswered question in the evaluation of a possible causal relationship.

Since the publication of this meta-analysis, Longnecker has updated his review of 1988 (Longnecker 1994) to include 38 studies that passed his methodological criteria, more than double the number in his previous review. He concludes that the estimated slope of the dose-response curve (using a random effects model) was modest, that no explanation for the marked variation in estimates across studies could be found, and that these two observations leave the causal explanation for this association in question. The variations reported in this analysis across studies are the equivalent of an estimate of the RR per drink per day from about 0.55 to 2.05 (both highly significantly different from unity), with a pooled weighted average of 1.11 (Table 2). The test for heterogeneity (not usually a very powerful test) between studies was significant at $P< 0.001$.

Smith-Warner et al. (1998) have performed a meta-analysis of 6 cohort studies from Canada, the Netherlands, Sweden and the USA, each including more than 200 cases of breast cancer. Each study attempted to adjust for nutrient intake, using a validated dietary assessment instrument. The adjusted relative risks for breast cancer are shown in Table 3.

The authors claim that the data represent a significant (*P*<0.001) trend of risk with increasing alcohol use, but there is actually no evidence for an excess risk at "normal" levels of consumption. Only one category (30-60 g/day) is itself significant, and the risk up to 30 g/day shows neither any effect nor trend whatsoever. (In this respect statistical tests for trend among large numbers of subjects are almost always significantly different from no trend.) There was no detectable difference according to type of alcoholic beverage consumed. These data are hardly compelling and could be attributable to confounding; yet the authors conclude that the estimated linear association of consumption with risk is causal and that a reduction in alcohol use would decrease the risk of breast cancer.

Table 2
Relative risk of breast cancer from Longnecker (1994)

Drinks per day	Pooled RR	95% CI
None	reference	
One	1.11	(1.07–1.16)
Two	1.24	(1.15–1.34)
Three	1.38	(1.23–1.55)

Table 3
Relative risk of breast cancer from Smith-Warner (1998): meta-analysis of 6 cohort studies

Alcohol (g/day)	RR	95% CI
none	Reference	
0–1.5	1.07	(0.96–1.19
1.5–5.0	0.99	(0.90–1.10)
5.0–15.0	1.06	(0.96–1.17)
15.0–30.0	1.16	(0.98–1.38)
30.0–60.0	1.41	(1.18–1.69)
60.0 +	1.31	(0.86–1.98)

Relative Risk

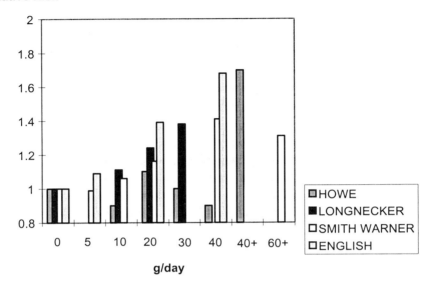

g/day

Figure 1
Estimated relative risks of breast cancer from four overviews

English et al. (1995) reviewed 7 cohort studies and 22 case control studies that met their methodological criteria. They estimated, in a meta-analysis, odds ratios for "hazardous" drinking levels (21–40 g/day) of 1.31 and for "harmful" levels of 1.68. These estimates seem, for no obvious reason, to be higher than those of other overviews. They conclude that "a causal interpretation of the evidence is credible, but in the absence of strong corroborating evidence, it is premature to rule out a non-causal explanation with certainty".

Overall, the estimated relative risks from four overviews (including English et al. 1995) illustrated in Figure 1 demonstrate the variation in the epidemiological consensus. Most of these estimates are not significantly different from unity, several achieve a degree of biological coherence by modelling linear dose-response relationships but nonetheless these estimates are not consistent at any level of alcohol consumption.

Examining Particular Associations

Nature of Consumption

TYPE OF ALCOHOL

Some investigators have reported that the risk of breast cancer is associated with a specific beverage type, such as wine or beer, whereas others did not find such a specific association. Two studies were mainly concerned with use of wine. Most data on alcohol use are expressed as quantity of alcohol per unit of time. The data on specific beverages do not allow any clear conclusions about specific risks, in spite of many attempts to identify such a relationship.

Van den Brandt et al. (1995) found no association with beer, whereas elevated risks were described for higher drinking levels for wine and spirits. In contrast, Katsouyanni et al. (1994), in Greece, found a significantly elevated risk for beer. A uniformly high risk for all kinds of alcohol was reported in a Swiss case-control study (Levi et al. 1996). However, in New York, Freudenheim et al. (1995) found little evidence for any association, but some weak support for an association with beer consumption. By contrast, Viel et al. (1997), in France, discerned a strong association with the consumption of red wine: an unusually large relative risk of about 4 with more than 4 litres per month (a little over 1 drink per day). But here, as in so much else in this literature, such an effect appears only among premenopausal women with breast cancer, and one is left to speculate about the consequence of subgroup analyses.

For instance, data from the most positive large combined study (Howe et al. 1991) estimate the adjusted RR of breast cancer per 10 g alcohol a day by type of beverage as 1.08 for beer, 1.06 for wine, and 1.13 for spirits. Only the figure of 1.07 per 10 g total alcohol is significantly different from unity, because of the overall increased RR of 1.7 for more than 40 g/day.

QUANTITY OF CONSUMPTION

As mentioned above, the definitions of alcohol use in the literature are variable, and it appears impractical for anyone to provide exact quantitative data on the consumption of alcoholic beverages. In addition, there is probably much underreporting, as illustrated by Rathje et al. (1992) who compared reported alcohol use with the contents of collected empty bottles in the garbage among several communities, and found underreporting of

60%. Friedenreich et al. (1990) report a study on recall bias in a nested case-control study in the National Breast Screening Study. Many authors mention the possibility of a recall bias, especially in case-control studies, where the cases might be influenced by the recent diagnosis. Further, the use of alcoholic drinks is often dependent on social occasions, such as parties or holidays, and on personal situations such as conflicts, depression or loneliness.

For several reasons it is difficult to form a conclusion about an association in a number of studies. For instance, Kato et al. (1989) used categories for drinking like "ever" and "occasional" and performed comparisons between daily versus occasional use. Zaridze et al. (1991), in Russia, reported a very high risk of breast cancer with consumption as low as less than 0.1 g/day, compared to abstinence. Ewertz (1991) described an increasing risk of breast cancer with increasing use of alcohol in a subgroup of women aged 50–59 and with lowest fat intake. With an alcohol intake of more than 24 g/day the relative risk was an astonishing 18, but this subgroup contained only 14 cases and 2 controls.

Van 't Veer et al. (1989) did perform a case-control study, but the small number of cases was divided over several subgroups (quantity of consumption, pre/postmenopausal, age at first consumption). Data on past drinking were obtained for only 120 cases. There is, however, a rather strong association with breast cancer in premenopausal women drinking more than 30 g/day, compared with 1–4 g/day (not in post-menopausal women). In pre- and postmenopausal women, the relative risk is not increased with consumption of less than 30 g/day.

Katsouyanni et al. (1994) make a strong circumstantial argument that observed associations with moderate drinking are a manifestation of confounding, whereas high levels more plausibly represent a causal association. They argue that such consumption may be acting as a late-stage growth-enhancing factor. However, just to confuse the issue, among women in the UK under 36, Smith et al. (1994) found a significant protective effect for consumption of more than 15 g/day. Royo-Bordonada et al. (1997) found, in five European countries, no association with the amount of alcohol consumed, but a significant risk among ex-drinkers. On the other hand, Martin-Moreno et al. (1993), in Switzerland, reported a RR of 1.7 for consumption of less than 8 g per day.

For the reasons discussed above, the consensus cannot reach far enough to cover a relationship, supported by evidence, between the risk of breast cancer and a particular dose or range of doses of alcohol.

AGE AT CONSUMPTION

Four studies have found drinking prior to the age of 25–30s to be associated with an increased risk (Hiatt et al. 1988a, Harvey et al. 1987, Young 1989, van 't Veer et al. 1989), but one study found no such association (La Vecchia et al. 1989).

Levi et al. (1996), in a case-control study in Switzerland, reported a stronger association among premenopausal than among postmenopausal women, but no effect of duration of drinking. By contrast, Bowlin et al. (1997), in New York, found no effect for age at onset of drinking, but the total duration of drinking was related to the incidence of breast cancer. Pawlega (1992), studying women in Cracow, described a significant effect on the risk for drinking vodka 20 years earlier among women under 50. Longnecker et al. (1995b), in a large case-control study of cases aged 55–64 conducted in Los Angeles, investigated the time of consumption and concluded that lifetime alcohol use was the best indicator of alcohol-associated risk.

In principle, all of this work might be important if the postulated biological mechanism for a causal hypothesis involves early- or late-stage carcinogenesis or particular constituents of alcoholic beverages associated with particular beverage types. Swanson et al. (1997), examining this hypothesis, found little association with drinking in early adulthood and concluded, therefore, that alcohol might act at a late stage in breast carcinogenesis. Effects on early-stage carcinogenesis exclusively would be expected to be detected on the basis of alcohol use measured over a long period of time, possibly as much as 20 years (McPherson et al. 1986), before diagnosis. The extent to which such consumption predicts more recent alcohol use will determine the relevance of empirical associations of recent consumption with breast cancer. However, Longnecker et al. (1995a), in a study of nearly 7000 cases, again found no association with drinking before age 30, but with recent use only. Like Katsouyanni et al. (1994), these authors suggest a late-stage effect. However, an association of recent drinking with breast cancer risk can only exclude an association with distant use if the latter is independent of recent use patterns, a most unlikely situation. The associations reported are far too weak and variable to inform conclusively.

Nature of Breast Cancer

Willett et al. (1987b), Hiatt et al. (1988b) and Rohan et al. (1988) report from subgroup analyses that alcohol is associated with a stronger effect among (essentially) premenopausal women. These particular effect modifications are not themselves significant, but demonstrating such effects usually lacks power. If anything, a consistently stronger association between alcohol and breast cancer among premenopausal women is shown. But Ranstam et al. (1995), in Sweden, report a protective effect of alcohol consumption on the occurrence of breast cancer among postmenopausal women, whereas Katsouyanni et al. (1994) find no such interaction. Van den Brandt et al. (1995), studying postmenopausal women in the Netherlands, found a significant trend of breast cancer risk with alcohol use, particularly among those who drink more than 30 g/day. We have already noted the study of Viel et al. (1997), in France, who found an implausibly strong association with wine among premenopausal women.

Swanson et al. (1997), when studying premenopausal women, noted a particularly strong effect of alcohol on advanced disease, that is with regional or distant metastases on diagnosis. Nasca et al. (1994), in New York State, found an association with alcohol to be present among oestrogen receptor-positive tumours and absent among those whose tumour was receptor-negative. These data offer, at best, only weak support for any particular hypothesis.

Nature of the Association

The possibility of confounding the putative relationship between alcohol and breast cancer requires serious examination. Broadly speaking, any association can be deemed causal if, and only if, (1) chance is an unlikely explanation, (2) aspects of selection of the subjects in the study cannot explain the association, and (3) confounding cannot be responsible for the finding.

All published studies report the extent to which chance is a plausible explanation for the observed association, and most make attempts to avoid selection bias. Hence, for this discussion it can be assumed that the literature consists of studies for which the role of chance is well quantified and the problem of subject selection is minimal. Decarli et al. (1997) attempted to remove possible confounding with dietary factors and found a residual effect of alcohol of around a 7% increased risk with each additional 0.4 MJ of alcohol per day. The equivalent increased risk for breast cancer from the consumption of saturated fat was 22%, a factor essentially ignored in the interpretation of the public health consequences.

Confounding is present if a known or unknown risk factor for breast cancer is correlated with alcohol consumption. Whether such confounding can explain the association must, therefore, depend on the extent of the breast cancer risk associated with the confounding variable and its correlation with alcohol use. The problem is, of course, that confounding can involve an unknown risk factor, including aspects of diet as yet unrelated to breast cancer risk. In breast cancer this is particularly important because its aetiology is poorly understood. Variation in known risk factors does not explain a large proportion of the variation in incidence of the disease. This implies that unknown potent risk factors remain, and hence the ability to analyse the true role of confounding is compromised.

Finally, cigarette smoking must be mentioned in the context of this review because of the possibility of a strong correlation between tobacco and alcohol exposure among women. The evidence that might implicate tobacco in the aetiology of breast cancer is extremely weak, however. MacMahon (1990), for instance, in a review of the epidemiology, estimates the RR of breast cancer among smokers to be about 1.14. His review examines the role of alcohol as a confounder in this association and argues, firstly, that alcohol is weakly associated with breast cancer and, secondly, that in those studies of the role of tobacco in which an adjustment for alcohol is made, the relative risk associated with cigarettes is not consistently elevated. Hence, for this discussion, since tobacco is not apparently a risk factor for breast cancer, it cannot be an important confounder in the association of alcohol with breast cancer. Conceivably, tobacco could be a negative confounder if exposure to cigarettes reduces the risk of breast cancer (Baron 1984) and is associated strongly with alcohol use.

Most known risk factors for breast cancer bestow a relative risk of 3 or more. Clearly, in a complicated carcinogenic process, some exposures could be truly primary risk factors with a small RR. For instance, they might only affect the probability of a particular cellular change in a multistage carcinogenic process. However, in epidemiological investigations of breast cancer, RRs of less than 2 for some alleged risk factor should routinely be suspected of confounding by a more potent risk factor. Since the RR for alcohol is almost universally estimated to be about

1.5, confounding remains the strongest candidate for an explanation. These unproven yet plausible arguments in research interpretation are the main barriers to a complete consensus.

Thus, by utilizing the Bradford Hill criteria (1971) for a causal association, we find (and these arguments are strongly supported by Steinberg et al. 1991) that:

1. There is a lack of consistency in the evidence; quite a number of studies do not find any association. There is, however, at least a suggestion of higher risk associated with more than moderate drinking. The particular sub-hypotheses do not stand up to any consistent observation.

2. The associations found are not strong, with relative risks usually of the order of 1.5. For individual higher-point estimates, the confidence limits are often wide and always include low RRs close to unity. Moreover, publication bias or subgroup analyses are likely to explain many of the more extreme estimates of RR. Even the meta-analyses described above give rise to inconsistent RR estimates.

3. Dose-response gradients are observed in several studies, but the gradients are usually not monotonic, the maximum risk level being associated sometimes with intermediate drinking levels. Some of the better studies find an association only with excessive drinking. The one study that examined total alcohol exposure

(La Vecchia et al. 1989) found no dose relationship. On the other hand, the study of Longnecker et al. (1995a) clearly did.

There is certainly no evidence for a consistent pattern, which would be expected in a strong causal association. The key study by Howe et al. (1991) found an effect only at very high reported daily drinking levels. The argument of Smith-Warner (1998) for a linear association using a combination of six prospective cohort studies does not dwell on the demonstrated total absence of increased risk with alcohol use of up to 30 g/day. In the general interpretation of the effects of high drinking levels, it is often assumed that the only difference between these drinkers and their controls is in the level of regular alcohol use. Much evidence suggests, however, that many other aspects of behaviour and life-style are consistently different, and that these might be the actual cause of the observed difference in outcome.

4. Temporal relationships between exposure and risk were examined in five studies. Four found drinking prior to age 25-30 to be associated with risk (Hiatt et al. 1988a, Harvey et al. 1987, Young 1989, Toniolo et al. 1989), and one study found no association (La Vecchia et al. 1989). Several studies found a stronger association with recent use than for distant use of alcohol (Longnecker et al. 1995a, Swanson et al. 1997).

5. Alcohol use should make a contribution that is specific and unambiguously independent of other known risk factors; only a few studies (Schatzkin et al. 1987, Willet et al. 1987a, Rohan et al. 1988, La Vecchia et al. 1989, Rosenberg et al. 1990) adjusted as thoroughly as is feasible for dietary fat intake, which has been regarded as a risk factor. Of course, the meta-analysis by Howe et al. (1991) did adjust for dietary factors, but reported no confounding and inconsistent daily alcohol dose relationships. The role of confounding in the key study of Smith-Warner et al. (1998) remains unclear, since the effect of adjustment for dietary factors is not reported. Furthermore, it is not much discussed by Longnecker (1994). Adjustment for exposure to stress was not seriously attempted in any study.

6. Epidemiological consistency was found in the low breast cancer incidence and low drinking levels in Mormon women (Lyon et al. 1980) and in the findings of rising breast cancer incidence with increasing alcohol use in the USA (Smith 1989, Glass et al.

1988). International and national correlation studies (La Vecchia et al. 1982, 1988, Pochin 1976, Kono et al. 1979, Wynder et al. 1990, Tuyns 1990, Henderson 1990) gave conflicting results, as did studies of breast cancer mortality and alcohol use (Breslow et al. 1974, Pochin 1976, Kono et al. 1979, Monson et al. 1975).

7. If alcohol is accepted as having promotional or co-carcinogenic properties, it is conceivable that it would enhance a response to any direct-acting carcinogens also present in alcoholic beverages. Such compounds have been identified, but their occurrence is variable and always at low concentrations. On a geographical basis, certain beverages produced and consumed in excess in certain localities have been associated with an increased incidence of cancer, mainly of the oesophagus, larynx and pharynx. Usually, however, the increase is small, except in subjects who also smoke cigarettes. The coincidence of these tumour sites with those observed experimentally with diethylnitrosamine and dimethylnitrosamine makes some believe that these compounds might be the prime carcinogens in specific alcoholic beverages. However, the available evidence falls far short of proof (Tuyns et al. 1979). (The evidence for the association of alcohol and these other cancers is reviewed in Appendix 1.) Any extrapolation of such a mechanism to the breast would, therefore, be conjectural.

8. The association between excessive drinking and cancers of the tongue, mouth, larynx and oesophagus is rather strong, but these cancers are linked to a local effect, possibly in association with smoking. In the breast, the evidence for such a local effect cannot exist. Moreover, breast cancer shares no known risk factors with these other cancers.

9. Experimental evidence is not available and not likely to become available; it is difficult to postulate randomized controlled studies of alcohol use.

Conclusions

A causal relationship between alcohol use and breast cancer certainly cannot be confirmed, but also cannot be conclusively excluded. Only few authors conclude that a causal relation is the most plausible explanation for the observed association, although some assume it to be the case (often implicitly). However, the totality of evidence excludes a strong causal association. It is certainly possible that the weak link found is an association only, a consequence of alcohol being related to risk factors (most likely dietary or stress-related factors) that are as yet poorly understood or poorly measured. Although the weak association with moderate drinking is probably a manifestation of confounding, the stronger association at levels consistent with "excessive" drinking may represent a causal association (Katsouyanni et al. 1994), although even here the evidence is not strong.

Thus, research in the area of breast cancer and alcohol must concentrate on the identification of presently poorly understood risk factors that are most likely to explain this association. Of these, aspects of diet appear to be the most plausible, or some other life-style characteristic that is as yet unidentified. Tobacco is an implausible confounding variable.

Many in public health have seen alcohol as a strong contender for breast cancer risk. The common use of alcohol, even with a weak causal association with breast cancer, could explain an important part of the variation in tumour incidence. It is important, however, not to allow hope to triumph over the evidence. Several authors have suggested that some 15% of the incidence of breast cancer could be explained by alcohol use (e.g. Ferrarroni et al. 1998). But this is also misleading because it is based on all alcohol consumption, the majority of which is moderate. To anticipate any change in alcohol use by women to universal abstention is not only totally unrealistic, but also unwise. Counselling women who consume more than two drinks a day to reduce that level of drinking is advisable by any criterion, not least because of the known harmful effects of "excess" alcohol on the liver, pancreas, heart, and possibly some directly exposed cancers (Rubin et al. 1998). The American Cancer Society (ACS) study of half a million people, followed since 1982, is beginning to show a slow increase in all-cause mortality for women at 2 drinks per day (Thun et al. 1997). But if all such women did reduce consumption to below two drinks a day, the attributable effect on total breast cancer incidence, even if entirely causative, could not amount to a 15% reduction. The attributable effect of reducing alcohol use to 2 or 3 drinks a day would only be about 3–5%, even if all the associations at high levels of consumption were causative (McPherson 1998).

More studies are needed to rule out the possibility that the relation-ship between alcohol and breast cancer can be due to confounding; but, while waiting for such evidence, it is worth reflecting on why we are accumulating new epidemiological data, and how and if such evidence could be transferred into practice, in terms of feasible, real-life advice.

The health effects of moderate drinking are confused by a great deal of noise in the epidemiologal literature, whereas the interpretation of such studies is often more certain than the evidence warrants. Alcohol is such a rooted component in the way of life of most populations, that people's attitudes toward it are full of strong and controversial feelings. We should appreciate this situation if we are discussing alcohol risk for diseases such as breast cancer. In this respect, we appear to be not much worried by risks of similar attributable effects, for example, fat intake, with respect to breast cancer, or hormone replacement therapy with respect to cardiovascular disease. We assume that alcohol "per se" is a substance that has to be controlled and its use possibly avoided.

But this very situation should make us cautious when advising "correct" behaviour with respect to alcohol use. Such messages have to be carefully considered, as their implications for behaviour do not necessarily stem from scientific evidence, even if this evidence does point to a causal relationship. Drinking behaviour is not usually determined by the putative or real long-term health consequences.

In fact, what is the possibility of "modulating" alcohol use because of the anticipated risks, in view of (1) its protective effects on cardiovascular disease, (2) the fact that the very concepts of "normal", "moderate" and "excessive" drinking are so different in various countries, and (3) the fact that drinking is so deeply rooted in the culture of the many populations for millennia? On the other side, the emphasis that has been put on the positive effect of alcohol with respect to cardiovascular disease by scientists and by the media, instead of fostering a positive attitude toward moderate drinking, might have an "authorizing effect" on problematic and heavy drinkers, who are always looking for outside justifications for their negative behaviour.

Our investigational strategies might take more account of the behavioural implications of research findings and of the essential necessity to guarantee a reasonable, effective and appropriate use of them. "Pure" research is not affected so much, or so directly, by these problems. However, epidemiology is, by the very fact that it deals with populations and must feed back its results to these populations. It has, therefore, the responsibility to provide for an "added value" to its results: their immediate and concrete predicted usability.

The findings reviewed here do not depend on any particular piece of research, but rather the amalgamation of many studies. It is not clear to us that any hypothesis has received inadequate attention because of the biases of particular researchers, although it is fairly clear that alcohol, as a putative risk factor for serious disease, does attract more attention in some circles than might be appropriate, possibly because of its other social and health associations.

In summary, in spite of very intensive investigation, evidence for a causal relationship between moderate or "social" drinking and breast cancer in women is lacking. Moreover, the relative risks for a causal link at higher drinking levels never exceed 2 and, therefore, are most likely to be seriously compromised by unknown confounders. Hence, it is inappropriate at this time to make any recommendations to reduce moderate alcohol use simply on the basis of its alleged effect on the incidence of breast cancer.

References

Baron JA (1984) Smoking and oestrogen related disease. Am J Epidemiol 119: 9–22

Bowlin SJ, Leske MC, Varma A, et al. (1977) Breast cancer risk and alcohol consumption: results from a large case control study. Int J Epimiol 26: 915–23

Bradford Hill (1971) The environment and disease association or causation. Proc Roy Soc Med: 295–59

Breslow NE, Enstrom JE (1974) Geographic correlations between cancer mortality rates and alcohol-tobacco consumption in the United States. J Natl Cancer Inst 53: 631–39

Brooks PJ (1997) DNA damage, DNA repair and alcohol toxicity. Alcohol Clin Exp Res 21: 1073–82

Bryla CM (1996) The relationship between stress and the development of breast cancer: a literature review. Oncol Nurs Forum 90: 441–48

Casagrande JT, Hanisch R, Pike MC, et al. (1981) A case-control study of male breast cancer. Cancer Res 48: 1326–30

Decarli A, Favero A, La Vecchia, et al. (1997) Macronutrients, energy intake and breast cancer risk: implication for different models. Epidemiology 8: 425–28

Dellarco VL (1988) A mutagenicity assessment of acetaldehyde. Mutat Res 195: 1–20

Dickersin K, Chan S, Chalmers TC, et al. (1987) Publication bias and clinical trials. Contr Clin Trials 8: 343–53

Drife JO (1981) Breast cancer, pregnancy and the pill. Br Med J 283: 78

English DR, Holman CCDJ, Milne E, et al. (1995) The quantification of drug caused morbidity and mortality in Australia. AGPS, Canberra

Ewertz M (1991) Alcohol consumption and breast cancer risk in Denmark. Cancer Causes Control 2: 247–52

Ferraroni et al. (1998) Alcohol and breast cancer: a case control study in Italy. Eur J Cancer 34: 1403–09

Freudenheim JL, Marshall JR, Graham S, et al. (1995) Lifetime alcohol consumption and risk of breast cancer. Nutr Cancer 23: 1–11

Friedenreich CM, Howe GR, Miller AB (1990) Recall bias in the association of diet and breast cancer (abstract). Am J Epidemiol 132: 783

Garfinkel L, Boffetta P, Stellman SD (1988) Alcohol and breast cancer: a cohort study. Prev Med 17: 686–93

Glass A, Hoover RN (1988) Changing incidence of breast cancer. J Natl Cancer Inst 80: 1076–77

Graham S (1987) Alcohol and breast cancer. N Engl J Med 317: 1289

Hankinson SE, Willett WC, Manson, et al. (1995) Alcohol, height and adiposity in relation to estrogen and prolactin levels in postmenopausal women. J Natl Cancer Inst 87: 1297–1302

Harvey EB, Schairer C, Brinton LA, et al. (1987) Alcohol consumption and breast cancer. J Natl Cancer Inst 78: 657–61

Henderson B (1990) Summary report of the sixth symposium on cancer registries and epidemiology in the Pacific Basin. J Natl Cancer Inst 82: 1186–90

Henderson BE, Pike MC, Bernstein L, et al. (1997) Breast cancer. In: Schottenfeld D, Fraumeni JF (eds.), Cancer Epidemiology and Prevention, 2nd ed., Chapter 47. Oxford University Press, New York

Hiatt RA, Klatsky AL, Armstrong MA (1988a) Alcohol consumption and the risk of breast cancer in a prepaid health plan. Cancer Res 48: 2284–87

Hiatt RA, Klatsky AL, Armstrong MA (1988b) Alcohol and breast cancer. Prev Med 17: 683–85

Howe G, Rohan T, Decarli A, et al. (1991) The association between alcohol and breast cancer risk: evidence from the combined analysis of six dietary case-control studies. Int J Cancer 47: 707–10

Hunter DJ, Willett WC (1996) Nutrition and breast cancer. Cancer Causes Control 7: 56–68

Kato I, Tominaga S, Terao CH (1989) Alcohol consumption and cancers of hormone-related organs in females. Jpn J Clin Oncol 19: 202–07

Katsouyanni K, Trichopoulou A, Stuverm S, et al (1994) Ethanol and breast cancer: an association that may be both confounded and causal. Int J Cancer 58: 356–61

Key TJA, Pike MC (1988) The role of oestrogen and progestogens in the epidemiology and prevention of breast cancer. Eur J Cancer Clin Oncol 24: 29–43

Kono S, Ikeda M (1979) Correlation between cancer mortality and alcoholic beverage in Japan. Br J Cancer 40: 449–55

La Vecchia C, Franceschi S (1982) Alcohol and breast cancer (letter). Lancet i: 621

La Vecchia C, Harris RE, Wynder EL (1988) Comparative epidemiology of cancer between the United States and Italy. Cancer Res 48: 7285–93

La Vecchia C, Negri E, Parazzini F, et al. (1989) Alcohol and breast cancer: update from an Italian case control study. Eur J Cancer Clin Oncol 25: 1711–17

Levi F, Pasche C, Lucchini F, et al. (1996) Alcohol and breast cancer in the Swiss Canton of Vaud. Eur J Cancer 32A: 2108–13

Lindegard B (1987) Alcohol and breast cancer (letter). N Engl J Med 317: 1285

Longnecker MP. (1994) Alcoholic beverage consumption in relation to risk of breast cancer: meta-analysis and review. Cancer Causes Control 5: 73–82

Longnecker MP, Berlin JA, Orza MJ, et al. (1988) A meta-analysis of alcohol consumption in relation to risk of breast cancer. JAMA 260: 652–66

Longnecker MP, Berlin J, Orza M, et al. (1989) Meta-analysis of alcohol and risk of breast cancer (letter). JAMA 261: 383

Longnecker MP, Newcomb PA, Mittendorf R, et al. (1995a) Risk of breast cancer in relation to lifetime alcohol consumption. J Natl Cancer Inst 87: 923–29

Longnecker MP, Paganini-Hill A, Ross RK (1995b) Lifetime alcohol consumption and breast cancer risk among postmenopausal women in Los Angeles. Cancer Epidemiol Biomark Prev 1995: 721–25

Lyon JL, Gardner JW, West DW (1980) Cancer incidence in Mormons in Utah during 1917–75. J Natl Cancer Inst 65: 1055–61

MacMahon B (1990) Cigarette smoking and cancer of the breast. In: Wald N, Baron J (eds), Smoking and hormone related disorders. Oxford University Press, Oxford, UK

Martin-Moreno JM, Boyle P, Gorgojo L, et al. (1993) Alcoholic beverage consumption and risk of breast cancer in Spain. Cancer Causes Control 4: 345–53

McPherson K (1998) Editorial: Alcohol and breast cancer. Eur J Cancer 34: 1307–8

McPherson K, Coope P, Vessey M (1986) Early oral contraceptive use and breast cancer theoretical effects of latency. Br J Epidemiol Commun Health 40: 289–94

Monson RR, Lyon JL (1975) Proportional mortality among alcoholics. Cancer 36: 1077–79

Nasca PC, Baptiste MS, Field NA, et al. (1990) An epidemiological case-control study of breast cancer and alcohol consumption. Int J Epidemiol 19: 532–38

Nasca PC, Lui S, Baptiste MS, et al. (1994) Alcohol consumption and breast cancer: estrogen receptor status and histology. Am J Epidemiol 140: 980-87

Newcomb PA, Klein R, Klein BEK, et al. (1995) Association of dietary and life style factors with sex hormones in postmenopausal women. Epidemiology 6: 318–21

Pawlega J. (1992) Breast cancer and smoking, vodka drinking and dietary habits. A case control study. Acta Oncol 31: 387–92

Plant ML (1992) Alcohol and breast cancer: a review. Int J Addict 27: 107–28

Pochin EE (1976) Alcohol and cancer of breast and thyroid (letter). Lancet i: 1137

Ranstam J, Olsson H. (1995) Alcohol, cigarette smoking, and the risk of breast cancer. Cancer Det Prev 19: 487–93

Rathje W, Murphy C (1992) Rubbish: the archeology of garbage. Harper-Collins, London/Glasgow

Redd WH, Silverfarb PM, Anderson BL, et al. (1991) Physiological and psychobehavioural research in oncology. Cancer 67: 813–22

Ristow H, Obe G (1978) Acetaldehyde induces cross-links in DNA and causes sister-chromatid exchanges in human cells. Mutat Res 58: 115–19

Rohan TE, Cook MG (1989) Alcohol consumption and risk of benign proliferative epithelial disorders of the breast in women. Int J Cancer 43: 631–36

Rohan TE, McMichael AJ (1988) Alcohol consumption and risk of breast cancer. Int J Cancer 41: 695–99

Rosenberg L, Palmer JR, Miller DR, et al. (1990) A case-control study of alcoholic beverage consumption and breast cancer. Am J Epidemiol 131: 6–14

Roth HD, Levy PS, Shi L, et al. (1994) Alcoholic beverages and breast cancer: some observations on published case-control studies. J Clin Epidemiol 47: 207–16

Royo-Bordonada MA, Martin- Moreno JM, Guallar E, et al. (1997) Alcohol intake and the risk of breast cancer: the EURAMIC study. Neoplasia 44: 150–56

Rubin E (1996) The questionable link between alcohol intake and cancer. Clin Chim Acta 246: 143–48

Rubin E, Hutterer F, Lieber CS (1968) Ethanol increases hepatic smooth endo-plasmic reticulum and drug metabolising enzymes. Science 159: 1469–70

Rubin E, Farber JF (1998) Pathology. Lippincott-Raven, Philadelphia, PA

Schatzkin A, Jones DY, Hoover RN, et al. (1987) Alcohol consumption and breast cancer in the epidemiologic follow-up study of the first National Health and Nutrition Examination Survey. N Engl J Med 316: 1169–73

Schatzkin A, Longnecker MP (1994) Alcohol and breast cancer. Where are we now and where do we go from here? Cancer 74 (suppl): 1101–10

Schrauzer GN, McGuiness JE, Ishmael D, et al. (1979) Effects of long term exposure to alcohol on spontaneous mammary adenocarcinoma and prolactin levels in C3H/St mice. J Stud Alcohol 40: 240–46

Smith DI (1989) Relationship between alcohol consumption and breast cancer morbidity rates in Western Australia 1971. Drug Alcohol Depend 24: 61–65

Smith SJ, Deacon JM, Chilvers CED (1994) Alcohol, smoking, passive smoking and caffeine in relation to breast cancer risk in young women. Br J Cancer 70: 112–19

Smith-Warner SA, Spiegelman D, Yuan S, et al. (1998) Alcohol and breast cancer in women. A pooled analysis of cohort studies. JAMA 279: 535

Sneyd MJ, Paul C, Spears GFS, et al. (1991) Alcohol consumption and risk of breast cancer. Int J Cancer 48: 812–15

Steinberg J, Goodwin PJ (1991) Alcohol and breast cancer risk (review). Breast Cancer Res Treatm 19: 221–31

Swanson CA, Coates RJ, Malone KE, et al. (1997) Alcohol consumption and breast cancer risk among women under age 45 years. Epidemiology 8: 231–37

Talamini R, La Vecchia C, Decarli A, et al. (1984) Social factors, diet and breast cancer in a northern Italian population. Br J Cancer 49: 723–29

Thun MJ, Peto R, Lopez AD, et al. (1997) Alcohol consumption and mortality among middle aged and elderly US adults. New Engl J Med 337: 1705–14

Toniolo P, Riboli E, Protta F, et al. (1989) Breast cancer and alcohol consumption: a case-control study in northern Italy. Cancer Res 49: 5203–06

Tuyns AJ (1990) Alcohol-related cancers in Mediterranean countries. Tumori 76: 315–20

Tuyns AJ, Pequignot G, Abbatucci JS (1979) Oesophageal cancer and alcoholic consumption. Importance of the type of beverage. Int J Cancer 23: 443–47

van den Brandt PA, Goldbohm RA, van 't Veer P (1995) Alcohol and breast cancer: results from the Netherlands Cohort Study. Am J Epidemiol 141: 907–15

van 't Veer P, Kok FJ, Hermus RJJ, et al. (1989) Alcohol dose, frequency and age at first exposure in relation to the risk of breast cancer. Int J Epidemiol 18: 511–17

Viel JF, Perarnau JM, Challier B, et al. (1997) Alcoholic calories, red wine consumption and breast cancer among premenopausal women. Eur J Epidemiol 13: 639–43

Webster LA, Wingo PA, Layde P, et al. (1983) Alcohol consumption and risk of breast cancer. Lancet ii: 724–26

Willett WC, Stampfer MJ, Colditz GA, et al. (1987a) Moderate alcohol consumption and the risk of breast cancer. N Engl J Med 316: 1174–80

Willett WC, Stampfer MJ, Colditz GA, et al. (1987b) Alcohol and breast cancer (letter). N Engl J Med 317: 1288–89

Williams RR, Horm JW (1977) Association of cancer sites with tobacco and alcohol consumption and socioeconomic status of patients: interview study from the Third National Cancer Survey. J Natl Cancer Inst 58: 525–47

Wynder EL, Fujita Y, Harris RE, et al. (1990) Comparative epidemiology of cancer between the United States and Japan. Cancer 67: 746–63

Ylikahri RH, Huttunen MO, Harkman M (1976) Effect of alcohol on anterior-pituitary secretion of trophic hormones (letter). Lancet i: 1353

Young TH (1989) A case-control study of breast cancer and alcohol consumption habits. Cancer 64: 552–58

Zaridze D, Lifanova Y, Maximovitch D, et al. (1991) Diet, alcohol consumption and reproductive factors in a case-control study of breast cancer in Moscow. Int J Cancer 48: 493–501

Acknowledgement

The authors are very grateful for able research assitance and advice from Ms Annie Britton of the Health Promotion Sciences Unit at the London School of Hygiene and Tropical Medicine.

Chapter 8

Alcohol and Bone

P. Charles
Amtssygehus, Aarhus, Denmark

K. Laitinen
Nakinkaari, Finland

A. Kardinaal
TNO Nutrition and Food Research Institute,
Zeist, The Netherlands

Abstract

Osteoporosis is a disease with significant morbidity, mortality and economic impact. The incidence of osteoporotic fractures (such as hip fractures) has increased in most industrialized countries in recent years. Only part of this increase can be explained by the increase in mean age of the population. Thus, factors connected with life-style and nutrition have been suggested as being linked to this increase. Among these is alcohol which has been associated with osteoporosis and osteoporotic fractures; many studies suggest it can interfere with bone metabolism.

The aim of this review is to discuss critically the connection between alcohol use, bone and mineral metabolism, bone quality and fractures. A low-energy fracture may be considered as the ultimate event and an excellent surrogate measure for osteoporosis. However, fractures are not only caused by poor bone quality but also by the propensity to fall.

Animal studies have shown that alcohol can cause many kinds of disturbances in mineral metabolism; it affects the quality of bone and decreases bone strength in animals. In man, acute alcohol intoxication causes profound but short-term changes in bone and mineral metabolism. Long-term moderate drinking does not seem to impair bone or mineral metabolism or to increase fracture risk. Chronic alcohol abuse, on the other hand, causes profound changes in bone and mineral metabolism, decreases bone mineral content and increases fracture risk.

The effects of alcohol on human bone depend on the alcohol dose and the duration of its use. Acute alcohol intoxication causes dose-dependent changes in mineral metabolism and depresses bone formation. Moderate drinking does not change mineral metabolism, but it does decrease bone formation as evaluated by serum markers. The relation between moderate alcohol use and bone mass gives an inconsistent picture, and this also holds true for fracture risk. Chronic alcohol abuse causes profound changes in mineral metabolism, it leads to deranged bone quality ("low-turnover osteoporosis"), may adversely affect bone mass, and clearly increases propensity to fall and with subsequent fractures.

In alcoholics there are several confounding factors (such as vitamin D deficiency, hypogonadism, hypomagnesaemia, liver disease and myopathy) which have a variable impact on the status of bone in addition to the direct effect of alcohol. Some studies on the relationship between alcohol and bone have been poorly controlled for these confounders, and additional prospective human data are needed.

Introduction

A consensus development conference has defined osteoporosis as "a systemic skeletal disease characterized by low bone mass and micro-architectural deterioration with a consequent increase in bone fragility and susceptibility to fracture risk". This definition is very difficult to apply to the individual patient, and therefore a working group of the World Health Organization has defined osteoporosis as a bone mineral density (T-score) that is 2.5 SD below the mean peak value in young adult women (Kanis et al. 1994). This definition also has its limitations in clinical practice because it uses the risk factor for fracture as a diagnostic criterion and ignores the importance of other determinants of bone strength. Since the WHO definition there has been much discussion as to whether this definition should be used for the individual patient. Nonetheless, the clinical significance of osteoporosis lies in the fractures that arise, and in the following discussion on the connection between alcohol and osteoporosis, a fracture will be the ultimate event used to evaluate such a connection.

Osteoporosis affects an estimated 75 million people in Europe, the USA and Japan (Anonymous 1997). Common sites of fractures are the spine, the distal forearm and the hip. Osteoporotic fractures occurring at the spine and the forearm are associated with significant morbidity, but the most serious consequences arise in patients with hip fractures, which are associated with a decrease in life expectancy by up to 18%, mostly due to excessive mortality during the 6 months after the fracture (Cooper et al. 1993). The lifetime risk of sustaining a hip fracture has been estimated to be 15% for white women and 5% for white men (Cummings et al. 1985). The risk for other types of osteoporotic fractures are nearly as high, so that the combined risk is 40% (Melton et al. 1991). The total medical costs per patient in Sweden has been estimated to be around USD 10,000 (Borgquist et al. 1991). The number of hip fractures occurring in the world in 1990 has been estimated to be 1.7 million and is expected to reach 6.3 millions by the year 2025 (Cooper et al. 1992).

The risk of fracture depends on bone strength and trauma. Some of the different determinants for fractures are shown in Figure 1.

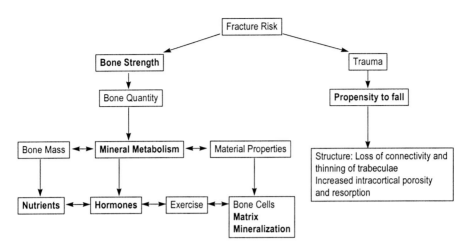

Figure 1
Risk factors for osteoporotic fractures
(factors influenced by alcohol are in bold).

Bone Metabolism

Normal Bone Metabolism

Bone is renewed throughout life through a process called remodelling. After peak bone mass has been attained about 10% on average is renewed every year. Remodelling ensures continuous removal of old bone and adapts its material properties to the mechanical demands placed on it. Remodelling also maintains the biomechanical competence of the skeleton by preventing the accumulation of microstructural damage. Moreover, bone constitutes a reservoir for mineral homeostasis.

The cells responsible for bone remodelling are the osteoclasts and the osteoblasts. Osteoclasts are the bone-resorbing cells formed in the bone marrow from cells of the monocyte lineage. The maturation of osteoclasts is under the influence of factors like vitamin D and parathyroid hormone (PTH) as well as many local growth factors (Figure 2). The bone-forming cells, the osteoblasts, are of mesenchymal origin and arise from stem cells in the bone marrow. Differentiation is stimulated by many hormones and growth factors including thyroid hormones, PTH and growth hormone.

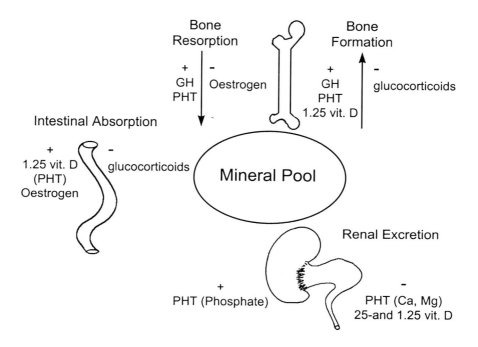

Figure 2
Effects of various hormones on bone mineral metabolism

The remodelling sequence is initiated by stimulation of osteoclasts resorbing bone for about 2 weeks. Later on, the bone is resorbed by macrophages which lasts for another 2 weeks. Resorption usually stops at a depth of 40 to 60 μm. After the resorption period of about 1 month, the resorption lacunae are invaded by the osteoblasts. These cells produce matrix which later mineralizes, and new bone is formed. The work of the osteoblasts lasts for about 3 months. The concept of bone remodelling, first described by Frost (1964, 1969), was based on the hypothesis that resorption is coupled to formation. Bone, compared to other organs, is characterized by relatively few cells and a preponderance of extracellular matrix. The matrix contains inorganic (mainly hydroxyapatite crystals) and organic (mainly collagen) components. Bone tissue is divided into cortical and trabecular bone. Of the skeletal mass in the young individual 80% is cortical bone and 20% is trabecular bone (Parfitt 1989).

The mechanisms underlying age-related bone loss and metabolic bone disease have been elucidated through histomorphometric studies (Eriksen et al 1989). In trabecular bone, a reversible loss of bone may occur if the activation frequency is increased, i.e. the number of active resorption lacunae is increased (increased remodelling space). Irreversible bone loss occurs in two ways, either through thinning of the trabeculae due to a negative balance in the remodelling sequence or through perforations of the trabeculae. In cortical bone, reversible bone loss (increased porosity) is seen when the number of remodelling Haversian canals increases due to an increased activation frequency. Irreversible bone loss in cortical bone occurs predominantly at the interface between cortical and trabecular bone, where cortical bone can be turned into trabecular bone (thinning of the cortex).

Peak bone mass is usually achieved around the age of 18 to 30 years. After the age of 35 bone is lost due to escalating changes in the balance between resorption and formation. The estimated loss is 0.5–1% per year with a tendency to a greater loss rate in women. Men lose 27% of trabecular bone volume before the age of 80 years whereas women lose 41%. The greater loss in women is caused by an increase in activation frequency of remodelling units and a more pronounced negative balance around the menopause (2–4% loss per year). The changes with increasing age are not of the same magnitude in cortical bone, but porosity increases and cortical width is either unchanged or reduced. The changes described are also reflected in measurements of bone mineral content (BMC). In normal women an age-related decrease in BMC occurs.

Biochemical Markers of Bone Metabolism

Osteocalcin is a vitamin K-dependent protein synthesized by osteoblasts and released into the circulation. Its concentration in serum is elevated in states of high osteoblastic activity and bone formation and reduced in states of diminished bone synthesis.

Alkaline phosphatase (ALP) is a marker of bone formation and can be separated into two fractions, a liver-related and a bone-related fraction. ALP levels are increased in metabolic bone diseases such as osteomalacia. In Paget's disease there is increased activity of osteoblasts.

Urinary excretion of hydroxyproline (HOP), pyridinoline (PYR) and deoxypyridinoline (DPYR) are the main markers of bone resorption. These proteins are excreted in urine during bone resorption processes and hence are a quantitative measure of bone resorption (Bilezikian et al 1996).

Effects of Alcohol on Bone

EFFECTS OF ALCOHOL ON BONE DENSITY AND FRACTURE RISK

The remodelling sequence may be affected by alcohol at different stages. Alcohol may affect osteoblast activity and numbers as well as osteoclast activity and numbers, thereby creating a negative, an unchanged or a positive balance per remodelling unit. Ethanol inhibits protein synthesis of rat bones (Preedy et al. 1991) and causes a reduced mineral content and decreased cortical thickness of bone (Preedy et al. 1991). The skeletal development of foetuses of rats consuming alcohol during gestation is delayed (Lee et al. 1983).

Chronic exposure to high alcohol doses adversely affects the bone of developing and adult animals (Keiver et al. 1996). In rats, alcohol reduces the development of foetal body weight and skeletal ossification (Keiver et al. 1996, 1997). Also in mice, alcohol lead to malformations of many organ systems including the skeleton (Padmanabhan et al. 1985). Moreover, alcohol delays bone and general growth of young rats (Saville et al. 1965, Lee et al. 1983, Weinberg et al. 1990, Sampson et al. 1996). One report on growing rats showed that moderate alcohol consumption had a beneficial effect on bone strength and mineral density (Yamamoto et al. 1997). Others have found moderate alcohol consumption not to augment ovariectomy-induced bone loss (Sampson et al. 1997b).

In rats treated chronically with ethanol an increased incidence of tibial fractures and decreased bone strength was reported (Peng et al. 1982, 1988, 1991, Kusy et al. 1989). The femurs of rats fed an alcohol-containing liquid diet for four weeks were not only weaker but also less energy-absorbing (Kusy et al. 1989). In another study (Hogan et al. 1997) bone stiffness, strength and energy absorbed to fracture were significantly lower in alcohol-fed rats but, obviously, data from animal studies do not necessarily apply to man.

In the past decade, determinants of bone density and fracture risk have been evaluated in amany population-based human studies, with populations ranging from just over a hundred to more than 80,000. In many of these studies, alcohol use has been included as one of the potential determinants (Table 1) In general, drinking levels in these studies were low to moderate and most study samples did not include large numbers of heavy drinkers. As the effect of moderate drinking may be different from the effect of excessive drinking, the population-based studies will be discussed separately from studies in alcoholics.

Table 1
Human studies of effects of alcohol on bone and mineral metabolism (only pure histomorphometric studies are included)

Study	Study design	Study population	Results attributable to alcohol
Linkola et al. 1979	cross-over	7 healthy volunteers	increase in CA and MG and decrease in cAMP excretion
Avery et al. 1983	prospective	alcoholics/non-alcoholics	decrease in total Ca and Ca^{2+}
Ljunghall et al. 1985	prospective	12 normal men	no change in serum PTH, Ca or Pi with an alcohol dose of 0.8 g/kg
Bjoerneboe et al. 1986, 1987	cross-sectional	13 alcoholics, 19 controls	decrease in α-tocopherol, selenium and 25-hydroxy-cholecalciferol
Bjoerneboe et al. 1988	cross-sectional	34 alcoholics, 35 controls	decrease in serum 25-hydroxy- and 1,25-dihydroxychole-calciferol
Diamond et al. 1989b	cross-sectional	28 drinkers, 12 abstainers, 35 controls	decrease in forearm and spinal BMD, decrease in cancellous bone areas and osteoblastic activity, decrease in osteocalcin
Nielsen et al. 1990	cross-sectional	6 normal volunteers	dose-dependent decerase in serum osteocalcin
Laitinen et al. 1990	cross-sectional, controlled	38 non-cirrhotic male alcoholics, 2 control groups	decrease in serum 25-hydroxy-, 1,25-dihydroxy- and 24,25-dihydroxycholecalciferol, no change in BMD
Laitinen et al. 1991a	cross-over	17 normal men, 7 normal women	transient decrease in PTH with a rebound increase, decrease in serum Ca^{2+} and Pi, increase in serum and urinary Mg, slight and delayed increase in urinary Pi
Laitinen et al. 1991b	prospective, controlled	10 normal men	decrease in osteocalcin during 3 weeks of alcohol use, increase in PTH
Lindholm et al. 1991	cross-sectional	20 alcohol abusers, 17 abstainers	no differences in bone mass, low-turnover osteoporosis in histomorphometry, lower PTH, 1,25-dihydroxycholecalciferol and osteocalcin
Laitinen et al. 1992b	cross-over	6 normal men	hypoparathyroidism, hyper-calciuria and hypermagnesuria are dose-dependent
Pepersack et al. 1992	prospective, controlled, 2-week follow-up	12 alcoholic men, 15 controls	decrease in osteocalcin, increase in HOP, increase in renal threshold of Pi excretion, rapid increase in osteocalcin during withdrawal

Table 1 (continued)

Laitinen et al. 1992a	cross-sectional, controlled, 2-week withdrawal	27 non-cirrhotic male alcoholics, three control groups	decrease in osteocalcin and PICP with normalization during withdrawal, increase in Ca^{2+} during withdrawal, decrease in BMD in parallel with length of drinking history
Laitinen et al. 1993	cross-sectional, controlled, 2-week withdrawal	19 non-cirrhotic female alcoholics, three control groups	decrease in serum 25-hydroxy- and 1,25-dihydroxycholecalciferol, decrease in osteocalcin with rapid normalization, increase in Ca^{2+} during withdrawal
Gonzalez-Galvin et al. 1993	cross-sectional, short follow-up	26 heavy drinkers, 13 moderate drinkers, 19 abstainers	decrease in ostocalcin and BMD
Laitinen et al. 1994	cross-sectional, controlled	26 alcohol-intoxicated men, 19 controls	decrease in Ca^{2+}, no difference in PTH, decrease in osteocalcin, increase in ICTP
Garcia-Sanchez et al. 1995	prospective	8 healthy volunteers	decrease in PTH and osteocalcin, increase in serum Pi, urinary Ca and urinary Mg
Nyquist et al. 1996	cross-sectional, 10-day follow-up	18 alcoholic men, 18 male abstainers, 29 male controls	decrease in osteocalcin at start of withdrawal, normalization during observation, high osteocalcin in abstainers, increase in urinary DPYR

cAMP, cyclic AMP; PTH, parathyroid hormone; BW, body weight; BMD, bone mineral density; HOP, hydroxyproline; PICP, procollagen I carboxy-terminal telopeptide; DPYR, deoxypyridinoline; Pi, inorganic phosphate.

A limited number of human follow-up studies have been reported (Hansen et al. 1991, Nguyen et al. 1996, Slemenda et al. 1992, Sowers et al. 1992, 1993) in which bone mineral density (BMD) was measured twice. This offered the opportunity to look at the relation between alcohol consumption and change in BMD. Sowers (1992, 1993) did not find an association between the quantity of alcohol drunk and the change in BMD of the radius during 5 years of follow-up, neither in pre- and perimenopausal women nor in postmenopausal women. Hansen et al. (1991) observed a reduced rate of radial bone loss among postmenopausal women who drank alcohol regularly compared to women who did not. A similar finding was reported by Nguyen et al. (1996) in a study among elderly men with bone loss in the femoral neck, but not in the spine. These studies (Hansen et al. 1991, Nguyen et al. 1996) did not mention whether there was a dose-reponse relationship among the subjects who used alcohol. The opposite finding has also been reported (Slemenda et al. 1992): higher alcohol consumption was associated with an increased rate of radial bone loss among elderly men.

Most studies have a cross-sectional design: alcohol consumption was measured at the same time as BMD. Generally, the questionnaires or interviews used to assess alcohol use aim at estimating habitual use over a long period of time. Most of these studies reported no association between alcohol use and BMD (Bauer et al.1993, Elders et al. 1989, Erdtsieck et al. 1994, Franceschi et al. 1996, Glynn et al. 1995, Krall et al. 1993, Kröger et al. 1992, Reid et al. 1992, Salamone et al. 1996, Shaw et al. 1993, Yano et al. 1985, Young et al. 1995). Several studies have found a positive association between alcohol use and BMD (Felson et al. 1995, Holbrook et al. 1993, May et al. 1995, Angus et al. 1988, Kröger et al. 1994, Laitinen et al. 1991c, New et al. 1997, Orwoll et al. 1996). The results of Angus et al. (1988) and Laitinen et al. (1991c) appear to be contradictatory; they both studied pre- and postmenopausal women in the same age range. Angus et al. (1988) reported a positive association between alcohol use and trochanter BMD in premenopausal, but not in postmenopausal women (after multivariate adjustment). Laitinen et al. (1991c) reported the opposite, namely a higher BMD of the lumbar spine and Ward's triangle being associated with alcohol in postmenopausal women, but not in premenopausal drinkers. In fact, the BMD of Ward's triangle was lower among premenopausal women who drank alcohol. Similarly, Stevenson et al. (1989) reported an inverse association between the amount of alcohol consumed and BMD of the lumbar spine and proximal femur among premenopausal women and no effect among postmenopausal women.

Several groups (Holbrook et al. 1993, Kröger et al. 1994, New et al. 1997, Orwoll et al. 1996) found a dose-dependent higher BMD of the lumbar spine in women who used alcohol, but no significant associations with femoral BMD (at least not after multivariate adjustment). In men (May et al. 1995, Holbrook et al. 1993) drinkers had a higher hip BMD, but not a higher BMD of the lumbar spine. In other studies in men (Glynn et al. 1995, Kröger et al. 1992, Nguyen et al. 1996), no association between alcohol use and BMD was found. In the Framingham study (Felson et al.

1995) women who drank more than 207 ml alcohol per week had higher bone densities at most sites than women in the lightest drinking category (<30 ml/week). Men who were heavy drinkers (>414 ml/week) also had higher bone densities than light drinkers, but the difference was less pronounced than in women. Lower levels of intake were not related to bone density, so a dose-reponse relationship could not be established. The Framingham study is one of the few in which relatively heavy drinkers were represented in reasonably large numbers. In most studies heavy drinkers form only a small part of the population. The absence of heavy drinkers may lead to the finding of a difference between drinkers and non-drinkers but no dose-response relationship among the drinkers. In many of the studies the average use of alcoholic beverages was less than 1 drink per day and only rarely did the quantity consumed in the high drinking categories exceed the average of 2 drinks per day (Stevenson et al. 1989, Kröger et al. 1994, Holbrook et al. 1993, Hernandez-Avila et al. 1991, Felson et al. 1995, Fehily et al. 1992, Elders et al. 1989), especially in studies among women.

Table 2 summarizes prospective and case-control studies which have evaluated the relation between moderate drinking and fracture risk. Most case-control studies performed in white populations found no association (Cumming et al. 1994, Grisso et al. 1991, Johnell et al. 1995, Kreiger et al. 1992, Paganini-Hill et al. 1981). An early case-control study in male patients with vertebral fractures found an increased risk among male drinkers (Seeman et al. 1983). Similarly, an increased risk of hip fracture was found for men having 3 or more drinks per day, compared to men drinking less or nothing at all (Grisso et al. 1991). Black women who had 7 or more drinks per week had a 4–5 times higher risk of hip fracture than non-drinkers (Grisso et al.1994). In a Japanese study (Suzuki et al. 1997), a decreased risk was observed for men and women who drank up to 27 g alcohol per day (roughly less than 3 drinks). The decreased risk at higher intakes was not statistically significant. In contrast, in a Hong Kong population, daily alcohol use was associated with an increased risk of hip fracture (Lau et al. 1988).

Table 2
Epidemiological studies on moderate alcohol use and fracture risk

Study	Design[a]	Study population	Drinking level	Fracture studied	Drinking category	RR (95% CI)[b]
Cummings et al. 1994	CC	women: 174 cases, 137 controls; men: 35 cases, 70 controls; mean age 65	?	hip	no alcohol	1.0
					<7 drinks/wk	0.7 (0.5–1.2)
					>7 drinks/wk	0.6 (0.3–1.3)
Cummings et al. 1995	PR (4.1 yrs)	9516 women, mean age 65 years	?	hip	abstainers	1.0
					drinkers	0.7 (0.5–0.9)
					<7 drinks/wk	0.7 (0.5–0.9)
					>7 drinks/wk	0.9 (0.5–1.4)
Felson et al. 1988	PR (35 yrs)	5209 men and women aged 68–96	light <30 ml/wk (men 26%, women 54%)	hip	light	1.0
			moderate 59–177 ml/wk (men 25%, women 15%)		moderate	men 0.8 (0.3–1.8), women 1.3 (0.9–1.9)
			heavy >207 ml/wk (men 25%, women 10%)		heavy	men 1.3 (0.6–2.5), women 1.5 (0.9–2.6)
Fujiwara et al. 1997	PR	1586 men and 2987 women aged 58±12	regular, 78% of men, 34% of women, mean use 35 g/day (men) and 9 g/day (women)	hip	regular	men+women 1.9 (1.1–3.4) women 2.4 (1.3–4.4)
Grisso et al. 1991	CC	women, 174 cases, 174 controls, aged 50–103	?	hip	no association with fractures	
Grisso et al. 1994	CC	women, 144 cases and 218 controls, mean age 45	86% 0–1 drinks/wk, 8% 2–6 drinks/wk, 6% ≥7 drinks/wk	hip	2–6 drinks/wk ≥7 drinks/wk	2.0 (0.8–5.0) 4.6 (1.5–14)

Table 2 (continued)

Hemenway 1988	PR (4 yrs)	96,508 women aged 30–55 in 1976	30% 0 g/d, 12% 0–1.5 g/d, 20% 1.5–5 g/d, 19% 5–15 g/d, 13% ≥15 g/d	hip and forearm	≥15 g/d, relative to abstainers and light drinkers	1.2 (1.0–1.5) 1.7 (1.3–2.3) for low BW combined with heavy drinking
Hemenway 1994b	PR (6 yrs)	49,895 men aged 40–75 in 1986	? 4% >50 g/d	wrist	no association with fractures	
Hemenway 1994a	PR (6 yrs)	51,529 men aged 40–75 in 1986	? 4% >50 g/d	hip	no association with fractures	
Hernandez-Avila et al. 1991	PR (6 yrs)	84,484 women aged 39–59 in 1980	32% 0 g/d, 34% 0.1–5 g/d, 20% 5–15 g/d, 7% 15–25 g/d, 7% ≥25 g/d	hip arm	≥25 g/d ≥25 g/d	2.3 (1.2–4.6) P for trend 0.04 1.4 (1.1–1.7) P for trend 0.08
Huang et al. 1996	PR	2513 women, mean age 45	14.3% 2–3 times/wk	hip	no association with fractures	
Johnell et al. 1995	CC	women, 2086 cases, 3532 controls, age 78±9	daily use 24.3%	hip	daily use moderate use of spirits in young adulthood	1.2 (0.9–1.3) 0.7 (0.6–0.8)
Nguyen et al. 1996	PR	820 men, mean age 60	?	low trauma	drinkers	0.7 (0.7–0.8) n.s. in multivariate analysis
Seeman et al. 1983	CC	men: 105 cases, 105 controls aged 44–85	drinkers: controls 70%, cases 82%	vertebral fracture	abstainers drinkers	1.0 2.4, dose-response relation
Suzuki et al. 1997	CC	249 cases, 498 controls, men/women, age 65–90	?	hip	abstainers <27 g/d ≥27 g/d	1.0 0.5 (0.3–0.9) 0.8 (0.3–1.8)
Tuppurainen et al. 1995	PR (2.4 yrs)	3140 women aged 53±3	32±84 g/wk	low trauma wrist all fractures wrist	drinkers ≥100 g/wk vs. <100 ≥100 g/wk	1.4 (1.0–2.0) no assoc. 1.7 (1.1–2.7) 2.1 (1.0–4.6)

[a] CC, case-control study; PR, prospective (cohort study). In parenthesis: number of follow-up years.

[b] Relative risk (95% confidence interval).

Prospective studies are inconclusive as well. Some studies found no association with either hip fracture (Hemenway et al. 1994b, Huang et al. 1996), wrist fracture (Hemenway et al. 1994a) or all fractures (Nguyen et al. 1996) and some reported a positive association (Felson et al. 1988, Hemenway et al. 1988, Hernandez-Avila et al. 1991, Fujiwara et al. 1997, Tuppurainen et al. 1995). However, Felson et al. (1988) report an increased risk of hip fractures at moderate and heavy drinking levels among men and women younger than 65, but not in older subjects.

There are two reports from the Nurses' Health Study. The first (Hemenway et al. 1988) reported a 24% increased combined risk of hip and forearm fractures among women who consumed more than 15 g of alcohol daily and had a low body weight. This study, reported after 4 years of follow-up, was replicated by Hernandez-Avila et al. (1991) after 6 years of follow-up, with separate analyses for hip and forearm fractures. In the highest drinking category (25 g/day), compared to abstainers, there was a significantly increased risk of both hip (RR 2.33) and forearm fractures (RR 1.38), with a significant linear trend with drinking categories for hip fracture. This study included only women under 65 years of age. A Finnish study (Tuppurainen et al. 1995) also reported an increased risk of fractures among drinking perimenopausal women. The only study reporting a reduced risk of hip fractures for women consuming 7 drinks per week or less in comparison with abstainers was performed among white women over 65 years of age (Cummings et al. 1985).

The relation between alcohol abuse and either bone density or fracture risk has been investigated in two different types of studies. In a few studies (Nilsson 1970; Horak et al. 1975, Hutchinson et al. 1979, Nordqvist et al. 1996), fracture incidence has been compared with healthy controls with respect to the prevalence of alcoholism. In these studies, which were true case-control studies, an odds ratio (or relative risk) can be calculated for the risk of fracture in alcohol abusers, but not the absolute risk of fracture. In the other type of study, alcoholics are cross-sectionally compared with controls (moderate drinkers) with respect to differences in (absolute) prevalence of fractures or bone mass. Nilsson (1970) reported a relatively high number of alcoholics among male patients with hip fracture (19%), compared to 2% in the control group. A somewhat smaller but significant difference was reported for women with hip or wrist fracture: 11.5% alcoholics among the cases and 3.2% among the controls (Hutchinson et al. 1979). In a large study in male and female patients with fractures of the upper humerus (Horak et al. 1975) smaller but still significant differences were observed: severe alcoholism in 1.4% of the cases and 0% of control subjects, the differences being greater in men under 65. A recent study (Nordqvist et al. 1996) showed that 12% of all patients with shoulder fractures and dislocations abused alcohol, compared to 3% of age- and sex-matched controls. For men in the same study, the proportions were 24% and 7%, respectively.

A number of studies have shown that the risk of fractures is increased among alcoholics (Crilly et al. 1988, Israel et al. 1980, Johnson et al. 1984, Kristensson et al. 1980, Lindsell et al. 1982, Wilkinson et al. 1985, Peris et al. 1995a). Kristensson et al. (1980) found that fractures were about four times more common among alcoholics than in an age-matched control group. Israel et al. (1980) found that 29% of male alcoholics had fractures of ribs or thoracic spine, against only 2% in the control group. On the other hand, in a study by Johnson et al. (1984) only 9% of cirrhotic alcoholics and 3% of other liver patients had rib fractures. More recently, Peris et al. (1995b) reported a prevalence of 61% for peripheral fractures in 76 male alcoholics compared to 3% in the age-matched control group.

The evidence from these studies clearly indicates that alcoholics have an increased risk of fractures in general. To evaluate whether this is mediated by an adverse effect on bone mineral density, studies on alcoholism and bone density will be considered. Many studies report reduced bone mass or bone density among male alcoholics compared to healthy controls, but the relation was not conclusively established. In the past decade, several well-designed studies did not find any differences in bone density between alcoholics and healthy controls (Bjoerneboe et al. 1988, Harding et al. 1988, Lindholm et al. 1991, Laitinen et al. 1990, 1992a, Odvina et al.1995). Bikle (1993) suggested that this absence of any differences may be attributed to the relatively young age of the subjects in most of these studies. This was supported by the observation that, although bone density in alcoholics was not different from controls, bone density decreased with increasing duration of alcohol abuse in the groups of alcoholics (Laitinen et al. 1992a, b, Odvina et al. 1995).

The impact of chronic alcohol abuse on bone density in women has been studied by a few groups. Clark (1996) reported a 7% decrease in BMD of the femoral neck and lumbar spine in 25 premenopausal alcoholic women compared to an equal number of control subjects matched for age, height and weight. However, this difference disappeared when the analysis was restricted to subjects matched for smoking status. Laitinen et al. (1993a) did not observe differences in BMD of the spine and proximal femur, or in BMC of the forearm, between premenopausal alcoholics and healthy controls. In contrast to the relationship of BMD with history of alcohol abuse among men, BMD was similar in female alcoholics with a drinking history of less than 5 years and more than 5 years. In general, the duration of alcohol abuse in men was longer than in women. Monegal et al. (1997) compared BMD in patients with cirrhosis from other causes and in alcoholics; alcoholics had a significantly lower BMD of the proximal femur than patients with cirrhosis.

Another question is whether loss of BMD by alcohol abuse is reversible. Lindholm et al. (1991) compared BMC of the distal forearm and lumbar spine in 11 men who had drunk at least 72 g of ethanol per day for at least 5 years and in 9 men who had drunk the same amount but had abstained for the last 2 years. No differences were observed. However, Peris et al. (1994) performed a follow-up study in 30 alcoholic men, who drank 140–400 g alcohol daily for an average of 27 years. Lumbar spine BMD was lower in the alcoholics than in age-matched controls. After 2 years of abstinence, BMD (both in the spine and femur) had significantly increased in the ex-alcoholics, while it had decreased in the control group.

EFFECTS OF ALCOHOL ON BIOCHEMICAL MARKERS OF BONE METABOLISM

Markers of Bone Formation

There are few data on the effect of ethanol on markers of bone metabolism in animals. Acute or more prolonged alcohol intoxication decreased serum level of osteocalcin in rats (Diez et al. 1997, Peng et al. 1991,Keiver et al. 1996). Lowering of osteocalcin has not, however, been found consistently in all studies (Thomas et al. 1990, Sampson et al. 1996).

Serum levels of alkaline phosphatase (ALP), have been reported to be higher in alcoholics (Verbanck et al. 1977,de Vernejoul et al. 1983) and osteoporotic alcoholics (Crilly et al. 1988) than in control subjects or non-osteoporotic alcoholics. However, high serum levels of ALP have not been found in all studies of alcoholics (Lindholm et al. 1991). The increased ALP levels may be due to other factors such as liver disease or vitamin D deficiency.

Suppressed serum levels of osteocalcin during acute alcohol intoxication (Laitinen et al. 1991a, b, Nielsen et al. 1990,Garcia-Sanchez et al. 1995) and even during more prolonged moderate alcohol use in normal volunteers (Laitinen et al. 1991a) may indicate that alcohol even acutely reduces osteoblastic activity. Low serum levels of osteocalcin have repeatedly also been reported in alcoholics (Rico et al. 1987, Labib et al. 1989, Lindholm et al. 1991, Laitinen et al. 1992a, 1993a, b, Mori et al. 1992, Pepersack et al. 1992, Peris et al. 1992, 1994, Gonzalez-Calvin et al. 1993, Diez et al. 1994,Nyquist et al. 1996) and patients with alcoholic cirrhosis of the liver (Diamond et al. 1989a, Resch et al. 1990, Pietschmann et al. 1990, Laitinen et al. 1994, Monegal et al. 1997). These studies of an alcohol-induced decrease in serum osteocalcin are supported by histomorphometric data showing decreased osteoblastic activity in alcoholics (Schnitzlet et al. 1994, Crilly et al. 1988, Lindholm et al. 1991, Bikle et al. 1993,Diez et al. 1994) and with investigations *in vitro* showing that alcohol directly inhibits bone cell function (Farley et al. 1985, Friday et al. 1991, Chavassieuz et al. 1993, Klein et al. 1995, 1996, Klein 1997). However, as osteocalcin is cleared through the kidneys, it is possible that alcohol might affect serum osteocalcin levels by increasing renal clearance.

Markers of Bone Resorption

Alcohol feeding for 3 months (Mezey et al. 1979) or 42 days (Preedy et al. 1991b) resulted in increased urinary excretion of HOP in rats. Six weeks of alcohol feeding decreased urinary PYR and DPYR in rats, indicating a reduction in bone resorption or ethanol-induced derangement in collagen or cross-link formation (Preedy et al. 1990, 1991a, b).

Urinary excretion of HOP has been reported to be increased in alcoholics (Crilly et al. 1988,Pepersack et al. 1992). This finding is not consistent, however (Lindholm et al. 1991). Nyquist et al. (1996) reported a more specific marker of bone resorption, urinary DPYR, to be elevated in alcoholics. Another resorption marker, serum cross-linked carboxy-terminal telopeptide of human type I collagen (ICTP), was 9% higher in alcohol-intoxicated drinkers than in controls (Laitinen et al. 1994).

EFFECTS OF ALCOHOL ON BONE HISTOMORPHOMETRY

Ethanol has been reported to acutely decrease both bone formation and resorption in animals (Diez et al. 1997). Chronic alcohol administration to growing rats resulted in decreased trabecular bone volume and thinner trabeculae despite a normal rate of skeletal mineralisation (Sampson et al. 1997a, Baran et al. 1980, Peng et al. 1988, Turner et al. 1988). Ethanol also inhibited bone matrix synthesis and mineralization in rats (Turner et al. 1987).

The first human study on bone biopsies from alcoholics was done by

Saville (1965b), who found a decrease in fat-free dry weight of the biopsies. Several histomorphometric studies have since been published on the effect of alcohol on bone. Most studies found that the bone changes in alcoholics are due to osteoporosis, not osteomalacia, when confounding factors such as liver disease and gastric resection were excluded. Most studies have found reduced bone formation and reduced bone turnover in bone biopsies from alcoholics, with reduced or unchanged bone resorption (Crilly 1988, Diamond 1989a,b, Lindholm 1991, Diez 1994). In contrast, Bikle et al (1993) found a pronounced increase in bone resorption. This might be due to differences in age of the study groups, as Bikle found higher bone turnover in younger than in older alcoholics. Schnitzler et al (1984) also found increased bone resorption. The inhibitory effect of alcohol on bone formation has been confirmed by studies on the effect of alcohol on human osteoblastic cells (Friday et al. 1991, Chavassieux et al. 1993), in which there was an inhibition of osteoblast proliferation and activity. The bone changes seemed to be reversible after a period of abstinence (Crilly et al. 1988, Diamond et al. 1989a, b, Lindholm et al. 1991).

Mineral Metabolism

Calcium Metabolism

NORMAL CALCIUM METABOLISM

Serum levels of calcium are regulated within narrow limits. Changes in calcium homeostasis are mainly regulated through intestinal absorption, renal calcium reabsorption and control of calcium efflux from bone.

Calcium is absorbed in the small intestine by an active, saturable cellular process, stimulated by vitamin D via calcium-binding protein (calbindin) but also by vitamin D-independent proteins (calmodulin) and a passive unsaturable concentration and voltage-dependent paracellular process which is independent of vitamin D. Normally, around 20–40% of dietary calcium is absorbed, but in calcium-deficient diets or in a state of increased calcium need absorption can be increased up to 60% (Nordin 1976, Parfitt 1992).

Calcium is secreted into the gut in the digestive juices and at very low calcium intakes the net intestinal calcium absorption may become negative. A high-calcium diet tends to increase intestinal calcium absorption by diffusion, thus increasing the absolute amount absorbed but decreasing fractional absorption as the saturable mechanism reaches its maximum.

Calcium absorption is not directly dependent on luminal phosphate or magnesium content but at increased luminal pH, the formation of unabsorbable calcium-phosphate complexes increases. Some studies have shown results supporting an inverse relationship between calcium and magnesium absorption, while others have provided evidence against this hypothesis (Wilkinson 1976).

The main regulator of calcium metabolism may be the kidneys (Nordin et al.1969). The kidneys quickly regulate the urinary output of calcium in response to hormonal stimuli, mainly PTH and vitamin D. Several studies have found that vitamin D is necessary for or potentiates the effect of PTH on renal calcium reabsorption (Harrison et al. 1964, Yamamoto et al. 1984). Renal tubular reabsorption of calcium is regulated by concentration-dependent reabsorption with no maximum and is independent of hormonal regulation (Bouhtiauy et al.1991, Frick et al. 1965). It is a rate-limiting process with a maximum value (Need et al.1985, Shaw et al. 1992) and is stimulated by PTH, 25-hydroxychole-calciferol and 1,25-dihydroxycholecalciferol (Bouhtiauy et al. 1991, Frick et al. 1965, Kanis et al. 1992, Norman et al. 1979, Yanagawa et al. 1992).

Bone tissue acts, besides its supportive function, as a reservoir capable of changing the in- and out-flux of minerals to extracellular fluid (ECF), notably calcium and phosphate but also magnesium. This is done by the slow bone remodelling process and the rapidly changing blood-bone-mineral exchange system (Dempster et al.1992, Parfitt 1976a, b, Parfitt 1989, Talmage 1969). The two systems are regulated by a variety of hormones (PTH, 1,25-dihydroxycholecalciferol, calcitonin, thyroid hormones, sex hormones, corticosteroids and growth hormone) and cytokines (Huffer 1988, Parfitt 1976 a, b, Reichel et al. 1989, Stern 1990).

EFFECTS OF ALCOHOL ON CALCIUM METABOLISM

In rats (Peng et al. 1974, Chanard et al. 1980, Hemmingsen et al. 1980, Baran et al. 1982, Krishnamra et al. 1983, Garcia-Sanchez et al. 1995, Keiver et al. 1996, 1997), dogs (Money et al, 1989, Peng et al. 1972) and rabbits (Mahboob et al. 1988) a rapid and sustained fall of both total and ionized calcium follows the ingestion of alcohol in doses of 1.0 g per kg body weight or more. The hypocalcaemic effect of ethanol is not caused by increased urinary calcium loss (Peng et al. 1972, Sargent et al. 1974), suppression of PTH secretion (Peng et al. 1972, Shan et al. 1978, Keiver et al. 1997) or increased secretion of calcitonin (Krishnamra et al. 1983, Peng et al. 1972). Alcohol decreases intestinal absorption of calcium (Krawitt 1975, Krawitt et al. 1975, Krishnamra et al. 1986) and urinary calcium excretion in rats (Krishnamra et al. 1983, Peng et al. 1972, Alho et al. 1988).

Hypocalcaemia is frequently encountered in heavy drinkers (Laitinen et al. 1991a, 1993) and in alcoholic cirrhosis, and it cannot be explained by hypoalbuminaemia alone (Pitts et al. 1986).

Previous studies in healthy human subjects have shown no consistent acute effect of alcohol on blood levels of calcium. Alcohol increased (Laitinen 1993) or decreased (Avery et al. 1983, Ylikahri et al. 1974) serum calcium levels in man, or it had no effect at all (Ljunghall et al. 1985). These inconsistent results may partly be explained by different routes of alcohol administration and by different doses. Additionally, only a few studies have analysed serum levels of ionized calcium (Ca^{2+}), which is the physiologically active calcium form in body fluids. In the studies where alcohol lowered serum calcium levels (Avery et al. 1983, Ylikari et al. 1974), the alcohol dose was 1.2–1.5 g/kg and resulted in serum alcohol concentrations of 26–33 mmol/l (1.2–1.6 g/l). In most of the (rather old) studies with no effect of alcohol on serum calcium levels the alcohol dose did not exceed 0.8 g/kg with resulting modest serum levels of 17 mmol (0.8 g/l).

Other groups have studied the effects of alcohol on serum ionized calcium (Ca^{2+}) in man (Every et al. 1983, Laitinen et al. 1991). In the first paper, alcohol (with a mean dose of 1.0 g/kg) was consumed in 2 h and during a 5 h follow-up a decrease by 3% of ionized calcium was found. However, this study had no control group, and Ca^{2+} was determined indirectly. The most recent findings, however, consistently show that alcohol acutely decreases Ca^{2+} levels and also increases urinary calcium excretion (Laitinen et al. 1991, 1992b). In contrast to animals, in man an acute alcohol intake of 0.6 g/kg or more increases urinary calcium excretion (Lonkola et al. 1979, Laitinen et al. 1991).

Intestinal absorption of calcium is reduced in both cirrhotic (Dechavanne et al. 1974, Luisier et al. 1977) and non-cirrhotic alcoholics (Luisier et al. 1977), possibly as a result of low serum levels of 1,25-dihydroxycholecalciferol (Bjorneboe et al. 1988, Lalor et al. 1986, Lund et al. 1977). However, the reducing effect of alcohol on intestinal calcium absorption (as measured by stable strontium) has not been found in more recent studies (Laitinen et al. 1991, 1992, 1993).

Magnesium Metabolism

NORMAL MAGNESIUM METABOLISM

Magnesium homeostasis is not well understood. Short-term control of magnesium homeostasis is regulated by the effects of both vitamin D and PTH on renal excretion. Long-term regulation of magnesium homeostasis is regulated mainly by intestinal absorption, via vitamin D and possibly PTH. Some magnesium is exchanged from bone and released during bone resorption.

Magnesium is absorbed in the small intestine, and normally 35–40% of dietary magnesium is absorbed. Intestinal magnesium absorption is regulated by a saturable active process, stimulated by 1,25-dihydroxycholecalciferol and a passive voltage-dependent process along a concentration gradient (Karbach et al. 1987, 1990). Whether the active process is regulated by PTH is a matter for debate.

Magnesium is reabsorbed in the kidneys, and in magnesium deficiency urinary excretion can be nearly zero (Rude 1980). Reabsorption is stimulated by vitamin D and PTH (Dirks 1983, Shafik 1992).

EFFECTS OF ALCOHOL ON MAGNESIUM METABOLISM

In animals (Hemmingsen et al. 1980, Mahboob et al. 1988, Peng et al. 1974, Ramp et al. 1975) acute alcohol administration of 0.6 g/kg or more increases serum magnesium concentration.

Magnesium deficiency and low serum magnesium are typical findings in alcoholics (Bohmer et al. 1982, McIntyre 1984, Berkelhammer et al. 1985, Rico 1990). The low serum magnesium levels during withdrawal can be explained by the shift of magnesium to the intracellular space because of respiratory alkalosis (Pitts et al. 1986, Laitinen 1993) and by the elevated serum levels of free fatty acids (FFA) (Flink et al. 1979), the magnesium salts of FFA being insoluble. Other possible causes of magnesium deficiency in alcoholics include inadequate magnesium intake, malabsorption, pancreatitis and diminished intestinal absorption of magnesium due to low vitamin D levels, as well as renal magnesium excretion (Posner et al. 1978, Flink 1986, Abbott et al. 1994).

Hypomagnesaemia and magnesium deficiency may contribute to the hypocalcaemia of alcoholics (Medalle et al. 1976) through reduced PTH secretion, PTH resistance (Laitinen et al. 1994, Laitinen 1993) or vitamin D resistance (Medalle et al. 1976). Thus alcohol increases urinary magnesium excretion (Dick et al. 1969, Linkola et al. 1979, Laitinen et al.

1991a, b, 1992a, b) in man independently of glomerular filtration and renal blood flow (Abbott et al. 1994). The elevated urinary excretion of magnesium has been considered as the primary cause of magnesium deficiency in alcoholism, and magnesium deficiency may contribute to osteoporosis in alcoholics (Abbott et al. 1994).

Phosphate Metabolism

NORMAL PHOSPHATE METABOLISM

Serum phosphate levels are not as tightly regulated as are calcium levels. Rapid changes in phosphate homeostasis are followed by PTH-mediated changes in renal reabsorption and probably also by PTH-mediated regulation of the rapidly exchangeable blood-bone pool. The long-term regulation of phosphate homeostasis is dominated by intestinal absorption, mainly stimulated by vitamin D, but there may also be an effect from bone remodelling and mineral exchange.

Phosphate is absorbed mainly from the jejunum. Increased luminal pH will increase formation of unabsorbable phosphate complexes with calcium and magnesium. Intestinal phosphate absorption is regulated by an active saturable cellular process which, under normal conditions, is the more important, and also by an unsaturable, concentration-dependent paracellular process. Absorption is stimulated by vitamin D (Reichel 1989).

Phosphate is reabsorbed mainly in the proximal tubules of the kidney by an active, rate-limited process with a maximum value (Amiel 1992, Yanagawa et al. 1992). It is inhibited by PTH (Walker et al. 1977) and stimulated by 25-hydroxy- and 1.25-dihydroxycholecalciferol (Puschett et al. 1972).

EFFECTS OF ALCOHOL ON PHOSPHATE METABOLISM

In some (Avery et al. 1983,Matsubara et al. 1982) but not all animal studies (Adler et al. 1985) acute alcohol ingestion had an effect on serum phosphate levels. Short-term oral administration of alcohol decreases serum phosphate levels in rabbits (Matsubara et al 1982) and chicks (Ramp et al. 1975) with a rebound increase following this decrease after a few hours. The alcohol doses in these animal studies were high (3 to 6 g/kg). In a study with rabbits (Matsubara et al. 1982) hypophosphataemia was related to the metabolism of ethanol by alcohol dehydrogenase.

As in animals, short-term oral alcohol administration decreases serum phosphate levels in man (Avery et al. 1983, Laitinen et al. 1991a), and a rebound increase follows this decrement in a few hours.

Hypophosphataemia is common in alcoholics (Berkelhammer et al. 1984, Pitts et al. 1986) and in hospitalized patients alcoholism is one of the most commonly recognized causes of severe hypophosphataemia (Territo et al. 1974, King et al. 1987). Alcoholic hypophosphataemia is present either on admission to the hospital or occurs within 1 to 4 days (Ryback et al. 1980, Stein et al. 1966).

Apart from dietary causes, malabsorption and use of antacids (which bind phosphate and prevent its absorption), there are many other causes of alcohol-associated hypophosphataemia. Respiratory alkalosis during alcoholic withdrawal stimulates glycolysis and increases the entry of phosphate into cells, often resulting in profound hypophosphataemia. Similarly, the resumption of an adequate diet during withdrawal results in an intracellular shift of phosphate (King et al. 1987).

After alcohol intoxication, urinary excretion of phosphate increases in healthy volunteers (Laitinen et al. 1991a) which is explained by the rebound increase in serum PTH levels. The hyperphosphaturia in alcoholics (Adler et al. 1984) has also been postulated to be a result of alcohol-induced renal tubular injury which leads to decreased tubular reabsorption of phosphate (Angeli et al. 1991, Labib et al. 1989b, Lalor et al. 1986, McDonald et al. 1979). Impairment of liver function is not responsible for this tubular dysfunction (Angeli et al. 1991).

Parathyroid Hormone Function

NORMAL PARATHYROID HORMONE FUNCTION

PTH is produced as a 115 amino acid preprohormone in the parathyroid glands and is secreted into the circuation as an 84 amino acid single-chain peptide hormone. PTH secretion is pulsatile and exhibits a diurnal rhythm with higher levels during the night (Jubiz et al. 1972). PTH secretion is inversely related to serum calcium levels and is very sensitive to changes in serum calcium, following a sigmoid curve form (Mundy 1989). Secretion of PTH is inversely regulated by serum magnesium, but on a molar basis magnesium is a 2–3 times less potent stimulator than is calcium (Habener et al. 1978, Mayer et al. 1978). In severe hypomagnesaemia PTH secretion and receptor sensitivity to PTH are decreased (Habener et al. 1976, 1984, Mayer et al. 1978). Parathyroid glands have receptors for 1,25-dihydroxycholecalciferol, which inhibit

PTH secretion (Habener et al. 1984, 1990, Reichel et al. 1989).

The parathyroid glands have a small storage capacity; in normal conditions the secretion reserve is sufficient for about 7 h but it lasts only for ca. 1.5 h when secretion is maximally stimulated. The half-life of PTH in serum is a few minutes (Habener et al. 1984, 1990).

PTH acts by binding to hormone-specific receptors on cell surfaces, which activate several second messenger systems. PTH does not enter the cell, and a direct effect of PTH on calcium channels has been postulated. How the cell "chooses" response mechanisms when stimulated by PTH is not exactly known (Fitzpatrick et al. 1992, Habener et al. 1978, 1984, 1990). PTH is necessary for stimulation of renal 1-α-hydroxylase activity, being the main stimulator of the conversion of 25-hydroxycholecalciferol into 1,25-dihydroxycholecalciferol (Fraser et al. 1973, Mawer et al. 1975). PTH is metabolized by cleavage and by clearance in the liver and kidneys (Habener et al. 1984).

EFFECTS OF ALCOHOL ON PARATHYROID HORMONE

Previously, alcohol (2.5 g/kg) has been reported to increase acutely (Shan et al. 1978) serum levels of PTH in rats and also to release PTH from bovine parathyroid cells (Williams et al. 1978). However, Chanard et al. (1980) found a suppressive effect of ethanol (with doses as high as 6 g/kg) on parathyroid activity in rats and on incubated rat parathyroid glands (concentrations of 0.05%, 0.5% and 5%). Ethanol also blunted the PTH response to hypocalcaemia in rats (Thomas et al. 1990) and directly inhibited the calcium-raising effect of exogenously administered PTH in rats (Peng et al. 1974). These results point to PTH resistance produced by alcohol and to inhibited PTH release from dispersed bovine parathyroid cells (Magliola et al. 1986).

Acute alcohol ingestion (0.8 g/kg) increased the serum PTH levels in human subjects in one study (Williams et al. 1986). In another trial the same dose of alcohol had no effect on serum PTH levels (Ljunghall et al. 1985). In a third study, acute ingestion of 25 or 50 g alcohol decreased serum PTH levels for 3 h, although the decrement was not statistically significant (Nielsen et al. 1990). This diminished PTH activity was further supported by a study (Linkola et al. 1979) where alcohol decreased urinary adenosine 3′,5′ cyclic adenosine monophosphate (cAMP), the cellular messenger for PTH.

According to Laitinen et al. (1991a, 1993), hypocalcaemia and hypercalciuria during acute alcohol intoxication may be due to a transient decrease in serum PTH concentration. The phase of hypoparathyroidism was followed by a rebound increase in serum level of PTH resulting in a decrease of the urinary excretion of calcium, and increase in phosphate excretion (Laitinen et al. 1991a).

The serum levels of PTH in alcoholics are normal (Angeli et al 1991, Bjoerneboe et al. 1987) or high (Bikle et al. 1985, Feitelberg et al. 1987, Johnell et al. 1982), the latter suggesting it is a compensatory mechanism to the diminished intestinal absorption of calcium (Dechavanne et al. 1974, Luisier et al. 1977). However, Chiba et al. (1987) reported a patient with alcoholic fatty liver whose hypocalcaemic crisis was attributed to transient hypoparathyroidism due to magnesium deficiency. In addition, in another study (Lindholm et al. 1991), serum PTH was low in men who abused alcohol relative to abstaining alcoholics. Although alcohol intoxication brings about transient hypoparathyroidism in healthy volunteers (Laitinen et al. 1991a), in alcohol-intoxicated alcoholics serum PTH was similar to that in the control group. This was true in spite of the fact that serum Ca^{2+} was 12% lower (Laitinen et al. 1994). This means that the parathyroid glands do not respond normally to a hypocalcaemic stimulus during alcohol intoxication.

Vitamin D Function

NORMAL VITAMIN D FUNCTION

Vitamin D is a steroid hormone formed by a transformational pathway starting with irradiation (ultraviolet light) of the skin causing transformation of 7-dehydrocholesterol (or its plant analogue ergosterol) into cholecalciferol (vitamin D_3) or ergocalciferol (vitamin D_2). Vitamin D is transported by vitamin D-binding serum proteins to the liver, where it is 25-hydroxylated by microsomal and mitochondrial 25-hydroxylase into 25-hydroxycholecalciferol. This metabolite is the most abundant vitamin D metabolite in blood. The half-life of 25-hydroxycholecalciderol in blood is around 31 days and it is less potent than 1,25-dihydroxycholecalciferol. *In vitro* studies have shown that both 25-hydroxy- and 1,25-dihydroxycholecalciferol stimulate bone resorption, 1,25-dihydroxycholecalciferol being roughly 100 times more potent than 25-hydroxycholecalciferol (Raisz et al. 1972). The 1,25-dihydroxycholecalciferol levels are not very tightly regulated. In vitamin D deficiency 25-hydroxycholecalciferol is considered to be the best indicator of vitamin D status (Mundy 1989, Robertson 1976). 25-hydroxycholecalciferol is 1-α-hydroxylated in the proximal convoluted tubules of the kidney into 1,25-dihydroxycholecalciferol. This hormone is considered to be the main active vitamin D metabolite, with a half-life of around 6 h (Norman 1979). With sufficient amounts of 1,25-dihydroxycholecalciferol in the system the kidneys produce other metabolites by hydroxylation. The renal enzyme 1-α-hydroxylase is mainly stimulated by PTH but also by low serum phosphate. Normally, the kidney is considered to be the main site of 1-hydroxylation of vitamin D (Reichel 1989). However, extrarenal hydroxylation has been observed in various diseases (Dusso et al. 1990, Mawer et al. 1991), and several studies have shown 1,25-dihydroxycholecalciferol production in nephrectomized rats and in uraemic patients (Dusso et al. 1990, Fraher et al. 1986). More than thirty different metabolites of active vitamin D are now known, but it is not certain if they are all inactive degradation products or if they represent hormonal metabolites with more specific effects. Vitamin D metabolites are degradated by the kidney and liver, and although the metabolites excreted by bile are reabsorbed to a certain extent, most are lost in faeces (Ikekawa 1987).

Receptors for vitamin D have been found in many tissues. Vitamin D has a general stimulating effect on cells and increases cell differentation. The nuclear vitamin D receptor is a high-affinity receptor, which regulates gene expression and alters cell function. It is in this way that the production of proteins, for example calbindins (calcium-binding proteins), is regulated (DeLuca et al. 1990, Haussler 1986). Furthermore, a non-genomic effect of vitamin D has been demonstrated in intestinal calcium absorption, "transcaltachia" (Lieberherr et al. 1991, Nemere 1991), causing a rapid effect, which can be inhibited by calcium blockers.

EFFECTS OF ALCOHOL ON VITAMIN D

Results of animal studies on vitamin metabolism are inconsistent. In rats alcohol use leads to unchanged (Mezey et al. 1979, Baran et al. 1980, Turner et al. 1987, Keiver et al. 1996,Sampson et al. 1996), increased (Gascon-Barre 1982, Turner et al. 1988) or decreased (Keiver et al. 1997) serum levels of 25-hydroxycholecalciferol. The results relating to the most active vitamin D metabolite, 1,25-dihydroxycholecalciferol, are also inconsistent, with unchanged (Turner et al. 1987), increased (Turner et al. 1988) and decreased (Keiver et al. 1987) serum levels being reported.

In alcoholics serum levels of 25-hydroxycholecalciferol (Luisier et al. 1977, Lund et al. 1977, Verbanck et al. 1977, de Vernejoul et al. 1983, Mobarhan et al. 1984, Bjoerneboe et al. 1986, 1987, 1988, Lalor et al. 1986, Feitelberg et al. 1987, Laitinen et al. 1990, 1993) and 1,25-dihydroxycholecalciferol (Lalor et al. 1986, Bjoerneboe et al. 1988, Laitinen et al. 1990, 1993, Lindholm et al. 1993) are low. It has been suggested that this depressed level is the result of deficient dietary intake, reduced sunlight, malabsorption, increased biliary excretion of 25-hydroxycholecalciferol-derived compounds or reduced reserves of vitamin D metabolites in the diminished muscle and adipose tissue of alcoholics. However, intestinal absorption of cholecalciferol is normal in alcoholic liver disease (Barragry et al. 1979, Lund et al. 1977). It has been postulated that low levels of vitamin D metabolites in alcoholics result from the decreased concentration of circulating vitamin D-binding protein (DBP) (Bikle 1988, Bikle et al. 1984), but this has been observed only in cirrhotics (Bikle et al. 1984, 1986b).

A plausible explanation for the reduced serum levels of vitamin D metabolites in human subjects appears to be the induction of the cytochrome P450 system by ethanol and the subsequent increase in degradation of vitamin D metabolites in the liver. Use of antiepileptic drugs also induces the cytochrome P450 system leading to low circulating 25-hydroxycholecalciferol levels (Christiansen et al. 1983). The reduced levels of 25-hydroxy- and 1,25-dihydroxycholecalciferol could also be due to an inhibitory effect of ethanol on the hydroxylase activities in the liver or kidney. However, even in cirrhotic alcoholics a normal hepatic 25-hydroxylation of vitamin D is found (Barragry et al. 1979, Lund et al. 1977, Posner et al. 1978).

Effects of alcohol on calcitonin

Ethanol raises serum levels of calcitonin in normal subjects (Williams et al. 1978) and in patients with medullary carcinoma of the thyroid (Dymling et al. 1976, Emmertsen et al. 1980, Wells et al. 1975). Since hypercalcaemia does not precede the increase in calcitonin (Williams et al. 1978) and because administration of alcohol does not increase serum levels of gastrin, a potent stimulator of calcitonin secretion (Wells et al. 1975), the mechanism for the increase in serum calcitonin is presumably a direct stimulation of calcitonin release by ethanol from thyroid C-cells, although mediators like histamine have been suggested to mediate calcitonin release after alcohol ingestion. It is also interesting that ethanol-induced elevation of serum calcitonin can be prevented by β-antagonists (Heynen et al. 1977, Kanis et al. 1979).

Table 3
Factors contributing to alcohol associated bone disease

Nutritional deficiencies
   calcium
   vitamin D
   other nutrients
Liver disease
Hypogonadism
Hypercortisolism
Direct effect of alcohol on bone
Age
Duration of alcohol use
Cigarette smoking
Heavy coffee use
Low physical activity
Gastrectomy
Medication
   prolonged use of anticids
   antiepileptic drugs

Confounding factors

There are several confounding factors which have a variable impact on bone in addition to the direct effect of alcohol (Table 3). However, it is not always relevant to separate the indirect effects of alcohol from the direct ones, because the end result (irrespective of the exact mechanisms) is the most important issue.

Irrespective of its cause, liver damage (alcoholic or non-alcoholic) affects bone and calcium metabolism. As to markers of bone metabolism, alcohol-associated diseases cause difficulties in the interpretation of markers of bone metabolism. The elevated urinary excretion of HOP in liver disease has been suggested to be due to changes in collagen turnover during the development of cirrhosis. ALP was also increased in liver diseases (Conte et al. 1989, Pietschmann et al. 1990, Diamond et al. 1989a) and because of its non-specificity ALP is not a very good marker of bone metabolism in alcoholics. Serum osteocalcin levels are low in liver cirrhosis independent of its cause (Pietschmann et al. 1990).

Histologically defined osteoporosis is common in alcoholic liver cirrhosis (Conte et al. 1989, Diamond et al. 1989b, Jorge-Hernandez et al. 1988, Chappard et al., 1989, 1991, McCaughan et al. 1994, Mobarhann et al. 1984) and in liver cirrhosis from other causes (Conte et al. 1989, Diamond et al. 1989b, 1990). In some clinical studies the pathological findings in the histomorphometry of bone from alcoholics could have been explained by liver cirrhosis alone (Lalor et al. 1986, Diamond et al. 1989a), but osteoporosis has also been found in studies where marked liver failure was excluded (de Vernejoul et al. 1983, Crilly et al. 1988, Verbanck et al. 1977, Lindholm et al. 1991).

Axial (Diamond et al. 1989, Conte et al. 1989, Monegal et al. 1997) and appendicular (Resch et al. 1990) bone mass is also decreased, even in non-alcoholic liver cirrhosis. Thus, liver disease is probably an important confounding factor in most, but perhaps not in all studies of alcoholics (Roginsky et al. 1976, Bikle et al. 1985, Feitelberg et al. 1987, Crilly et al. 1988, Bjoerneboe et al. 1988, Laitinen et al. 1990, 1992a, 1993, Lindholm et al. 1991, Golzalez-Calvin et al. 1993, Odvina et al. 1995).

Blood levels of 25-hydroxycholecalciderol are decreased in 40–50% of patients with a variety of liver diseases, including non-alcoholic cirrhosis (Dibble et al. 1982). As a possible result of low levels of vitamin D, intestinal absorption of calcium is reduced in cirrhosis (Dechavanne et al. 1974, Luisier et al. 1977). PTH levels measured by old methodology have often been found to be elevated in cirrhosis from all causes. If not a true response to hypovitaminosis D, they may be due to impaired liver capacity in removing PTH fragments from blood. Serum calcitonin is also elevated in hepatoma and liver cirrhosis (Conte et al. 1984), perhaps as a result of its ectopic secretion.

Nutritional deficiencies of vitamin D and other vitamins, certain minerals and protein are common in alcoholics (Ryle et al. 1984). These deficits have been suggested as a cause of bone disease in alcoholics (Mezey 1985). However, poor nutrition alone does not induce osteoporosis in experimental animals (Mezey et al. 1979), and in many of the histomorphometric studies with low-turnover osteoporosis in alcoholics, no nutritional deficiencies have been found. The impact of widely different calcium intakes, in different countries, on osteoporosis is not known but it is noteworthy that, for example, in Finland, where alcohol-associated bone disease is rare, dietary calcium intake exceeds by far that in most other countries.

Hypogonadism is a risk factor for osteoporosis and osteoporotic fractures (Swarz et al. 1988, Baillie et al. 1992, Kelepouris et al. 1995, Peris et al. 1995a, Seeman 1997b). Men suffering from chronic alcoholism often suffer from impotence, sterility and testicular atrophy (Välimäki et al. 1984) and have a reduced level of plasma testosterone (Van Thiel et al. 1974, 1975, 1981). Alcohol administration may stimulate secretion of cortisol (Välimäki et al. 1984), and result in hypercortisolism and pseudo-Cushing syndrome.

Myopathy is found in many alcoholics, and also in persons with no spontaneous muscle complaints. Myopathy of both skeletal type 2B muscle fibres and of cardiac fibres is a dose-dependent consequence of alcoholism (Urbano-Marquez et al 1989). The atrophy of the muscle fibres is reversible if alcohol abuse stops. The atrophy is found even in alcoholics with no signs of malnutrition, vitamin deficiency or neuropathy (Peters et al. 1985, Duane et al. 1988, Urbano-Marquez et al. 1989).

Most of the studies of alcohol and bone mass have been poorly controlled with respect to confounding factors and hence cannot be used to describe the direct effects of alcohol on bone.

Conclusions

Although animal data are somewhat inconclusive (because most studies have been performed in growing animals), both markers of bone formation and resorption as well as results from histomorphometric studies point to a "low-turnover" osteoporosis, where both bone formation and bone resorption are reduced with alcohol consumption. Data on formation are conclusive, but those on resorption are less consistent. In animals alcohol causes decreased bone strength and an increased tendency to fractures.

There is a large body of evidence showing that alcohol decreases serum total and ionized calcium in several animal species. This hypocalcaemic effect does not depend on changes in urinary calcium excretion or calcium regulating hormones like PTH, calcitonin or vitamin D. Some studies show that alcohol diminishes intestinal calcium absorption by a mechanism independent of vitamin D.

Contrary to calcium, acute alcohol intoxication causes serum magnesium levels to increase in animals. There are also some data showing that serum phosphate is decreased by alcohol and that this decrement

Table 4
Effects of alcohol on bone and mineral metabolism

Acute intoxication
>   transient hypoparathyroidism followed by a rebound increase in
>   serum PTH
>   hypocalcaemia
>   hypercalciuria (hypocalciuria in a later phase)
>   transient hypermagnesaemia
>   hypermagnesuria
>   suppressed osetocalcin levels
>   vitamin D metabolism not affected

Moderate drinking
>   suppressed osteocalcin levels
>   elevated PTH levels
>   vitamin D metabolism not affected

Chronic abuse
>   magnesium deficiency with hypomagnesaemia and hypomagnesuria-
>   hypocalcaemia
>   PTH levels normal or elevated
>   suppressed osteocalcin levels
>   low serum levels of 25-hydroxy-, 1,25-dihydroxy- and 24,25-
>   dihydroxycholecalciferol

is linked to alcohol metabolism. Most animal studies on PTH excretion show increased levels. Animal studies on the effect of alcohol on vitamin D metabolism have produced incompatible results.

Alcohol may have differential effects on human mineral metabolism depending on the dose and duration used. Acute effects differ from those of moderate drinking, and also chronic alcohol abuse brings about changes that are different from those of acute use or moderate drinking (Table 4).

Acute Effects

Acute alcohol intake elevates serum levels of calcitonin. Serum osteocalcin levels decrease as an index of the bone-depressing effect of alcohol.

In man acute alcohol intoxication causes hypocalcaemia and hypermagnesaemia and brings about hypercalciuria and hypermagnesuria. Hypocalcaemia and hypercalciuria during acute alcohol intoxication may be due to a transient decrease in the mean PTH concentration, and a decrease in the urinary excretion of calcium after recovery may be due to the rebound increase in serum level of PTH. Both serum magnesium and its urinary excretion are increased after alcohol ingestion, which also has a short-term hypophosphataemic effect. Alcohol intoxication is followed by an increase in urinary phosphate excretion. The alcohol-induced changes in mineral metabolism are dose-dependent. The decrease in serum PTH may contribute to hypercalciuria but not to hypermagnesuria. Vitamin D metabolites and intestinal absorption of calcium (as measured by stable strontium) do not change during acute alcohol intake.

Moderate Drinking

As evaluated by serum markers, moderate drinking decreases bone formation. The markers of bone formation consistently point to decreased bone formation, while data on markers of bone resorption are inconsistent.

The relation between moderate alcohol consumption and BMD at different sites has been investigated in a large number of studies, the results of which are inconsistent. Evaluating the studies according to BMD site, male or female population, pre- or postmenopausal women or level of alcohol consumption does not help to resolve the conflicting results. However, with the exception of a few studies, the overall conclusion must be that moderate drinking is not likely to have adverse effects on bone density. Studies finding a possibly higher BMD among alcohol consumers compared to abstainers are cited more frequently than studies finding no association. In several prospective studies a positive association has been observed between moderate alcohol consumption and risk of hip and forearm fracture, but these results are not confirmed in other studies. There is some indication that interaction with age may play a role, particularly in women. Increased risk of fracture in alcohol consumers seems to be restricted to populations under 65, while no inverse associations are seen in older populations.

Moderate drinking does not change serum calcium, magnesium, phosphate or their urinary excretion. The serum levels of vitamin D metabolites as well as intestinal absorption of calcium (at least when measured by stable strontium) also remain unchanged. However, the serum level of PTH may increase somewhat.

Chronic alcohol abuse

Although the available evidence suggests that chronic alcohol abuse adversely affects bone mineral density, it may well be that clinically meaningful effects only become apparent after a very long period of abuse. Chronic alcohol abuse seems to be associated with an increased risk of fractures.

Chronic alcohol abuse brings about profound changes in mineral metabolism. It may cause hypocalcaemia, hypophosphataemia and magnesium deficiency. One of the main reasons for these findings is the increase in urinary excretion of these ions.

Studies on serum PTH levels in alcoholics have produced contradictory findings, although there is current evidence that the response of the parathyroid glands to the hypocalcaemic stimulus is impaired by alcohol. In alcoholics serum levels of 25-hydroxy- and 1,25-dihydroxycholecalciderol are low. A possible cause of reduced levels of vitamin D metabolites is increased degradation in the liver.

Future Research

Although acute alcohol intoxication has a short-term effect on bone metabolism, it seems to be conclusive that moderate alcohol use does not derange mineral metabolism. Similarly, alcohol abuse easily leads to fracture. However, there are inconclusive human data on the effect of moderate or heavy alcohol use on bone mass and quality. Therefore, good prospective studies (on variable levels of alcohol use) on the development of bone mass and histomorphometric variables of bone are needed in the future. Moreover, a reliable biochemical marker of the amount of alcohol taken is needed. During the past decade an increasing intake of alcohol has been seen among teenagers, and the effects of this on peak bone mass and fracture later in life are still to be elucidated.

References

Abbott L, Nadler J, Rude RK (1994) Magnesium deficiency in alcoholism: possible contribution to osteoporosis and cardiovascular disease in alcoholics. [Review]. Alcohol Clin Exp Res 18: 1076–82

Adler AJ, Gudis S, Berlyne GM (1984) Reduced renal phosphate threshold concentration in alcoholic cirrhosis. Miner Electrolyte Metab 10: 63–66

Adler AJ, Fillipone EJ, Berlyne GM (1985) Effect of chronic alcohol intake on muscle composition and metabolic balance of calcium and phosphate in rats. Am J Physiol 249: E584–88

Alho A, Hoiseth A, Husby T (1988) Bone density and bone strength: an ex vivo study on cadaver femora. Rev Chir Orthop Réparatrice Appar Mot 74 (Suppl 2): 333–34

Amiel C, Bailly C, Escoubet B, et al. (1992) Hypo- and hyperphosphataemia. In: Cameron S et al (eds) Oxford textbook of clinical nephrology. Oxford University Press, Oxford, pp. 1782–1801

Angeli P, Gatta A, Caregaro L, et al. (1991) Hypophosphatemia and renal tubular dysfunction in alcoholics. Are they related to liver function impairment? Gastroenterology 100: 502–12

Angus RM, Sambrook PN, Pocock NA, et al. (1988) Dietary intake and bone mineral density. Bone Miner 4: 265–77

Anonymous: Consensus Development Statement: Who are candidates for prevention and treatment for osteoporosis? Osteoporosis Int 1997: 1–6

Avery DH, Overall JE, Calil HM, et al. (1983) Plasma calcium and phosphate during alcohol intoxication. Alcoholics versus nonalcoholics. J Stud Alcohol 44: 205–14

Baillie SP, Davison CE, Johnson FJ, et al. (1992) Pathogenesis of vertebral crush fractures in men. Age Ageing 21: 139–41

Baran DT, Teitelbaum SL, Bergfeld MA, et al. (1980) Effect of alcohol ingestion on bone and mineral metabolism in rats. Am J Physiol 238: E507-10

Baran DT, Bryant C, Robson D (1982) Alcohol-induced alterations in calcium metabolism in the pregnant rat. Am J Clin Nutr 36: 41–44

Barragry JM, Long RG, France MW, et al. (1979) Intestinal absorption of cholecalciferol in alcoholic liver disease and primary biliary cirrhosis. Gut 20: 559–64

Bauer DC, Browner WS, Cauley JA, et al. (1993) Factors associated with appendicular bone mass in older women. Ann Intern Med 118: 657–65

Berkelhammer C, Bear RA (1984) A clinical approach to common electrolyte problems. 3. Hypophosphatemia. Can Med Ass J 130: 17–23

Berkelhammer C, Bear RA (1985) A clinical approach to common electrolyte problems. 4. Hypomagnesemia [Review]. Can Med Ass J 132: 360–68

Bikle DD (1988) Effects of alcohol abuse on bone [Review]. Comp Ther 14: 16–20

Bikle DD (1993) Alcohol-induced bone disease. In: Simopoulos AP, et al. (eds) Osteoporosis: nutritional aspects. World Rev Nutr Diet 73: 53–79

Bikle DD, Gee E, Halloran B, et al. (1984) Free 1,25-dihydroxyvitamin D levels in serum from normal subjects, pregnant subjects, and subjects with liver disease. J Clin Invest 74: 1966–71

Bikle DD, Genant HK, Cann C, et al. (1985) Bone disease in alcohol abuse. Ann Intern Med 103: 42–48

Bikle DD, Gee EA, Munson SJ (1986a) Effect of ethanol on intestinal calcium transport in chicks. Gastroenterology 91: 870–76

Bikle DD, Halloran BP, Gee E, et al. (1986b) Free 25-hydroxyvitamin D levels are normal in subjects with liver disease and reduced total 25-hydroxyvitamin D levels. J Clin Invest 78: 748–52

Bikle DD, Stesin A, Halloran B, et al. (1993) Alcohol-induced bone disease: relationship to age and PTH levels. Alcohol Clin Exp Res 17: 690–95

Bilezikian JP, Raisz LG, Rodan GA (eds) (1996) Principles of bone biology. Academic Press, San Diego, CA, pp. 127–206

Bjoerneboe GE, Johnsen J, Bjoerneboe A, et al. (1986) Effect of alcohol consumption on serum concentration of 25-hydroxyvitamin D3, retinol, and retinol-binding protein. Am J Clin Nutr 44: 678–82

Bjoerneboe GA, Johnsen J, Bjoerneboe A, et al. (1987) Effect of heavy alcohol consumption on serum concentrations of fat-soluble vitamins and selenium. Alcohol Alcoholism (Suppl) 1: 533–37

Bjoerneboe GE, Bjoerneboe A, Johnsen J, et al. (1988) Calcium status and calcium-regulating hormones in alcoholics. Alcohol Clin Exp Res 12: 229–32

Bohmer T, Mathiesen B (1982) Magnesium deficiency in chronic alcoholic patients uncovered by an intravenous loading test. Scand J Clin Lab Invest 42: 633–36

Borgquist L, Lindelow G, Thorngren KG. (1991) Costs of hip fracture. Rehabilitation of 180 patients in primary health care. Acta Orthop Scand 62: 39–48

Bouhtiauy I, Lajeunesse D, Brunette MG (1991) The mechanism of parathyroid hormone action on calcium reabsorption by the distal tubule. Endocrinology 128:251–58

Chanard J, Lacour B, Drueke T, et al. (1980) Effect of acute ethanol loading on parathyroid gland secretion in the rat. Adv Exp Med Biol 128: 495–504

Chappard D, Plantard B, Fraisse H, et al. (1989) Bone changes in alcoholic cirrhosis of the liver. A histomorphometric study. Pathol Res Pract 184: 480–85

Chappard D, Plantard B, Petitjean M, et al. (1991) Alcoholic cirrhosis and osteoporosis in men: a light and scanning electron microscopy study. J Stud Alcohol 52: 269–74

Chavassieux P, Serre CM, Vergnaud P, et al. (1993) In vitro evaluation of dose-effects of ethanol on human osteoblastic cells. Bone Miner 22: 95–103

Chiba T, Okimura Y, Inatome T, et al. (1987) Hypocalcemic crisis in alcoholic fatty liver: transient hypoparathyroidism due to magnesium deficiency. Am J Gastroenterol 82: 1084–87

Christiansen C, Roedbro P, Tjellesen L (1983) Pathophysiology behind anticonvulsant osteomalacia. Acta Neurol Scand (Suppl) 94: 21–28

Clark K, Sowers MFR (1996) Alcohol dependence, smoking status, reproductive characteristics, and bone mineral density in premenopausal women. Res Nurs Health 19: 399–408

Conte N, Cecchettin M, Manente P, et al. (1984) Calcitonin in hepatoma and cirrhosis. Acta Endocrinol (Copenh) 106: 109–11

Conte D, Caraceni MP, Duriez J, et al. (1989) Bone involvement in primary hemochromatosis and alcoholic cirrhosis. Am J Gastroenterol 84: 1231–34

Cooper C, Campion G, Melton LJ (1992) Hip fracture in elderly: a world wide projection. Osteoporosis Int 2: 285–89

Cooper C, Atkinson EJ, Jacobsen SJ,et al. (1993) Population-based study of survival after osteoporotic fractures. Am J Epidemiol 137: 1001–05

Crilly RG, Anderson C, Hogan D, et al. (1988) Bone histomorphometry, bone mass, and related parameters in alcoholic males. Calcif Tissue Int 43: 269–76

Cumming RG, Klineberg RJ (1994) Case-control study of risk factors for hip fractures in the elderly. Am J Epidemiol 139: 493–503

Cummings SR, Kelsey JL, Nevitt MC, et al. 1985 Epidemiology of osteoporosis and osteoporotic fractures. Epidemiol Rev 7: 178–208

Cummings SR, Nevitt MC, Browner WS, et al. (1995) Risk factors for hip fracture in white women. N Engl J Med 332: 767–73

Dechavanne M, Barbier Y, Prost G, et al. (1974) Etude de l'absorption du 47 calcium dans la cirrhose éthylique. Effet du 25-hydroxycholecalciferol. [Calcium-47 absorption in alcoholic cirrhosis. Effect of 25-hydroxycholecalciferol] [French]. Nouv Presse Méd 3: 2549–51

DeLuca HF, Krisinger J, Darwish H (1990) The vitamin D system 1990. Kidney Int 38: S2–S8

Dempster DW (1992) Bone Remodeling. In: Coe FL et al. (eds) Disorders of bone and mineral metabolism. Raven Press, New York, pp. 355–82

de Vernejoul MC, Bielakoff J, Herve M, et al. (1983) Evidence for defective osteoblastic function. A role for alcohol and tobacco consumption in osteoporosis in middle-aged men. Clin Ort Rel Res: 107–15

Diamond TH, Stiel D, Lunzer M, et al. (1989a) Hepatic osteodystrophy. Static and dynamic bone histomorphometry and serum bone Gla-protein in 80 patients with chronic liver disease. Gastroenterology 96: 213–21

Diamond T, Stiel D, Lunzer M, et al. (1989b) Ethanol reduces bone formation and may cause osteoporosis. Am J Med 86: 282–88

Diamond T, Stiel D, Lunzer M, et al. (1990) Osteoporosis and skeletal fractures in chronic liver disease. Gut 31: 82–87

Dibble JB, Sheridan P, Hampshire R, et al. (1982) Osteomalacia, vitamin D deficiency and cholestasis in chronic liver disease. Q J Med 51: 89–103

Dick M, Evans RA, Watson L (1969) Effect of ethanol on magnesium excretion. J Clin Pathol 22: 152–53

Diez A, Puig J, Serrano S, et al. (1994) Alcohol-induced bone disease in the absence of severe chronic liver damage. J Bone Min Res 9: 825–31

Diez A, Serrano S, Cucurull J, et al. (1997) Acute effects of ethanol on mineral metabolism and trabecular bone in Sprague-Dawley rats. Calcif Tissue Int 61: 168–71

Dirks JH (1983) The kidney and magnesium regulation. Kidney Int 23: 771–77

Duane P, Peters TJ (1988) Nutritional status in alcoholics with and without chronic skeletal muscle myopathy. Alcohol Alcoholism 23: 271–77

Dusso A, Finch J, Delmez J, et al. (1990) Extrarenal production of calcitriol. Kidney Int 38: S36–S40

Dymling JF, Ljungberg O, Hillyard CJ, et al. (1976) Whisky: a new provacative test for calcitonin secretion. Acta Endocrinol (Copenh) 82: 500–09

Elders PJM, Netelenbos JC, Lips P, et al. (1989) Perimenopausal bone mass and risk factors. Bone Miner 7: 289–99

Emmertsen KK, Nielsen HE, Mosekilde L, et al. (1980) Pentagastrin, calcium and whisky stimulated serum calcitonin in medullary carcinoma of the thyroid. Acta Radiologica–Oncology 19: 85–89

Erdtsieck RJ, Pols HA, Algra D, et al. (1994) Bone mineral density in healthy Dutch women: spine and hip measurements using dual-energy X-ray absorptiometry. Neth J Med 45: 198–205

Eriksen EF, Moesekilde M, Mehlsen F. (1989) Histomorphometric analysis of bone in metabolic bone diseases. Endocrinol Metab Clin North Am 18: 919–54

Farley JR, Fitzsimmons R, Taylor AK, et al. (1985) Direct effects of ethanol on bone resorption and formation in vitro. Arch Biochem Biophys 238: 305–14

Fehily AM, Coles RJ, Evans WD, et al. (1992) Factors affecting bone density in young adults. Am J Clin Nutr 56: 579–86

Feitelberg S, Epstein S, Ismail F, et al. (1987) Deranged bone mineral metabolism in chronic alcoholism. Metabolism 36: 322–26

Felson DT, Kiel DP, Anderson JJ, et al. (1988) Alcohol consumption and hip fractures: the Framingham Study. Am J Epidemiol 128: 1102–10

Felson DT, Zhang Y, Hannan MT, et al. (1995) Alcohol intake and bone mineral density in elderly men and women: the Framingham Study. Am J Epidemiol 142: 485–92

Fitzpatrick LA, Coleman DT, Bilezikian JP (1992) The target tissue actions of parathyroid hormone. In: Coe FL, Favus MJ (eds) Disorders of bone and mineral metabolism. Raven Press, New York, pp. 123–49

Flink EB (1986) Magnesium deficiency in alcoholism [Review]. Alcohol Clin Exp Res 10: 590–94

Flink EB, Shane SR, Scobbo RR, et al. (1979) Relationship of free fatty acids and magnesium in ethanol withdrawal in dogs. Metabolism 28: 858–65

Fraher LJ, Adami S, Papapoulos SE, et al. (1986) Evidence for extrarenal metabolism of 25-hydroxyvitamin D in man. Clin Sci 71: 89–95

Franceschi S, Schinella D, Bidoli E, et al. (1996) The influence of body size, smoking, and diet on bone density in pre- and postmenopausal women. Epidemiology 7: 411–14

Fraser DR, Kodicek E (1973) Regulation of 25-hydroxycholecalciferol-1-hydroxylase activity in kidney by parathyroid hormone. Nature New Biol 241: 163–66

Frick A, Rumrich G, Ullrich KJ, et al. (1965) Microperfusion study of calcium transport in the proximal tubule of the rat kidney. Pflügers Archiv 286: 109–17

Friday KE, Howard GA (1991) Ethanol inhibits human bone cell proliferation and function in vitro. Metabolism 40: 562–65

Frost HM (1964) Dynamics of bone remodeling. In: Frost HM (ed) Bone dynamics. Little Brown & Co., Boston

Frost HM (1969) Tetracyclin- based histological analysis of bone remodeling. Calcif Tissue Res 3: 211–37

Fujiwara S, Kasagi F, Yamada M, et al. (1997) Risk factors for hip fracture in a Japanese cohort. J Bone Mineral Res 12: 998–1004

Garcia-Sanchez A, Gonzalez-Calvin JL, Diez-Ruiz A, et al. (1995) Effect of acute alcohol ingestion on mineral metabolism and osteoblastic function. Alcohol Alcoholism 30: 449–53

Gascon-Barre M (1982a) Interrelationships between vitamin D3 and 25-hydroxyvitamin D3 during chronic ethanol administration in the rat. Metabolism 31: 67–72

Glynn NW, Meilahn EN, Charron M, et al. (1995) Determinants of bone mineral density in older men. J Bone Mineral Res 10: 1769–77

Gonzalez-Calvin JL, Garcia-Sanchez A, Bellot V, et al. (1993) Mineral metabolism, osteoblastic function and bone mass in chronic alcoholism. Alcohol Alcoholism 28: 571–79

Grisso JA, Kelsey JL, Strom BL, et al. (1991) Risk factors for falls as a cause of hip fracture in women. N Engl J Med 324: 1326–31

Grisso JA, Kelsey JL, Strom BL, et al. (1994) Risk factors hip fracture in black women. N Engl J Med 330: 1555–59

Habener JF, Potts JT (1976) Relative effectiveness of magnesium and calcium on the secretion and biosynthesis of parathyroid hormone in vitro. Endocrinology 98: 197–202

Habener JF, Potts JT Jr (1978) Parathyroid physiology and primary hyperparathyroidism. In: Avioli LV et al. (eds) Metabolic bone disease, vol II. Academic Press, New York, pp. 1–132

Habener JF, Rosenblatt M, Potts JT Jr (1984) Parathyroid hormone: biochemical aspects of biosynthesis, secretion, action, and metabolism. Physiol Rev 64: 985–1053

Habener JF, Potts JT Jr (1990) Fundamental considerations in the physiology, biology and biochemistry of parathyroid hormone. In: Avioli LV, Krane SM (eds) Metabolic bone disease, 2nd ed. W. B. Saunders Comp., Philadelphia, Ch. 3

Hansen MA, Overgaard K, Riis BJ, et al. (1991) Potential risk factors for development of postmenopausal osteoporosis--examined over a 12-year period. Osteoporosis Int 1: 95–102

Harding A, Dunlap J, Cook S, et al. (1988) Osteoporotic correlates of alcoholism in young males. Orthopedics 11: 279–82

Harrison HE, Harrison HC (1964) The interaction of vitamin D and parathyroid pormone on calcium phosphorous and magnesium homeostasis in the rat. Metabolism 13: 952–58

Haussler MR (1986) Vitamin D receptors: nature and function. Annu Rev Nutr 6: 527–62

Hemenway D, Colditz GA, Willett WC, et al. (1988) Fractures and lifestyle: effect of cigarette smoking, alcohol intake and relative weight on the risk of hip and forearm fractures in middle-aged women. Am J Publ Health 78: 1554-58

Hemenway D, Azrael DR, Rimm EB, et al. (1994a) Risk factors for wrist fracture: effect of age, cigarettes, alcohol, body height, relative weight, and handedness on the risk for distal forearm fractures in men. Am J Epidemiol 140: 361–67

Hemenway D, Azrael DR, Rimm EB, et al. (1994b) Risk factors for hip fracture in US men aged 40 through 75 years. Am J Publ Health 84: 1843–45

Hemmingsen R, Kramp P (1980) Effects of acute ethanol intoxication, chronic ethanol intoxication, and ethanol withdrawal on magnesium and calcium metabolism in the rat. Psychopharmacology (Berl) 67: 255–59

Hernandez-Avila M, Colditz GA, Stampfer MJ, et al. (1991) Caffeine, moderate alcohol intake, and risk of fractures of the hip and forearm in middle-aged women. Am J Clin Nutr 54: 157–63

Heynen G, Cecchettin M, Gaspar S, et al. (1977) The effect of beta-blockade on ethanol-induced secretion of calcitonin in chronic renal failure. Calcif Tissue Res 22 (Suppl): 137–41

Ho SC, Chan SSG, Woo J, et al. (1995) Determinants of bone mass in the Chinese old-old population. Osteoporos Int 5: 161–66

Hogan HA, Sampson HW, Cashier E, et al. (1997) Alcohol consumption by young actively growing rats: a study of cortical bone histomorphometry and mechanical properties. Alcohol Clin Exp Res 21: 809–16

Holbrook TL, Barrett-Connor E (1993) A prospective study of alcohol consumption and bone mineral density. Br Med J 306: 1506–09

Horak J, Nilsson BE (1975) Epidemiology of fracture of the upper end of the humerus. Clin Orthop 112: 250–53

Huang Z, Himes JH, MacGovern PG (1996) Nutrition and subsequent hip fracture risk among a national cohort of white women. Am J Epidemiol 144: 124–34

Huffer WE (1988) Morphology and biochemistry of bone remodeling: possible control by vitamin D, parathyroid hormone, and other substances. Lab Invest 59: 418–42

Hutchinson TA, Polansky SM, Feinstein AR (1979) Post-menopausal oestrogens protect against fractures of hip and distal radius. Lancet ii: 705–09

Ikekawa N (1987) Structures and biological activities of vitamin D metabolites and their analogs. Med Res Rev 7: 333–66

Israel Y, Orrego H, Holt S, et al. (1980) Identification of alcohol abuse: thoracic fractures on routine chest X-rays as indicators of alcoholism. Alcohol Clin Exp Res 4: 420–22

Johnell O, Kristensson H, Nilsson BE (1982) Parathyroid activity in alcoholics. Br J Addict 77: 93–95

Johnell O, Gullberg B, Kanis JA, et al. (1995) Risk factors for hip fracture in European women: the MEDOS study. J Bone Mineral Res 10: 1802–15

Johnson RD, Davidson S, Saunders JB, et al. (1984) Fractures on chest radiography as indicators of alcoholism in patients with liver disease. Br Med J 288: 365–66

Jorge-Hernandez JA, Gonzalez-Reimers CE, Torres-Ramirez A, et al. (1988) Bone changes in alcoholic liver cirrhosis. A histomorphometrical analysis of 52 cases [Review]. Dig Dis Sci 33: 1089–95

Jubiz W, Canterbury JM, Reiss E, et al (1972) Circadian rhythm in serum parathyroid hormone concentration in human subjects: correlation with serum calcium, phosphate, albumin and growth hormone levels. J Clin Invest 51: 2040–46

Kanis JA (1994) Assesment of fracture risk and its application to screening for postmenopausal osteoporosis: synopsis of a WHO report. Osteoporosis Int 4: 368–81

Kanis JA, Adams ND, Cecchettin M, et al. (1979) Ethanol induced secretion of calcitonin in chronic renal disease. Clin Endocrinol (Oxf) 10: 155–61

Kanis JA, Hamdy NAT, McCloskey (1992) Hypercalcaemia and hypocalcaemia. In: Cameron S, Davison AM, Grünfeld J, et al. (eds) Oxford textbook of clinical nephrology. Oxford University Press, Oxford, pp. 1753–82

Karbach U, Ewe K (1987) Calcium and magnesium transport and influence of 1,25-dihydroxyvitamin D₃ Digestion 37: 35–42

Karbach U, Rummel W (1990) Cellular and paracellular magnesium transport across the terminal ileum of the rats and its interaction with the calcium transport. Gastroenterology 98: 985–92

Keiver K, Herbert L, Weinberg J (1996) Effect of maternal ethanol consumption on maternal and fetal calcium metabolism. Alcohol Clin Exp Res 20: 1305–12

Keiver K, Ellis L, Anzarut A, et al. (1997) Effect of prenatal ethanol exposure on fetal calcium metablism. Alcohol Clin Exp Res 21: 1612–18

Kelepouris N, Harper KD, Gannon F, et al. (1995) Severe osteoporosis in men [Review]. Ann Intern Med 123: 452–60

King AL, Sica DA, Miller G, et al. (1987) Severe hypophosphatemia in a general hospital population. South Afr Med J 80: 831–35

Klein RF (1997) Alcohol-induced bone disease: impact of ethanol on osteoblast proliferation [Review]. Alcohol Clin Exp Res 21: 392–99

Klein RF, Carlos AS (1995) Inhibition of osteoblastic cell proliferation and ornithine decarboxylase activity by ethanol. Endocrinology 136: 3406–11

Klein RF, Fausti KA, Carlos AS (1996) Ethanol inhibits human osteoblastic cell proliferation. Alcohol Clin Exp Res 20: 572–78

Krall EA, Dawson-Hughes B (1993) Heritable and life-style determinants of bone mineral density. J Bone Mineral Res 8: 1–9

Krawitt EL (1975) Effect of ethanol ingestion on duodenal calcium transport. J Lab Clin Med 85: 665–71

Krawitt EL, Sampson HW, Katagiri CA (1975) Effect of 1,25-dihydroxycholecalciferol on ethanol mediated suppression of calcium absorption. Calcif Tissue Res 18: 119–24

Krishnamra N, Limlomwongse L (1983) The acute hypocalcaemic effect of ethanol and its mechanism of action in the rat. Can Physiol Pharmacol 61: 388–94

Krishnamra N, Boonpimol P (1986) Acute effect of ethanol on intestinal calcium transport. J Nutr Sci Vitaminol 32: 229–36

Kristensson H, Lunden A, Nilsson BE (1980) Fracture incidence and diagnostic roentgen in alcoholics. Acta Orthop Scand 51: 205–07

Kröger H, Laitinen K (1992) Bone mineral density measured by dual-energy X-ray absorptiometry in normal men. Eur J Clin Invest 22: 454–60

Kröger H, Tuppurainen M, Honkanen R, et al. (1994) Bone mineral density and risk factors for osteoporosis: a population-based study of 1600 perimenopausal women. Calcif Tissue Int 55: 1–7

Kusy RP, Hirsch PF, Peng TC (1989) Influence of ethanol on stiffness, toughness, and ductility of femurs of rats. Alcohol Clin Exp Res 13: 185–89

Labib M, Abdel-Kader M, Ranganath L, et al. (1989a) Bone disease in chronic alcoholism: the value of plasma osteocalcin measurement. Alcohol Alcoholism 24: 141–44

Labib M, Abdel-Kader M, Ranganath L, et al. (1989b) Impaired renal tubular function in chronic alcoholics. J R Soc Med 82: 139–41

Laitinen K (1993) Alcohol and Bone. Helsinki University, Helsinki, Finland.

Laitinen K, Valimaki M, Lamberg-Allardt C, et al. (1990) Deranged vitamin D metabolism but normal bone mineral density in Finnish noncirrhotic male alcoholics. Alcohol Clin Exp Res 14: 551–56

Laitinen K, Lamberg-Allardt C, Tunninen R, et al. (1991a) Transient hypoparathyroidism during acute alcohol intoxication. N Engl J Med 324: 721–27

Laitinen K, Lamberg-Allardt C, Tunninen R, et al. (1991b) Effects of 3 weeks' moderate alcohol intake on bone and mineral metabolism in normal men. Bone Miner 13: 139–51

Laitinen K, Välimäki M, Keto P (1991c) Bone mineral density measured by dual-energy x-ray absorptiometry in healthy Finnish women. Calcif Tissue Int 48: 224–31

Laitinen K, Lamberg-Allardt C, Tunninen R, et al. (1992a) Bone mineral density and abstention-induced changes in bone and mineral metabolism in noncirrhotic male alcoholics. Am J Med 93: 642–50

Laitinen K, Tahtela R, Välimäki M (1992b) The dose-dependency of alcohol-induced hypoparathyroidism, hypercalciuria, and hypermagnesuria. Bone Miner 19: 75–83

Laitinen K, Kärkkäinen M, Lalla M, et al. (1993) Is alcohol an osteoporosis-inducing agent for young and middle-aged women? Metabolism 42: 875–81

Laitinen K, Tahtela R, Luomanmäki K, et al. (1994) Mechanisms of hypocalcemia and markers of bone turnover in alcohol-intoxicated drinkers. Bone Miner 24: 171–79

Lalor BC, France MW, Powell D, et al. (1986) Bone and mineral metabolism and chronic alcohol abuse. Q J Med 59: 497–511

Lau E, Donnan S, Barker DJP, et al. (1988) Physical activity and calcium intake in fracture of the proximal femur in Hong Kong. Br Med J 297: 1441–43

Lee M, Leichter J (1983) Skeletal development in fetuses of rats consuming alcohol during gestation. Growth 47: 254–62

Lieberherr M, Grosse B, Bourdeau A, (1991). Non-gene-mediated effects of calcitriol: a possible involvment of membrane receptor. In: Norman AW, Bouillon R, Thomasset M (eds) Vitamin D: gene regulation, structure-function analysis and clinical application. Walter de Gruyter, Berlin, pp. 368–75

Lindholm J, Steiniche T, Rasmussen E, et al. (1991) Bone disorder in men with chronic alcoholism: a reversible disease? J Clin Endocrinol Metab 73: 118–24

Lindsell DR, Wilson AG, Maxwell JD (1982) Fractures on the chest radiograph in detection of alcoholic liver disease. Br Med J 285: 597–99

Linkola J, Fyhrquist F, Ylikahri R (1979) Adenosine 3′,5′ cyclic monophosphate, calcium and magnesium excretion in ethanol intoxication and hangover. Acta Physiol Scand 107: 333–37

Ljunghall S, Lundin L, Wide L (1985) Acute effects of ethanol intake on the serum concentrations of parathyroid hormone, calcium and phosphate. Exp Clin Endocrinol 85: 365–68

Luisier M, Vodoz JF, Donath A, et al. (1977) Carence en 25-hydroxyvitamine D avec diminution de l'absorption intestinale de calcium et de la densité osseuse dans l'alcoolisme chronique. [25-hydroxy vitamin D deficiency with reduction of intestinal calcium absorption and bone density in chronic alcoholism]. [French]. Schweiz Med Wochenschr 107: 1529–33

Lund B, Sorensen OH, Hilden M, et al. (1977) The hepatic conversion of vitamin D in alcoholics with varying degrees of liver affection. Acta Med Scand 202: 221–24

Magliola L, Anast CS, Forte LR (1986) Vitamin D metabolites do not alter parathyroid hormone secretion acutely. Bone Miner 1: 495–505

Mahboob T, Haleem MA (1988) Effect of ethanol on serum electrolytes and osmolality. Life Sci 42: 1507–13

Matsubara K, Nakahara M, Takahashi S, et al. (1982) Acute effects of ethanol and acetaldehyde on plasma phosphate level. J Pharma Pharmacol 34: 373–76

Mawer EB, Backhouse J, Hill LF, et al. (1975) Vitamin D metabolism and parathyroid function in man. Clin Sci 48: 349–65

Mawer EB, Hayes ME, Still PE, et al. (1991) Evidence for nonrenal synthesis of 1,25-dihydroxyvitamin D in pateints with inflammatory arthritis. J Bone Min Res 6: 733-39

May H, Murphy S, Khaw K-T (1995) Alcohol consumption and bone mineral density in men. Gerontology 41: 152–58

Mayer GP, Hurst JG (1978) Comparison of the effects of calcium and magnesium on parathyroid hormone secretion rate in calves. Endocrinology 102: 1803–07

McCaughan GW, Feller RB (1994) Osteoporosis in chronic liver disease: pathogenesis, risk factors, and management [Review]. Dig Dis 12: 223–31

McDonald JT, Margen S (1979) Wine versus ethanol in human nutrition. III. Calcium, phosphorous, and magnesium balance. Am J Clin Nutr 32: 823–33

McIntyre N (1984) The effects of alcohol on water, electrolytes and minerals [Review]. Contemp Issues Clin Biochem 1: 117–34

Medalle R, Waterhouse C, Hahn TJ (1976) Vitamin D resistance in magnesium deficiency. Am J Clin Nutr 29: 854–58

Melton LJ III (1991) Epidemiology of osteoporosis. Clin Obstet Gynaecol 5: 785–805

Mezey E (1985) Metabolic effects of alcohol [Review]. Fed Proc 44: 134–38

Mezey E, Potter JJ, Merchant CR (1979) Effect of ethanol feeding on bone composition in the rat. Am J Clin Nutr 32: 25–29

Mobarhan SA, Russell RM, Recker RR, et al. (1984) Metabolic bone disease in alcoholic cirrhosis: a comparison of the effect of vitamin D2, 25-hydroxyvitamin D, or supportive treatment. Hepatology 4: 266–73

Monegal A, Navasa M, Guanabens N, et al. (1997) Osteoporosis and bone mineral metabolism disorders in cirrhotic patients referred for orthotopic liver transplantation. Calcif Tissue Int 60: 148–54

Money SR, Petroianu A, Kimura K, et al. (1989) Acute hypocalcemic effect of ethanol in dogs. Alcohol Clin Exp Res 13: 453–56

Mori S, Harada S, Okazaki R, et al. (1992) Hypomagnesemia with increased metabolism of parathyroid hormone and reduced responsiveness to calcitropic hormones. Intern Med 31: 820–24

Mundy GR (1989) Calcium homeostasis: hypercalcemia and hypocalcemia. Dunitz, London

Naves Diaz M, O'Niell TW, Silman AJ (1997) The influence of alcohol consumption on the risk of vertebral deformity. Osteoporosis Int 7: 65–71

Need AG, Guerin MD, Pain RW, et al. (1985) The tubular maximum for calcium reabsorption: normal range and correction for sodium excretion. Clin Chim Acta 150: 87–93

Nemere I, Zhou L-X, Norman AW (1991) Vesicular calcium transport across the intestine and its initiation by 1,25-dihydroxyvitamin D during transcaltachia. In: Norman AW, Bouillon R, Thomasset M (eds) Vitamin D: gene regulation, structure, function analysis and clinical application. Walter de Gruyter, Berlin, pp. 360–67

New SA, Bolton-Smith C, Grubb DA, et al. (1997) Nutritional influences on bone mineral density: a cross-sectional study in premenopausal women. Am J Clin Nutr 65: 1831–39

Nguyen TV, Eisman JA, Kelly PJ, et al. (1996) Risk factors for osteoporotic fractures in elderly men. Am J Epidemiol 144: 255–63

Nielsen HK, Lundby L, Rasmussen K, et al. (1990) Alcohol decreases serum osteocalcin in a dose-dependent way in normal subjects. Calcif Tissue Int 46: 173–78

Nieves JW, Golden AL, Siris E, et al. (1995) Teenage and current calcium intake are related to bone mineral density of the hip and forearm in women aged 30–39 years. Am J Epidemiol 141: 342–51

Nilsson BE (1970) Conditions contributing to fracture of the femoral neck. Acta Chir Scand 136: 383–84

Nordin BEC (1976) Plasma calcium and plasma magnesium homeostasis. In: Nordin BEC (ed) Calcium, phosphate and magnesium metabolism. Churchill Livingstone, New York, pp. 186–216

Nordin BEC, Peacock M (1969) Role of kidney in regulation of plasma calcium. Lancet ii: 1280–83

Nordqvist A, Petersson CJ (1996) Shoulder injuries common in alcoholics: an analysis of 413 injuries. Acta Orthopaed Scand 67: 364–66

Norman AW (1979) Vitamin D, the calcium homeostatic steroid hormone. Academic Press, New York

Nyquist F, Ljunghall S, Berglund M, et al. (1996) Biochemical markers of bone metabolism after short and long time ethanol withdrawal in alcoholics. Bone 19: 51–54

Odvina CV, Safi I, Wojtowicz CH, et al. (1995) Effect of heavy alcohol intake in the absence of liver disease on bone mass in black and white men. J Endocrinol Metab 80: 2499–2503

Orwoll ES, Bauer DC, Vogt TM, et al. (1996) Axial bone mass in older women. Ann Intern Med 124: 187–96

Padmanabhan R, Muawad WM (1985) Exencephaly and axial skeletal dysmorphogenesis induced by acute doses of ethanol in mouse fetuses. Drug Alcohol Depend 16: 215–27

Parfitt A M (1976a) The Actions of parathyroid hormone on bone: relation to bone remodeling and turnover, cCalcium homeostasis and metabolic bone disease.I Mechanisms of calcium transfer between bood and bone and their cellular basis. Morphologic and kinetic approaches to bone turnover. Metabolism 25: 809–44

Parfitt AM (1976b) The actions of parathyroid hormone on bone: relation to bone remodeling and turnover, calcium homeostasis and metabolic bone disease. II PTH and bone cells: Bone turnover and plasma calcium regulation. Metabolism 25: 909–55

Parfitt AM (1989) Plasma calcium control at quiescent bone surfaces: A new approach to the homeostatic function of bone lining cells. Bone 10: 87–88

Parfitt AM (1992) Calcium homeostasis. In: Mundy GR, Martin JT (eds) Physiology and pharmacology of bone. Springer-Verlag, Berlin, pp. 1–65

Peng TC, Cooper CW, Munson PL (1972) The hypocalcemic effect of ethyl alcohol in rats and dogs. Endocrinology 91: 586–93

Peng TC, Gitelman HJ (1974) Ethanol-induced hypocalcemia, hypermagnesemia and inhibition of the serum calcium-raising effect of parathyroid hormone in rats. Endocrinology 94: 608–11

Peng TC, Garner SC, Frye GD, et al. (1982) Evidence of a toxic effect of ethanol on bone in rats. Alcohol Clin Exp Res 6: 96–99

Peng TC, Kusy RP, Hirsch PF, et al. (1988) Ethanol-induced changes in morphology and strength of femurs of rats. Alcohol Clin Exp Res 12: 655–59

Peng TC, Lian JB, Hirsch PF, et al. (1991) Lower serum osteocalcin in ethanol-fed rats. J Bone Min Res 6: 107–15

Pepersack T, Fuss M, Otero J, et al. (1992) Longitudinal study of bone metabolism after ethanol withdrawal in alcoholic patients. J Bone Mineral Res 7: 383–87

Peris P, Pares A, Guanabens N, et al. (1992) Reduced spinal and femoral bone mass and deranged bone mineral metabolism in chronic alcoholics. Alcohol Alcoholism 27: 619–25

Peris P, Pares A, Guañabens N, et al. (1994) Bone mass improves in alcoholics after 2 years of abstinence. J Bone Mineral Res 9: 1607–12

Peris P, Guanabens N, Monegal A, et al. (1995a) Aetiology and presenting symptoms in male osteoporosis. Br J Rheumatol 34: 936–41

Peris P, Guañabens N, Pares A, et al. (1995b) Vertebral fractures and osteopenia in chronic alcoholic patients. Calcif Tissue Int 57: 111–14

Peters TJ, Martin F, Ward K (1985) Chronic alcoholic skeletal myopathy: common and reversible. Alcohol 2: 485–89

Pietschmann P, Resch H, Muller C, et al. (1990) Decreased serum osteocalcin levels in patients with liver cirrhosis. Bone Miner 8: 103–08

Pitts TO, Van Thiel DH (1986) Disorders of divalent ions and vitamin D metabolism in chronic alcoholism. Recent Dev Alcohol 4: 357–77

Posner DB, Russell RM, Absood S, et al. (1978) Effective 25-hydroxylation of vitamin D2 in alcoholic cirrhosis. Gastroenterology 74: 866–70

Preedy VR, Marway JS, Salisbury JR, et al. (1990) Protein synthesis in bone and skin of the rat are inhibited by ethanol: implications for whole body metabolism. Alcohol Clin Exp Res 14: 165–68

Preedy VR, Sherwood RA, Akpoguma CI, et al. (1991a) The urinary excretion of the collagen degradation markers pyridinoline and deoxypyridinoline in an experimental rat model of alcoholic bone disease. Alcohol Alcoholism 26: 191–98

Preedy VR, Baldwin DR, Keating JW, et al. (1991b) Bone collagen, mineral and trace element composition, histomorphometry and urinary HOP excretion in chronically-treated alcohol-fed rats. Alcohol Alcoholism 26: 39–46

Puschett JB, Moranz J, Kurnick WS (1972) Evidence for a direct action of cholecalciferol and 25-hydroxycholecalciferol on the renal transport of phosphate, sodium and calcium. J Clin Invest 51: 373–85

Raisz LG, Trummel CL, Holick MF, et al. (1972) 1,25-dihydroxy-cholecalciferol: a potent stimulator of bone resorption in tissue culture. Science 175: 768–69

Ramp WK, Demaree DN (1984) Inhibition of net calcium efflux from bone by ethanol in vitro. Am J Physiol 246: C30–36

Ramp WK, Murdock WC, Gommerman WA, et al. (1975) Effects of ethanol on chicks in vivo and on chick embryo tibiae in organ culture. Calcif Tissue Res 17: 195–203

Reichel H, Koeffler HP, Norman AW (1989) The role of the vitamin D endocrine system in health and disease. N Engl J Med 320: 980–91

Reid IR, Ames R, Evans MC, et al. (1992) Determinants of total body and regional bone mineral density in normal postmenopausal women: a key role for fat mass. J Clin Endocrinol Metab 75:45–51

Resch H, Pietschmann P, Krexner E, et al. (1990) Peripheral bone mineral content in patients with fatty liver and hepatic cirrhosis. Scand J Gastroenterol 25: 412–16

Rico H, Cabranes JA, Cabello J, et al. (1987) Low serum osteocalcin in acute alcohol intoxication: a direct toxic effect of alcohol on osteoblasts. Bone Miner 2: 221–25

Rico H (1990) Alcohol and bone disease. [Review]. Alcohol Alcoholism 25: 345–52

Riesenfeld A (1985) Growth-depressing effects of alcohol and nicotine in two strains of rats. Acta Anat (Basel) 122: 18–24

Robertson WG (1976) Urinary excretion. In: Nordin BEC (ed) Calcium, phosphate and magnesium metabolism. Churchill Livingstone, New York, pp. 113–61

Roginsky MS, Zanzi I, Cohn SH (1976) Skeletal and lean body mass in alcoholics with and without cirrhosis. Calc Tissue Res 21 (Suppl): 386–91

Rude RK, Bethune JE, Singer FR (1980) Renal tubular maximum for magnesium in normal, hyperparathyroid and hypoparathyroid man. J Clin Endocrinol Metab 51: 1425–31

Ryback RS, Eckardt MJ, Pautler CP (1980) Clinical relationships between serum phosphorus and other blood chemistry values in alcoholics. Arch Intern Med 140: 673–77

Ryle PR, Thomson AD (1984) Nutrition and vitamins in alcoholism [Review]. Contemp Issues Clin Biochem 1: 188–224

Salamone LM, Glynn NW, Black DM, et al. (1996) Determinants of premenopausal bone mineral density : the interplay of genetic and lifestyle factors. J Bone Mineral Res 11: 1557–65

Sampson HW, Perks N, Champney TH, et al. (1996) Alcohol consumption inhibits bone growth and development in young actively growing rats. Alcohol Clin Exp Res 20: 1375–84

Sampson HW, Chaffin C, Lange J, et al. (1997a) Alcohol consumption by young actively growing rats: a histomorphometric study of cancellous bone. Alcohol Clin Exp Res 21: 352–59

Sampson HW, Shipley D (1997b) Moderate alcohol consumption does not augment bone density in ovariectomized rats. Alcohol Clin Exp Res 21: 1165–68

Sargent WQ, Simpson JR, Beard JD (1974) The effects of acute and chronic ethanol administration on divalent cation excretion. J Pharmacol Exp Ther 190: 507–14

Saville PP (1965) Changes in bone mass with age and alcoholism. J Bone Joint Surg 47: 492–99

Saville PD, Lieber CS (1965) Effect of alcohol on growth, bone density and muscle magnesium in the rat. J Nutr 87: 477–84

Schnitzler CM, Solomon L (1984) Bone changes after alcohol abuse. S Afr Med J 66: 730–34

Seeman E (1997a) Do men suffer with osteoporosis? Aust Fam Physician 26: 135–43

Seeman E (1997b) Osteoporosis in men. Bailliere's Clin Rheumatol 11: 613–28

Seeman E, Melton LJ III, O'Fallon WM, et al. (1983) Risk factors for spinal osteoporosis in men. Am J Med 75: 977–83

Shafik IM, Dirks JH (1992) Hypo- and hypermagnesaemia. In: Cameron S et al. (eds) Oxford textbook of clinical nephrology. Oxford University Press, Oxford, pp. 1802–21

Shan JH, Bowser EN, Hargis GK, et al. (1978) Effect of ethanol on parathyroid hormone secretion in the rat. Metabolism 27: 257–60

Shaw NJ, Wheeldon J, Brocklebank JT (1992) The tubular maximum for calcium reabsorption: a normal range in children. Clin Endocrinol 36: 193–95

Shaw CK (1993) An epidemiologic study of osteoporosis in Taiwan. Ann Epidemiol 3: 264–71

Slemenda CW, Christian JC, Reed T, et al. (1992) Long-term bone loss in men: effects of genetic and environmental factors. Ann Intern Med 117: 286–91

Sowers MR, Clark MK, Hollis B, et al. (1992) Radial bone mineral density in pre- and perimenopausal women: a prospective study of rates and risk factors for loss. J Bone Mineral Res 7: 6471–57

Sowers MR, Clark MK, Jannausch ML, et al. (1993) Body size, estrogen use and thiazide diuretic use affect 5-year radial bone loss in postmenopausal women. Osteoporosis Int 3: 314–21

Stein JH, Smith WO, Ginn HE (1966) Hypophosphatemia in acute alcoholism. Am J Med Sci 252: 78–83

Stern P (1990) Vitamin D and bone. Kidney Int 38 (S29): S17–S21

Stevenson JC, Lees B, Devenport M, et al. (1989) Determinants of bone density in normal women: risk factors for future osteoporosis? Br Med J 298: 924–28

Suzuki T, Yoshida H, Hashimoto T, et al. (1997) Case-control study of risk factors for hip fractures in the Japanese elderly by a Mediterranean osteoporosis study (MEDOS) questionnaire. Bone 21: 461–67

Swartz CM, Young MA (1988) Male hypogonadism: risks for myocardial infarction and bone fracture [Review]. Compr Ther 14: 21–24

Talmage RV (1969) Calcium homeostasis–calcium transport–parathyroid action: the effect of parathyroid hormone on the movement of calcium between bone and fluid. Clin Orthop 67: 210–24

Territo MC, Tanaka KR (1974) Hypophosphatemia in chronic alcoholism. Arch Intern Med 134: 445–47

Thomas S, Movsowitz C, Epstein S, et al. (1990) The response of circulating parameters of bone mineral metabolism to ethanol- and EDTA-induced hypocalcemia in the rat. Bone Miner 8: 1–6

Tuppurainen M, Kröger H, Honkanen R, et al. (1995) Risks of perimenopausal fractures: a prospective population-based study. Acta Obstet Gynecol Scand 74: 624–28

Turner RT, Aloia RC, Segel LD, et al. (1988) Chronic alcohol treatment results in disturbed vitamin D metabolism and skeletal abnormalities in rats. Alcohol Clin Exp Res 12: 159–62

Turner RT, Greene VS, Bell NH (1987) Demonstration that ethanol inhibits bone matrix synthesis and mineralization in the rat. J Bone Mineral Res 2: 61–66

Urbano-Marquez A, Estruch R, Navarro-Lopez F, et al. (1989) The effect of alcoholism on skeletal and cardiac muscle. N Engl J Med 320: 409–15

Välimäki M, Ylikahri R (1981) Alcohol and sex hormones [editorial]. Scand J Clin Lab Invest 41: 99–105

Välimäki MJ, Harkonen M, Eriksson CJ, et al. (1984) Sex hormones and adrenocortical steroids in men acutely intoxicated with ethanol. Alcohol 1: 89–93

Van Thiel DH, Lester R, Sherins RJ (1974) Hypogonadism in alcoholic liver disease: evidence for a double defect. Gastroenterology 67: 1188–99

Van Thiel DH, Gavaler JS, Lester R, et al. (1975) Alcohol-induced testicular atrophy. An experimental model for hypogonadism occurring in chronic alcoholic men. Gastroenterology 69: 326–32

Van Thiel DH, Gavaler JS, Eagon PK, et al. (1981) Hypogonadism and feminization in alcoholic men: the past, present and future [Review]. Curr Alcohol 8: 29–40

Verbanck M, Verbanck J, Brauman J, et al. (1977) Bone histology and 25-OH vitamin D plasma levels in alcoholics without cirrhosis. Calc Tissue Res 22 (Suppl) 538–41

Walker DA, Davies SJ, Siddle K, et al. (1977) Control of renal tubular phosphate reabsorption by parathyroid hormone in man. Clin Sci 53: 431–438

Weinberg J, D'Alquen G, Bezio S (1990) Interactive effects of ethanol intake and maternal nutritional status on skeletal development of fetal rats. Alcohol 7: 383–88

Wells SA Jr, Cooper CW, Ontjes DA (1975) Stimulation of thyrocalcitonin secretion by ethanol in patients with medullary thyroid carcinoma-an effect apparently not mediated by gastrin. Metabolism 24: 1215–19

Wilkinson R (1976) Absorption of calcium, phosphate and magnesium. In: Nordin BEC (ed) Calcium, phosphate and magnesium metabolism. Churchill Livingstone, New York, pp.36–112

Wilkinson G, Cundy T, Parsons V, et al. (1985) Metabolic bone disease and fractures in male alcoholics: a pilot study. Br J Addict 80: 65–68

Williams GA, Bowser EN, Hargis GK, et al. (1978) Effect of ethanol on parathryroid hormone and calcitonin secretion in man. Proc Soc Exp Biol Med 159: 187–91

Yamamoto M, Kawanobe Y, Takahashi H, et al. (1984) Vitamin D deficiency and renal calcium transport in the rat. J Clin Invest 74: 507–13

Yanagawa N, Lee DBN (1992) Renal handling of calcium and phosphate. In Coe FL et al. (eds) Disorders of bone and mineral metabolism. Raven Press, New York, pp. 3–41

Yano K, Heilbrun LK, Wasnich RD, et al. (1985) The relationship between diet and bone mineral content of multiple skeletal sites in elderly Japanese-American men and women lining in Hawaii. Am J Clin Nutr 42: 877–88

Ylikahri RH, Poso AR, Huttunen MO, et al. (1974) Alcohol intoxication and hangover: effects on plasma electrolyte concentrations and acid-base balance. Scand J Clin Lab Invest 34: 327–36

Young D, Hopper JL, Nowson CA, at al. (1995) Determinants of bone mass in 10- to 26-year-old females: a twin study. J Bone Mineral Res 10: 558–67

Chapter 9

Alcohol and the Central Nervous System

B. Tabakoff
University of Colorado, Denver, CO, USA

K.A. Grant
Wake Forest University School of Medicine,
Winston-Salem, NC, USA

P.L. Hoffman
University of Colorado, Denver, CO, USA

H.J. Little
Durham University, UK

Abstract

The behavioural manifestations of ethanol ingestion are a result of ethanol's interactions with the neuronal systems of the brain. Ethanol can produce a reduction in anxiety and a feeling of pleasure as well as sedation, motor incoordination, aggression, changes in other forms of social interaction, and aberrations in cognition as part of its spectrum of action. Ethanol produces its effects at significantly higher concentrations (in the millimolar range) than most of the other psychoactive drugs, and specific binding sites for ethanol, such as receptors characterized for other drugs and neurotransmitters, have not been identified. However, recent research has established that certain neurotransmitter systems of the brain are more or less sensitive to ethanol. The main excitatory and inhibitory systems of the brain (glutamate and GABA (γ-aminobutyric acid) systems, respectively) seem to be the targets of ethanol's actions, but even within these systems, different subtypes of receptors for glutamate and GABA show differential sensitivity to ethanol's effects. Particularly sensitive components of the neurotransmission process are certain receptor-gated ion channels including the $GABA_A$ receptor, the N-methyl-D-aspartate (NMDA) subtype of glutamate receptor, the nicotinic cholinergic receptor, and the serotonin-3 receptor. Ethanol also alters the release of a number of transmitter substances in particular areas of the brain. A notable example of this effect is the increase in release of dopamine in the nucleus accumbens. This event has been proposed to influence alcohol intake and is associated with increased firing of dopaminergic neurons, most probably mediated by ethanol's actions on systems that impinge on and modulate the activity of the mesolimbic dopamine system. Depending on dose and increasing concentrations of ethanol in the brain, additional systems that participate in the conduction and transmission of information become involved in ethanol's actions. Some of these systems alter their function (adapt) during periods of chronic drinking and such (mal)adaptation may generate manifestations of tolerance, physical dependence, and craving upon cessation of alcohol ingestion. Maladaptations in the NMDA receptor system and the other systems that gate calcium ion entry into neurons can also contribute to brain damage noted in some alcoholics.

Introduction

Beverage alcohol (ethanol) is a psychoactive compound that produces a spectrum of behavioural effects ranging from an increase in gregariousness to sedation and motor incoordination, from reduction in anxiety to increase in aggression, from instances of enhanced recall of events to significant cognitive deficits. Overlaid on such overt (objective) behavioural manifestations of alcohol ingestion is the ability of this compound to activate neural pathways and to generate subjective responses that produce reinforcement of behaviours associated with alcohol use (i.e. certain individuals find alcohol use pleasurable). From the very beginning, it should be emphasized that individuals differ extensively in their responses to alcohol. These differences in response are dictated by both inherited genetic factors and environmental/experiential factors. For instance, certain individuals find even low doses of ethanol aversive, and many choose not to drink alcohol, even when it is freely available to them. It should also be emphasized that although the behavioural manifestations of ethanol's actions are a result of the effects of ethanol in the brain, pharmacokinetic factors (absorption, distribution of ethanol in tissues, and rates of alcohol metabolism) contribute to the character, intensity and duration of ethanol's actions. Finally, the dose (quantity) of alcohol ingested and the rapidity of ingestion certainly modulate qualitatively, as well as quantitatively, the spectrum of ethanol's actions. The issue of the dose of alcohol needed to produce a particular manifestation of ethanol's actions on behaviour is frequently further blurred by the use of terms such as "light", "moderate" or "heavy" drinking without further definition (see Chapter 1). A recent review (Eckardt et al. 1998) on the effect of "moderate" alcohol use on brain function attempted to define the term "moderate drinking". In that review, it was concluded that an individual's alcohol intake (e.g. in "standard" drinks or even in g per kg body weight) cannot *per se* provide an adequate definition of moderate "doses" due to individual variability in pharmacokinetic parameters. To consider the CNS effects of moderate drinking, it is instead necessary to define a range of blood and brain ethanol concentrations, and duration of exposure, that is considered moderate. The upper range of moderate exposure proposed in the earlier review was a brain ethanol level of ≤ 0.92 g/l, which is equivalent to a concentration of ≤ 20 mM ethanol. The guidelines proposed in the earlier review will guide the terminology in this chapter.

When one confronts the myriad of ethanol's effects on brain function and on behaviour, one is struck by the simplicity of the chemical structure of ethanol and the significant difference in the doses required for the manifestation of ethanol's actions compared to other psychoactive compounds. Many of the other psychoactive compounds (opiates, cannabinoids, cocaine, nicotine, etc.) are taken in milligram (or even lower) quantities, while alcohol is imbibed in gram quantities. These differences in chemical structure and dose indicate that ethanol's molecular mode of action in the brain is inherently different from other psychoactive drugs. The difference seems to be primarily in how ethanol initiates its effects. Specific recognition sites (receptors) are utilized by most psychoactive drugs to initiate biochemical/biophysical changes in the brain. No such receptors have yet been identified for ethanol. As will be detailed later in this chapter, ethanol does selectively affect certain systems in brain, and some of these systems are also affected by other psychoactive drugs. The mode of ethanol's action seems to be more that of a modulator of the function of endogenous neurotransmitter substances, rather than of an independent instigator of receptor-mediated events.

Behavioural Manifestations of Alcohol's Actions

Acute Effects of Alcohol on Behaviour

Alcohol, when imbibed or otherwise administered, produces a constellation of physiological and behavioural effects in human beings and laboratory animals. The spectrum of ethanol's effects is related to the dose ingested and to individual differences in susceptibility to ethanol's actions. The most obvious overt behavioural effects occurring at moderate brain ethanol levels are those that involve activation or sedation and motor incoordination. There are also other subsets of alcohol-induced effects, including subjective effects, i.e. the individual's perception of how alcohol makes him/her feel, and cognitive effects, such as the effect of alcohol on the recall of recently learned material. Although the very first exposure to alcohol may elicit unlearned, reflexive responses, most behavioural effects of alcohol in human beings are the result of repeated administration and involve a process of learning and other forms of neuroadaptation (e.g. functional tolerance). In this way, the behavioural responses of an individual to alcohol are continually evolving, allowing for new patterns of behaviours to be established in relation to the presentation and ingestion of alcohol. The learned responses are either strengthened or weakened, depending on the context in which alcohol is consumed, the individual's predisposition to find particular aspects of alcohol's actions reinforcing (pleasurable), and the overall consequences of having drunk alcohol.

Because alcohol's effects are continually being influenced by experience, it is often difficult to assign absolute dose-response relationships to the behavioural effects of alcohol. For example, the question "what dose of alcohol impairs motor performance?" will not generate a single number, but a range of values. Alcohol's ability to impair performance is also directly proportional to the complexity of the task. A task that requires a person to recognize and classify an object is more sensitive to perturbation by alcohol than a task that only requires responding if an object is present or absent (Hindmarch et al. 1991). An equally important influence appears to be the characteristics of an individual's personal history with alcohol, such as his/her current level of alcohol consumption, family history of alcoholism and expectancies regarding alcohol's effects. Most studies with human subjects find significant effects of alcohol on a variety of subjective and performance measures when the blood alcohol concentration (BAC) reaches 0.4 g/l or higher (Nixon 1995). These studies also provide a general consensus that the most sensitive measure is self-report of feeling "intoxicated", which occurs at BACs in the range of 0.1–0.3 g/l. This lower dose range of ethanol is often reported to be stimulating, to decrease anxiety and to increase social interaction and induce a feeling of euphoria. In general, animal models have confirmed these effects of alcohol, although there are animal strains, like human individuals, that do not show the low-dose activating effects of alcohol. Rather, some animals only show sedation, and/or signs of stress when given alcohol. The variability in individual reactions to the effects of alcohol is probably reflected in the epidemiological data showing that an appreciable proportion (16-33%) of the population in Europe and North America choose not to drink alcohol (Hupkens et al. 1993, WHO 1995, Brewers Association of Canada 1995, NIAAA 1994).

Activating Effects of Alcohol

The ability of psychoactive drugs to induce motor stimulation in laboratory animals has been suggested to be a characteristic of drug-mediated reward (Wise et al. 1987). In human beings, the stimulating effect of alcohol has been measured in the context of performance of tasks or in social contexts. In very well learned tasks, low doses of alcohol can increase reaction times, although this effect is not always beneficial to the overall performance of complex tasks. An underlying mechanism may be the ability of low doses of alcohol to increase impulsivity (Mulvihill et al. 1997). Low doses of alcohol also increase locomotor and other activity in rats. Although it has been suggested that the increase in motor activity in animals may be a model for human novelty-seeking or risk-taking behaviour (Cloninger 1988), there are difficulties in this analogy and in the direct extrapolation of the motor-activating effects of alcohol to the rewarding effects of alcohol. Studies investigating both the stimulant and rewarding effects of alcohol found that the motor-activating effects of alcohol could be blocked or attenuated by various drugs without altering the expression of alcohol reward (Risinger et al. 1992, Risinger 1997). In addition, mice selectively bred to have high motor activation in response to alcohol (FAST mice) do not show enhanced preference for alcohol (Phillips et al. 1991). Thus, the motor-activating effects of alcohol can be dissociated from alcohol's rewarding effects.

One of the better known activating effects of alcohol on human beings is an increase in social interaction and conversation. Alcohol increases social conversation in both alcoholics and social drinkers (Stitzer et al. 1981, Babor et al. 1983, Samson et al. 1984). Alcohol, up to 4 drinks during one session, also increased speaking even in isolated individuals, whereas the same doses decreased performance on a non-verbal behavioural task (Higgins et al. 1988). There is evidence that the increase in speech is restricted to the rising limb of the BAC curve and occurs at the same doses that produce the euphorigenic effects in humans. In human beings, positive social interactions may also act as a secondary reinforcer to promote alcohol use. Several studies in humans have shown that initial drug use can be associated with peer interactions and friendship groups (Jessor et al. 1972, 1975, Kandel et al. 1978). Drinking initially maintained by peer approval can be conceived of as being a conditioned reinforcer, also serving to expose individuals to alcohol and allowing for development of tolerance to certain (aversive?) actions of alcohol. Animal models have confirmed that alcohol self-administration can be established by conditioned reinforcement. Animals that have to drink alcohol in order to gain access to a sweet solution or to avoid shock (see Grant 1995) will later drink significant quantities of alcohol without the initial reinforcer being present, strengthening the possibility that conditioned reinforcement can indeed play a role in the initiation of alcohol drinking that is later maintained by other factors.

It should be re-emphasized that alcohol may not produce the same spectrum of effects in all individuals. For example, there are many demonstrations that some individuals within a group of experimental animals consistently consume more alcohol than others in a particular induction procedure. This suggests that genetically determined factors, as well as other factors, modulate the expression of alcohol-seeking behaviour. The interaction between genetic and environmental factors in determining alcohol-seeking behaviours appears to be a robust finding, as noted in studies of the aetiology of alcoholism (Marlatt et al. 1988, Tarter 1988). Presumably both factors and their interaction contribute to individual risk for developing a pattern of behaviour that can escalate into heavy drinking resulting in alcohol abuse or alcoholism (Pickens et al. 1991).

AVERSIVE EFFECTS OF ALCOHOL

Interestingly, depending on the species and strain of animals used in experiments, the doses that produce evidence of aversive consequences of ethanol ingestion overlap those that produce evidence of reward (reinforcement). Aversive effects of alcohol are present even in rats that are genetically selected to prefer alcohol solutions to water; however, their aversion to alcohol is less apparent (Froehlich et al. 1988, Schechter et al. 1992). It has also been shown that mice with a genetic predisposition to drink large amounts of alcohol show reduced sensitivity to the aversive effects of ethanol (Risinger et al. 1994). However, the correlation between high preference for alcohol and low sensitivity to its aversive effects does not hold in all cases. "Knock-out" mice lacking the gene for a single protein in the brain (the serotonin-1B [5-HT_{1B}] receptor; see below) drank significantly more alcohol than mice (wild-type) that had this protein (Crabbe et al. 1996), but wild-type and knock-out mice were equally sensitive to ethanol-induced taste aversion. These results suggest that aversive and rewarding properties of alcohol may be separable and mediated by different neural mechanisms. The balance between the aversive and rewarding properties of ethanol does, however, impact alcohol consumption, and this impact is influenced by associations formed by prior experiences. Tolerance to the aversive effects of alcohol may also develop and further allow the positive reinforcing effects of alcohol to become evident. An intriguing hypothesis is that alcohol initially produces a spectrum of effects from aversive to rewarding, but that with repeated alcohol exposure, animals become less sensitive to the aversive effects while remaining sensitive to the positive reinforcing effects of alcohol. This hypothesis has support from data indicating that a period of prior alcohol exposure (an induction procedure) is needed to generate alcohol self-administration in animals (see Grant et al. 1990a). These induction procedures are methods for gradually exposing animals to the effects of alcohol while strengthening the expression of behaviours that will propagate further alcohol use.

ALCOHOL AND STRESS/ANXIETY

It has been hypothesized for many years that the ability of alcohol to reduce stress underlies its ability to serve as a reinforcer (Williams 1966, Pohorecky 1981). Indeed, accumulating clinical evidence indicates a high degree of co-occurrence of anxiety disorders and alcohol dependence (Langenbucher et al. 1990, Crum et al. 1995). Two mechanisms are likely to be responsible for this comorbidity. First, excessive alcohol use may be due to the anxiolytic (anxiety-reducing) properties of alcohol, which could alleviate a constant, high "basal" state of anxiety in some individuals. Second, abstinence after excessive use of alcoholic beverages gives rise to dysphoric effects, including exacerbation of anxiety, that may be relieved by subsequent alcohol use.

Evidence for alcohol's anxiolytic effect is derived from human and, particularly, from animal studies (Tornatzky et al. 1995). In animals, the anxiolytic effect of alcohol occurs at low-to-moderate alcohol doses, and is not always separable from other behavioural effects of alcohol. Caution is necessary, however, in extrapolating from the demonstrated anxiolytic effect of alcohol in animals, under certain conditions, to the contention that a reduction in anxiety is one of the reinforcing effects of alcohol in man. Important caveats are the generally weak anxiolytic effect of alcohol noted in human subjects as well as the role of expectancies in the alcohol-induced reduction of anxiety in humans. When human social drinkers *believe* they have consumed alcohol, even when ingesting a non-alcoholic drink, a decreased level of anxiety can be experienced (Abrams et al. 1979). There are also several studies that have failed to show any anxiolytic effect of alcohol in human subjects (Stritzke et al. 1996). Although the anxiolytic effect of alcohol seems to be most apparent in human subjects with high basal levels of anxiety, it is also not clear that this anxiolytic effect, despite being apparent to the drinker, promotes alcohol consumption. For example, after reporting an anxiolytic effect of alcohol, a subset of highly anxious individuals did not choose to drink alcohol (Chutuape et al. 1995), suggesting a distinction between the anxiolytic effect and the reinforcing effect of alcohol. On the other hand, higher innate levels of anxiety have been detected in selectively bred alcohol-preferring rats compared to rats that do not prefer to ingest alcohol (Stewart et al. 1993, Colombo et al. 1995). In these selected lines of animals, the simultaneous occurrence of higher baseline levels of anxiety and higher alcohol consumption supports a link between the anxiolytic effect of alcohol and a higher drinking level.

As mentioned above, anxiety can also arise as a *consequence* of alcohol consumption. "Hangovers" are a common occurrence after ingestion of large amounts of alcohol, and are characterized by tremors, nausea, sweating, sleep disruption and a state of anxiety. Animal models show that a state of anxiety can be produced by a single large dose of alcohol or after chronic drinking for several days (Lal et al. 1988, Emmett-Oglesby et al. 1990, Gauvin et al. 1989, 1992).

ALCOHOL AND AGGRESSION

The association of acts of aggression with alcohol intake varies widely across individuals, dose ranges and situations in which ethanol is ingested/administered. The effect of alcohol on aggression is dose-dependent, with low doses increasing aggressive acts and higher doses decreasing aggression, probably due to sedation (see Miczek et al. 1993, Blanchard et al. 1987). However, increased aggression is not found in every animal or human being tested (White et al. 1993). In fact, some animals show reduced aggression after consuming doses of alcohol that produce aggressive behaviour in other animals. There is evidence that the social context can determine the direction and magnitude of ethanol's effects on aggression, particularly in monkeys (Weertz et al. 1996) and humans (Gustafson 1993). Factors that appear to increase an aggressive outcome during alcohol intoxication are provocation, the alcohol dose, the level of frustration, cognitive function and the ability to engage in alternative, non-aggressive behaviours.

COGNITIVE EFFECTS OF ALCOHOL

In general, the cognitive effects of acute ethanol ingestion reflect ethanol's actions on information processing and actions on the ability to perceive, learn and remember information. Sophisticated techniques have been developed to separate and quantify different aspects of cognitive ability in human beings, including measures of overall mental ability, verbal/visuospatial learning, conceptual learning and perceptual/motor abilities. Human studies have also correlated physiological measures of brain function with the cognitive effects of alcohol (e.g. electroencephalographic measures and functional imaging techniques such as PET and SPECT). As discussed earlier, complex tasks are very sensitive to the effect of alcohol and can be disrupted at BACs in the range of 0.4 g/l. In contrast, simple reaction time tasks may require higher BACs before disruption. The disruption of memory by alcohol appears to require a relatively high alcohol dose (e.g. a BAC higher than 1.5 g/l).

Chronic alcohol use at levels associated with alcohol dependence can result in lasting cognitive deficits in explicit memory processing such as those associated with Korsakoff's syndrome (Lister et al. 1991) and deficits in visuospatial abilities (Schandler et al. 1988). Although many alcoholics do not develop Korsakoff's syndrome, many develop alcoholic dementia, which is associated with cerebral atrophy. In many respects, the decline in cognitive function associated with alcoholism is similar to the decline noted in ageing (Oscar-Berman et al. 1996). These correlations suggest that alcoholism can cause premature ageing. Although there is evidence to support this hypothesis, there are also data to suggest that alcohol-induced neuropathology and related functional deficits are distinct from changes associated with ageing. An important factor believed to be associated with development of alcohol-induced dementia is nutritional status, particularly thiamine deficiency. In addition, it appears that some brain regions are more vulnerable to alcohol-induced neuropathological processes than other areas, although there are widespread neuropathological deficits associated with alcoholism. The issue of recovery in structure and function of the brain in abstinence is still under debate, with some divergent data that generate difficulty in drawing firm conclusions (e.g. Cala 1985, Birnbaum et al. 1983, Hannon et al. 1987, Carey et al. 1987, Volkow et al. 1994). An interesting addition to the recent literature on alcohol's effects on cognition are the studies of Orgogozo et al. (1997). These epidemiological studies examined the effects of moderate, as opposed to heavy drinking (wine) in a French population and noted a protective effect of alcohol with regard to development of dementia of the Alzheimer type.

Summary of the Behavioural Effects of Alcohol

In summary, the effects of alcohol on behaviour are varied and depend on environmental, genetic and pharmacological factors. The intoxicating effects of alcohol are clearly reinforcing to a subset of animal species (including human subjects) exposed to alcohol. The most positive effects of ethanol appear to be associated with the early stages of ethanol's actions and are evidenced on the ascending limb of the BAC curve after ethanol ingestion. Through repeated consumption of alcohol, behaviours pivotal in obtaining alcohol become associated with particular environmental cues, and these cues can influence the desire to drink. In addition, anxiety and stress appear to be contributors to alcohol use, but the interactions between stress, anxiety and drinking are complicated. Likewise, alcohol has been found to influence aggressive and violent behaviour; however, this relationship is also complicated and a number of mediating factors may influence outcome. Alcohol's effects on learning and memory are clearly demonstrable at higher drinking levels. Attention appears to be more sensitive to impairment by alcohol than are memory functions, and within memory functions, explicit and working memory appear to show the greatest vulnerability. Long-term alcohol use associated with alcohol dependence can result in long-term deficits in cognitive function, which may impair the individual's ability to respond to treatment. On the other hand, recent evidence provides some initial information that moderate alcohol (wine) intake may be neuroprotective. The physiological and biochemical mechanisms that underlie these behavioural actions of alcohol are being identified (see below), and this information is generating an understanding of how alcohol produces behavioural changes.

Acute Biochemical and Electrophysiological Effects of Alcohol

Introduction to Neurotransmission

Nerve cells (neurons) and the connections among them are integral for the cognitive functions of the brain and the generation of behavioural repertoires. Thus, to understand the behavioural effects of alcohol it is necessary to determine the effects of ethanol on the neuronal systems that underlie the behaviours. These neuronal systems have been studied with electrophysiological and biochemical techniques.

A typical neuron has four morphologically defined regions: the cell body or soma, two types of processes (dendrites and axons) and terminals. Usually a neuron has numerous dendrites, which receive input from other neurons, and one axon which is the main conducting unit of the neuron. The terminals of the axon are regions that provide for the transmission of information from one neuron to the next. The point of juxtaposition of the axon of one neuron and the dendrite of another is called the synapse. The cell sending out the information is the presynaptic neuron, and the one receiving it is the postsynaptic neuron.

Information is conducted along the axon in an all-or-none manner by means of a transient electrical signal called an action potential. Neurons maintain an electrical potential difference across their cell membrane that results from the unequal distribution of ions across the membrane. When a neuron is activated, the membrane potential is reduced to a defined degree (the membrane is "depolarized"), and an action potential is initiated. This action potential signal is then propa-gated along the axon ("conduction" of information). The mechanism of membrane potential changes involves the opening of specific pores (voltage-sensitive ion channels) in the neuronal membrane.

Transmission of information *between* neurons in the CNS is generally accomplished by a chemical, rather than electrical, mechanism. A number of molecules have been identified as neurotransmitters in the CNS; these include acetylcholine (ACh), γ-aminobutyric acid (GABA), glutamate, noradrenaline (norepinephrine), serotonin (or 5-hydroxytryptamine, 5-HT), dopamine and various neuropeptides. When the action potential reaches the terminal region of the axon, the depolarization of the terminal membrane results in the release of these neurotransmitters. This process is dependent on the influx of calcium ions into the terminals (presynaptic terminals) through voltage-sensitive calcium ion channels. The released transmitter diffuses across the synapse to the postsynaptic neuron, where it interacts with specific neurotransmitter receptors located in the neuronal membrane. Most neurotransmitter receptors have several structural variants (receptor subtypes), which can be distinguished from each other by pharmacological means (i.e. selective agonists and antagonists).

The neurotransmitter-receptor interaction produces a signal in the postsynaptic cell (the process of signal transduction). This signal transduction process may be mediated by an "ionotropic" receptor, i.e. a receptor that comprises a ligand binding site(s) and an ion channel, or by "metabotropic" receptors which stimulate the production of molecules known as "second messengers". The second (intracellular) messengers trigger a cascade of reactions within a cell that changes a cell's biochemical state. In many cases, these metabotropic effects are mediated by receptors that are coupled to enzymes through an intermediary protein called a guanine nucleotide-binding protein, or G protein.

Molecular Site of Action of Ethanol

There is still much controversy regarding the molecular targets of ethanol's actions, i.e. whether ethanol acts on the lipid of the cell membrane, or directly on proteins, or at sites where lipids and proteins interact. Early theories have suggested that the initial site of action of ethanol is the lipid of the cell membrane, but most of such studies were focused on the high-dose, general anaesthetic properties of ethanol rather than the effects seen at lower doses or concentrations more relevant to usual drinking levels. The anaesthetic effects of ethanol were suggested to be due to increased "fluidity" of the cell membrane lipids (the level of molecular motion within the lipid membrane bilayers) (Goldstein et al. 1981), while lower ethanol levels were suggested to have differential effects on fluidity within defined areas of the cell membrane (Wood et al. 1992). More recently, a direct action of ethanol on proteins has been suggested, and mutational and other analyses of certain receptor proteins have identified sites on these proteins that may act as hydrophobic "pockets" in which ethanol can bind and alter receptor function (Li et al. 1994, Peoples et al. 1995, Mihic et al., 1997). Although the molecular site and mechanism of ethanol's actions is still being debated, there is no question that ethanol affects interneuronal communication in the CNS.

Acute Effects of Ethanol on Neuronal Signalling

AXONAL CONDUCTION

The effects of ethanol on all aspects of neuronal function – i.e. conduction, transmission and signal transduction – have been studied. A general finding is that conduction of information by neurons (i.e. the action potential) is the aspect of neurotransmission that is least sensitive to ethanol. For example, the activity of voltage-activated sodium and potassium channels has been found to be insensitive to low levels of ethanol (Frenkel et al. 1997, Anantharam et al. 1992).

TRANSMISSION (PRESYNAPTIC EFFECTS)

Calcium Channels

Much research has focused on the effects of ethanol on transmission of information at the synapse, including presynaptic mechanisms related to neurotransmitter synthesis and release. As mentioned above, neurotransmitter release is regulated by calcium ions. Calcium enters the neuronal terminal through voltage-sensitive calcium ion channels, and the function of these channels has been studied with electrophysiological methods. The results show that ethanol can inhibit or block the activity of calcium channels. Some of these effects are seen at low to moderate ethanol levels (Wang et al. 1991a, b, Solem et al. 1997) and may contribute to the effects of ethanol on neurotransmitter release. One report, however, suggested that very low ethanol levels (<11 mM) can *increase* calcium currents (Oakes et al. 1982), and this action of ethanol may generate an increased neurotransmitter release under certain conditions. Such low-dose effects of ethanol may be responsible for some of the behavioural activating effects of ethanol (see above).

In addition, there have been many biochemical studies that use *in vitro* brain tissue preparations to investigate the effect of ethanol on the dynamics of calcium ion flux (see Hoffman et al. 1985). Low to moderate ethanol levels have been found to inhibit the uptake of calcium ions by neuronal preparations, similar to the results of some of the electrophysiological studies described above. Ethanol's effects on calcium ion uptake differs among brain regions, suggesting that the release of neurotransmitters in various parts of the brain could be affected differentially by ethanol. Higher levels of ethanol also increase the movement of calcium ions from storage sites within the neuronal terminals, which would lead to increases in intracellular calcium ion concentrations (Daniell et al. 1987, Shah et al. 1988). Therefore, the overall effect of ethanol on calcium ion levels in the neuron terminal depends on the ethanol level in brain tissue, the area of brain being studied and ethanol's differential actions on a number of processes that influence neuronal calcium ion dynamics. Consequently, the effect of ethanol on neurotransmitter release is not necessarily predictable from studies of calcium ion channels/dynamics.

Dopamine/Glutamate/Serotonin-Mediated Neurotransmission

A significant amount of research has also been carried out to study more directly the effect of ethanol on the release and/or turnover (i.e. synthesis, release and metabolism) of various neurotransmitters. Electrophysiological studies have shown that ethanol increases the activity of dopamine-containing neurons in the substantia nigra, a brain area involved in the control of movement. Doses of ethanol that would produce motor stimulation or ataxia increased the firing rate of dopamine neurons in the substantia nigra of unanaesthetized rats (Mereu et al. 1984). Low doses of ethanol also increased the firing rate of dopamine neurons in mesolimbic brain areas (ventral tegmental area, VTA) of unanaesthetized rats (Mereu et al. 1984). These mesolimbic brain areas are believed to be critical for the pleasurable, reinforcing effect of alcohol. *In vitro*, ethanol added to brain slices in concentrations of 20–320 mM also stimulated the activity of ventral tegmental dopamine neurons (Brodie et al. 1990, Brodie et al. 1998), an effect that was increased by co-application of serotonin (5-HT) (Brodie et al. 1995).

Increased activity of dopaminergic neurons is expected to result in increased release of the neurotransmitter, dopamine, from the neuron terminals. In fact, some of the most consistent effects of ethanol have been found in neurochemical studies of dopamine release. Ethanol has generally been found to increase the release of dopamine in the brain, with the regions of the brain thought to be involved in the reinforcing effect of ethanol (i.e. mesolimbic regions including the VTA and the nucleus accumbens) being particularly sensitive to this effect (Imperato et al. 1986, Wozniak et al. 1991, Yoshimoto et al. 1992, Blanchard et al. 1993,

Heidbreder et al. 1993). Interestingly, even ingestion of alcohol by rats selectively bred to prefer alcohol was found to result in increased dopamine release in the nucleus accumbens, in support of the hypothesis that dopamine release in this brain area is important for ethanol-induced reinforcement (Weiss et al. 1993). Other support for the hypothesis that activity of dopaminergic neurons influences the reinforcing properties of ethanol derives from findings that drugs that enhance or decrease the effects of dopamine, when injected directly into different sites of the mesolimbic dopaminergic circuit, can alter alcohol self-administration (see Hodge et al. 1996). Further, there is evidence that alcohol itself, injected directly into this circuit, supports alcohol self-administration (Gatto et al. 1994).

The mesolimbic dopamine pathway is intimately involved in reinforced responses in general (Salamone 1994, Hitchcott et al. 1997a, b), but the fact that dopaminergic tone in the mesolimbic pathways increases upon stressful events, as well as pleasurable stimuli, has led to the speculation that mesolimbic dopaminergic activity does not signal pleasure *per se*, but accentuates conditioned responses to significant stimuli (Salamone 1994). Thus, while activation of the mesolimbic dopamine system by ethanol is consistent with a positive reinforcing effect of ethanol, simply knowing that ethanol activates this pathway may be insufficient to understand the mechanisms underlying ethanol-induced feelings of pleasure and reinforcement.

Furthermore, there is substantial evidence that the effect of ethanol on dopamine release is indirect, i.e. ethanol interacts with other neurotransmitter systems that, in turn, control dopamine neuron activity and dopamine release in the brain. For example, increased activity of neurons that use glutamate as a neurotransmitter has been reported to *inhibit* the activity of dopaminergic neurons (Whitton 1997), leading to inhibition of dopamine release. Ethanol can block the action of glutamate at its postsynaptic receptors (discussed below), and thereby lead to an increase in dopamine release. The activity of neurons that release serotonin also influences dopamine release. As mentioned, co-application of serotonin enhances the effect of ethanol on the activity of ventral tegmental dopamine-containing neurons, and early studies suggested that high doses of ethanol can increase the turnover (synthesis and release) of serotonin (see Hoffman et al. 1985). Recent studies using the more sensitive technique of brain microdialysis also suggest that ethanol increases extracellular serotonin levels in the nucleus accumbens (Yoshimoto et al. 1992). In addition to the effects of ethanol on serotonin release, ethanol potentiates the actions of serotonin at one of its postsynaptic receptors (i.e. the 5-HT$_3$ receptor, see below), which could further influence dopamine release and possibly modulate alcohol drinking behaviour. It is of interest that a number of studies have indicated that *low* serotonin levels in the brain are associated with increased ethanol intake, and that drugs that *increase* the level of serotonin within the synapse result in decreased alcohol drinking in animals and man. Such results can be interpreted with postulates that drugs that increase serotonin within synapses may substitute for the effect of ethanol on serotonergic neurotransmission (Le Marquand et al. 1994a, b).

Serotonin systems in the brain are also involved in initiation of sleep and modulation of sleep patterns (Leonard 1996). Serotonin regulates slow-wave sleep, and serotonergic activity is suppressed during rapid-eye-movement (REM) sleep, the stage of sleep associated with dreaming; this stage of sleep is regulated by noradrenaline. Alcohol administration suppresses REM sleep (Mendelson 1979), which could be associated with an activation of serotonin neurons, or with depression of the activity of noradrenergic neurons (see below). Thus, an intoxicated individual lapses into slow-wave sleep, but during the night, as the BAC drops due to alcohol metabolism, the suppressed REM phase of sleep "rebounds" and vivid dreams occur. Since individuals are also easily awakened from REM sleep, sleep is many times interrupted during the later phases of the sleep cycle of a previously intoxicated individual.

Acetylcholine

Another neurotransmitter whose release is affected by low concentrations of ethanol is acetylcholine. A number of studies in the 1970s and 1980s have shown that ethanol inhibits electrically stimulated acetylcholine release *in vivo* and in brain slices *in vitro* (see Hoffman et al. 1985). As for dopamine release, this effect of ethanol was suggested to be mediated indirectly, by interactions of ethanol with other neurotransmitter systems that affect acetylcholine release. A very recent study, which used the sensitive microdialysis technique, provided evidence for a biphasic effect of ethanol on acetylcholine release in the hippocampus: a low concentration of ethanol (ca. 20 mM, ca. 0.90 g/l) *stimulated* acetylcholine release, while higher ethanol concentrations were inhibitory, in agreement with the earlier results (Henn et al. 1998). There is substantial evidence for a role of acetylcholine in facilitation of learning and memory (Jerusalinsky et al. 1997), so the effects of ethanol on acetylcholine release could play a role in the cognitive effects of alcohol.

Noradrenaline

The locus coeruleus is an area of the brain that consists of the cell bodies of noradrenergic neurons (which use noradrenaline as a neurotransmitter). The magnitude of electrophysiological responses evoked in the locus coeruleus of rats in response to sensory stimuli is reduced by alcohol (Aston-Jones et al. 1982). Shefner et al. (1985) found that the effect of lower alcohol levels depends on the inherent spontaneous firing rate of the locus coeruleus neurons prior to addition of ethanol. Ethanol (at concentrations below 10 mM) depressed, had no effect on, or increased the neuronal firing rate in a manner related to the basal firing rate of the noradrenergic neurons, while higher ethanol levels resulted in decreased firing of all the locus coeruleus neurons. In biochemical studies, ethanol has also been reported to have a biphasic effect on noradrenaline turnover in the brain, with low doses causing increased turnover and higher doses depressing turnover. The sensitivity to these effects of ethanol varies among brain regions, and the brainstem neuronal systems (i.e. the locus coeruleus) are most sensitive to the effects of ethanol (see Tabakoff et al. 1996a). Studies with animals selectively bred for sensitivity and resistance to the sedative/hypnotic effect of alcohol have suggested that the inhibitory effect of ethanol on the activity of noradrenergic neurons, and noradrenaline release, may relate to alcohol-induced sedation (Shefner et al. 1986). The importance of the noradrenergic systems for arousal and the control of REM sleep suggests noradrenergic neuron involvement in ethanol-induced sleep disturbances.

GABA and Glutamate Release

The main inhibitory and excitatory neurotransmitters in the brain are, respectively, the amino acids GABA and glutamic acid (glutamate). Most studies of the effects of ethanol on the actions of these neurotransmitters have focused on their postsynaptic effects, and are discussed below. However, some very recent studies of the electrophysiological responses to GABA (inhibitory postsynaptic potentials, or IPSPs) have suggested that ethanol may be acting pre-synaptically to increase GABA release (Siggins et al. 1998). Similarly, evaluation of the ability of ethanol to *decrease* responses to glutamate in the nucleus accumbens has shown that ethanol has both pre- and postsynaptic effects (Nie et al. 1994).

Neurotransmitter Transporters

Another aspect of presynaptic signalling that may be affected by ethanol is the reuptake of neurotransmitters after their release from the presynaptic neuron. In many cases, reuptake is the main mechanism for terminating the postsynaptic action of the neurotransmitter. Neurotransmitters have specific transporters that allow for their recycling into the presynaptic neuron, and the transporter system that has been studied most extensively with respect to ethanol's actions is the adenosine transporter. Adenosine is a neurotransmitter substance that acts through G-protein-coupled receptors to control cellular events. It has been suggested that adenosine is involved in certain motor effects of ethanol (Dar et al. 1983, Dar 1990), but the exact role of this neurotransmitter in brain is not clear at present. In cultured neurons and other cultured cells, ethanol has been found to inhibit adenosine reuptake (Nagy et al. 1989, 1990, 1991). However, recordings of electrical potentials in hippocampal cells sensitive to adenosine provided no evidence of effects due to changes in adenosine uptake by ethanol (Diao et al. 1996). Therefore, the effect of ethanol on adenosine transport may be restricted to certain cell types. The few studies of the effects of ethanol on the dopamine transporter have also produced some equivocal results (Samson et al. 1997, Wang et al. 1997, Wozniak et al. 1991), which indicate that if ethanol affects the function of the dopamine transporter, it does so only in very limited cases.

SIGNAL TRANSDUCTION (POSTSYNAPTIC EFFECTS)

After the neurotransmitter is released and crosses the synaptic cleft, it interacts with ionotropic or metabotropic receptors on the postsynaptic neuron, as described above.

Ionotropic Receptors: GABA_A Receptor

Because many effects of ethanol (e.g. sedative, anxiolytic) resemble those of barbiturates and benzodiazepines, both of which are believed to act by enhancing the action of GABA at its ionotropic $GABA_A$ receptor, the effects of ethanol on this receptor have been studied in detail. The $GABA_A$ receptor, like other "ligand-gated ion channels", is composed of several subunits that interact to produce the ligand binding sites and the pore that gates the chloride ion currents (Macdonald et al. 1994). Although it has become generally accepted that potentiation of GABA$_A$ receptor-mediated chloride ion conductance plays an important part in the behavioural effects of alcohol, in particular its sedative and anxiolytic actions, the action of ethanol at the GABA$_A$ receptor does not account for the full spectrum of alcohol's behavioural effects.

Biochemical studies of ethanol's effects on the GABA$_A$ receptor have used cultured neurons or brain preparations that contain pre- and postsynaptic membranes, and have measured GABA-stimulated uptake of chloride ions by these preparations. Low levels of ethanol have been found to potentiate the ability of GABA to increase chloride ion flux, but the effect varies among brain areas (Suzdak et al. 1986, Ticku et al. 1986, Mehta et al. 1988, Allan et al. 1987).

Electrophysiological studies of the effects of ethanol on the function of the GABA$_A$ receptor have been more controversial than biochemical studies. Ethanol, in a broad range of concentrations, has, in some studies, been shown to increase responses to GABA and to increase GABA-mediated inhibition in neurons of the cerebral cortex (Nestoros 1980), spinal cord (Celentano et al. 1988) and hippocampus (Takada et al. 1989, Procter et al. 1992), but other authors failed to see this effect (e.g. Carlen et al. 1982, Siggins et al. 1987).

Whether or not potentiation of GABA responses by ethanol is observed appears to be dependent on the species of animal, the brain area investigated, the subunit composition of the GABA$_A$ receptors, the post-translational modification of the receptor (for example, phosphorylation, which is the addition of phosphate groups to amino acids in the receptor protein), and the duration of application of ethanol. For example, Wafford et al. (1992) reported the initial evidence that the potentiation of GABA responses by ethanol depends on the subunit composition of the GABA$_A$ receptor, and occurs only when the γ2L subunit is present in the GABA$_A$ receptor complex. Although the necessity for having the γ2L subunit present as a prerequisite for ethanol's actions has not been totally substantiated by other data (Sigel et al. 1993, Marszala et al. 1994), it may be relevant to witnessing the effects of low concentrations of ethanol under certain conditions. Criswell et al. (1995) have provided evidence that GABA$_A$ receptors composed of the α1, β2 and γ2 subunits may be particularly sensitive to ethanol. The distribution of these receptors in various regions of brain has been proposed to determine the brain region-specific sensitivity of $GABA_A$ receptors to ethanol.

Although the interactions between ethanol and the $GABA_A$ receptor depend on a number of variables which have yet to be fully defined, there are several lines of evidence to support a role for the GABA system in certain of ethanol's behavioural actions. For example, a compound that has the opposite effect of benzodiazepines at the $GABA_A$ receptor (an "inverse agonist"), Ro15-4513, was found to reverse the ability of ethanol to potentiate biochemical and electrophysiological responses to GABA, as well as to attenuate a number of the behavioural effects of ethanol, including the sedative/hypnotic, anxiolytic, incoordinating, amnesic and anticonvuls-ant effects (see Tabakoff et al. 1996a). A caveat to these observations is that Ro15-4513 can have effects on its own that are opposite to those of ethanol, and these intrinsic effects could simply negate the effects of ethanol in an algebraically additive manner. A more "pure" antagonist of the benzodiazepine receptor (flumazenil), in fact, did not reverse these behavioural effects of alcohol (Barrett et al. 1985). On the other hand, the observation that ethanol enhanced the response to GABA (measured as chloride ion flux) in a brain preparation from a line of mice bred selectively for sensitivity to the sedative/hypnotic effect of ethanol, but not in brain tissue from mice bred for resistance to this effect, further implicated the role of the $GABA_A$ receptor in the sedative effect of ethanol (Allan et al. 1986).

Ionotropic Receptors: Glutamate Receptors

Glutamate receptors have also been studied intensively with respect to ethanol's effects. The actions of glutamate are mediated by two types of ionotropic receptors, the *N*-methyl-D-aspartate (NMDA) and the non-NMDA, or kainate and AMPA, receptors. All are multi-subunit, ligand-gated ion channels. The kainate and AMPA receptors mediate fast excitatory neurotransmission. When activated, the NMDA receptor-coupled ion channel is permeable to calcium ions, as well as to sodium and potassium ions, and the large increases in intracellular calcium ion concentration produced by activation of this receptor, as well as its property of voltage-dependent activation, contribute to its roles in learning and memory and neuronal development, as well as in the generation of epileptiform seizures and neuronal toxicity when the receptor is overactive (Collingridge et al. 1989, McBain et al. 1994).

It has been consistently demonstrated since the late 1980s that ethanol is a potent inhibitor of the function of the NMDA receptor. This inhibition was observed both in the original biochemical studies, i.e. by measures of NMDA-stimulated increases in intracellular calcium ion concentration or other downstream effects, and in electrophysiological studies (see review by Tabakoff et al. 1996b). Brain regional and local variations occur in the blockade of NMDA receptor responses by ethanol, however (Yang et al. 1996a, Froehlich et al. 1994).

The molecular mechanism by which ethanol inhibits NMDA receptor function is still not clear. As for the GABA$_A$ receptor, it has been suggested that the subunit composition of the NMDA receptor affects its sensitivity to ethanol (Kuner et al. 1993, Koltchine et al. 1993, Masood et al. 1994, Chu et al. 1995, Buller et al. 1995, Yang et al. 1996b). Phosphorylation, either of the receptor itself or of an associated protein, has also been suggested to influence the sensitivity of the receptor to ethanol inhibition (the evidence for this interaction is discussed below). Subunit composition and differential phosphoryla-tion may account, in part, for the brain regional variation in sensitivity of NMDA receptor responses to ethanol.

It should also be noted that one early report suggested that there may be a biphasic action of ethanol on NMDA receptor-mediated responses. Low concentrations of ethanol (1.74–8.65 mM, 0.05–0.4 g/l) *increased* the probability of NMDA-activated channel opening in cultured rat hippocampal cells (Lima-Landman et al. 1989). Since activation of NMDA receptors can accentuate neuronal depolarization and increase neuronal firing, these "low-dose" effects of ethanol on NMDA receptors may be related to the increases in neuronal firing seen with low concentrations of ethanol in certain brain areas (Shefner et al. 1985, and discussion above) and in the behavioural stimulant properties of ethanol.

The inhibitory action of ethanol (at concentrations >10 mM) on NMDA receptor function has also been linked to several alcohol-related behavioural and pharmacological effects. For example, the inhibition of NMDA receptor function is likely to contribute to the amnesic effects of alcohol or other alcohol-induced cognitive deficits. The NMDA receptor plays a key role in the induction of the electrophysiological phenomenon of long-term potentiation (LTP), a form of synaptic plasticity which is believed to be important for early stages of learning. Ethanol decreases LTP in hippocampal neurons at concentrations as low as 10–20 mM

(Sinclair et al. 1986, Blitzer et al. 1990), an effect apparently due to depression of NMDA receptor-mediated responses (Morrisett et al. 1993). If the effect of ethanol on LTP contributes to the amnesic actions of ethanol, the greater sensitivity to this effect of neurons from immature rats (Swartzwelder et al. 1995) may be important in the effects of alcohol on learning and memory in adolescents.

Inhibition of NMDA receptor function could also contribute to anxiolytic effects of ethanol, since specific NMDA receptor antagonists have been reported to be anxiolytic (e.g. Brandao et al. 1980, Chait et al. 1981, Faiman et al. 1994, Xie et al. 1995). There is also some evidence that the inhibition of NMDA receptor function by ethanol could be involved in ethanol-induced reinforcement and pleasurable effects of ethanol, since, as mentioned above, the activity of dopamine-containing neurons in the areas of the brain thought to be involved in reinforcement can be *inhibited* by the activity of glutamate-containing neurons (Whitton 1997). Inhibition by ethanol of the action of glutamate at the NMDA receptor would, therefore, lead to disinhibition and increased activity of the dopamine-containing neurons (Di Chiara et al. 1994). Finally, glutamate, acting at the NMDA receptor, can produce neuronal toxicity if the receptor is overstimulated. Ethanol, by inhibiting NMDA receptor function acutely, protects against such toxicity (Lustig et al. 1992, Chandler et al. 1991, Takadera et al. 1990).

Ethanol also inhibits the action of glutamate at the ionotropic kainate and AMPA receptors. These receptors are, in general, less sensitive than the NMDA receptor to the inhibitory effect of ethanol (Martin et al. 1995, Dildy-Mayfield et al. 1992a, b, Snell et al. 1994), but the effects of ethanol on AMPA/kainate receptor-mediated responses have been postulated to be involved in the sedative and general anaesthetic actions of ethanol.

Ionotropic Receptors: 5-HT$_3$ Receptor

Serotonin (5-HT), like glutamate and GABA, interacts with a large number of receptor subtypes. Most of these receptors are of the metabotropic type, but the 5-HT$_3$ receptor is a ligand-gated ion channel. Ligand binding, measured *in vitro*, to the various subtypes of serotonin receptors is not affected by ethanol (Buckholtz et al. 1989, Hellevuo et al. 1991). Electrophysiological studies, however, indicate that the responses of some serotonin receptors are decreased by ethanol, including the 5-HT$_{1C}$ and 5-HT$_{2A}$ receptors (Sanna et al. 1994, Minami et al. 1997a). A slowly developing *potentiation* by 30 mM ethanol of the actions of serotonin on currents in hippocampal neurons which are mediated by 5-HT$_{1A}$ and 5-HT$_4$ receptors has also been observed (Lau et al. 1996). The most robust effects of ethanol on serotonin receptors have, however, been witnessed in electrophysiological studies of 5-HT$_3$ receptors. These studies have shown that moderate to high levels of ethanol (25–100 mM) *potentiate* the action of serotonin at this receptor (Lovinger 1991, Lovinger et al. 1991, 1994). The 5-HT$_3$ receptor is found primarily in the mesolimbic areas of the brain of rats, and the importance of this receptor in the actions of ethanol was illustrated by the fact that an antagonist of serotonin's actions at the 5-HT$_3$ receptor was found to reduce ethanol-induced enhancement of dopamine release in the nucleus accumbens (Carboni et al. 1989, Wozniak et al. 1990). In addition, antagonists of this receptor have been found to reduce ethanol intake by selectively bred alcohol-preferring rodents (Costall et al. 1990, Fadda et al. 1991, Tomkins et al. 1995). This reduced intake of ethanol is presumably due to the ability of the 5-HT$_3$ receptor antagonist to block the dopamine-releasing, reinforcing effect of ethanol. Thus, the ability of ethanol to potentiate the action of serotonin at the 5-HT$_3$ receptor may be important for mediation of a particular component of the reinforcing effect of ethanol.

As was mentioned earlier, however, agents that *increase* the levels of serotonin in synapses, or agents that *activate* serotonin receptors, can also reduce alcohol intake. This phenomenon has been explained by postulating that these drugs do not block ethanol reinforcement, but instead *substitute* for ethanol (the animal "feels" as if it has taken alcohol, and therefore reduces its voluntary intake of ethanol). In part, the "feeling" of having ingested ethanol could reflect an anxiolytic effect of agents that increase serotonin within synapses. In particular, the activation of the 5-HT$_{1A}$ subtype of receptor has been found to modulate anxiety (Barrett et al. 1993). Alcohol was similar to benzodiazepines and 5-HT$_{1A}$ receptor agonists (e.g. buspirone) in decreasing signs of anxiety (Tornatzky et al. 1995), and 5-HT$_{1A}$ receptor agonists have been reported to significantly reduce voluntary alcohol intake in rats, mice and monkeys (see De Vry 1995), possibly by substituting for alcohol.

Another area in which the interactions of ethanol with serotonergic systems are important is alcohol-associated violent behaviour. As noted above, the serotonergic system has been implicated, under certain conditions, in aggressive behaviours (see Olivier et al. 1990). The serotonin receptor subtype most implicated in animal models of aggression is the 5-HT_{1B} receptor. Molecular genetic techniques have generated a "knock-out" mouse that does not have functional 5-HT_{1B} receptors, and these mice are highly aggressive (Saudou et al. 1994). On the other hand, drugs that increase 5-HT_{1B} receptor activity display remarkable anti-aggressive activity in animal models and have hence been termed "serenics" (Mann 1995). Although the 5-HT_{1B} receptor system has not been specifically studied in the context of alcohol-induced aggression, this receptor mediates a physiological effect that is perceived by the animal as being similar to the effect of low doses of ethanol (Grant et al. 1997). Interestingly, 5-HT_{1B} "knock-out" mice drink large quantities of alcohol and show enhanced conditioned place preference with alcohol (Crabbe et al. 1996).

Ionotropic Receptors: Cholinergic Receptors

Acetylcholine interacts with two classes of receptors, muscarinic and nicotinic cholinergic receptors, and each of these receptor classes has a number of subtypes. Effects of ethanol on cholinergic receptor responses, although less studied than effects on other receptors, may be of equal importance in the actions of ethanol as the more widely studied effects on $GABA_A$ and NMDA receptors. The cholinergic as well as NMDA receptor responses, for example, may be important in the cognitive actions of ethanol. Ethanol potentiated the excitatory responses of rat hippocampal neurons to acetylcholine (Mancillas et al. 1986). Low concentrations of ethanol *in vitro* (11–22 mM) also enhanced muscarinic cholinergic activation of hippocampal cells (Madamba et al. 1995), but depression of muscarinic receptor activation of the hippocampal neurons occurred with higher ethanol levels (Sanna et al. 1994, Minami et al. 1997b). Similarly, high ethanol levels (50-200 mM) inhibited the response of a recombinant muscarinic receptor studied in an expression system (Minami et al. 1997a). The depressant effects of high concentrations of ethanol on muscarinic cholinergic transmission may be involved in the amnesic actions of ethanol, while facilitation of memory at low ethanol doses has been reported in some instances (Alkana et al. 1979).

There is also evidence that ethanol can affect the function of nicotinic cholinergic receptors in the brain. The type of nicotinic receptor believed to be involved in nicotine addiction (the one containing the α-7 subunit) was inhibited by ethanol when the recombinant receptor was studied in an expression system (Yu et al. 1996), and ethanol has been reported to reduce the action of nicotine at nicotinic cholinergic receptors in the brain (Collins 1996, Yang et al. 1996a, Frohlich et al. 1994). However, there is one report of a synergistic potentiation by ethanol of nicotine effects on cerebellar neurons (Freund et al. 1997). Such differences may indicate that ethanol differentially affects various subtypes of nicotinic cholinergic receptors (Covernton et al. 1997), similar to results with $GABA_A$ and glutamate receptors.

Opiate Receptors

Opiate receptors have also been reported to be affected by ethanol. While high concentrations of ethanol were found to inhibit agonist binding to opiate receptors, a low ethanol concentration *increased* agonist binding to the µ subtype of opiate receptor (Tabakoff et al. 1983b). Activation of these receptors also promotes the release of dopamine from neurons in the mesolimbic areas of the brain. Interestingly, opioid receptor antagonists, as well as the $5-HT_3$ antagonists mentioned, have been found to block the ability of ethanol to release dopamine in the nucleus accumbens (Acquas et al. 1993, Benjamin et al. 1993). As discussed above, the effect of ethanol on dopamine release may also be mediated, in part, by ethanol-induced inhibition of responses to glutamate. Nie et al. (1993, 1994) found that naloxone, an opiate receptor antagonist, prevented the ethanol-induced reduction of glutamate responses in the nucleus accumbens. Their data suggest that activation of the endogenous opioid system by ethanol is part of the circuit that mediates ethanol's actions on dopamine neurons in the nucleus accumbens. Opioid receptor antagonists also decrease alcohol self-administration (see Froehlich et al. 1993, Gonzales et al. 1998).

It must be pointed out that alcohol is not unique in its ability to activate the endogenous opioid system; this system is believed to affect consumption behaviour in general. Therefore, opioid antagonists should not be expected to *specifically* attenuate the self-administration of alcohol. Nevertheless, naltrexone has efficacy in preventing relapse in alcoholics (O'Malley et al. 1992, Volpicelli et al. 1992) and recent animal studies have also begun to focus on the role of the endogenous opioid system in modulating aversive effects of alcohol (Cunningham et al. 1998, Froehlich et al. 1998).

Metabotropic Receptors: Interactions with Cyclic AMP Signalling Cascades

As described above, many neurotransmitter receptors are coupled through guanine nucleotide binding proteins (G proteins) to signalling cascades that result in the activation of protein kinases. Protein kinases are enzymes that add phosphate groups to proteins (phosphorylate proteins). The protein kinase pathways are affected by ethanol, and alterations in phosphorylation can play a role in modulating the sensitivity of other systems, such as ligand-gated ion channels, to the effects of ethanol.

One of the signalling cascades that has been found to be affected by ethanol is the adenylyl cyclase system. Adenylyl cyclase is the enzyme that converts ATP to $3',5'$-cyclic AMP, a ubiquitous intracellular second messenger molecule. Cyclic AMP (cAMP) activates a protein kinase (protein kinase A, PKA) that phosphorylates various proteins in the cell, including proteins in the cell nucleus that regulate gene expression (transcription factors). Ethanol has been found to enhance the stimulation of adenylyl cyclase activity by various neurotransmitters and hormones (see Tabakoff et al. 1998). There are currently nine known isoforms of adenylyl cyclase, and these different forms of the enzyme show differential sensitivity to ethanol, with Type VII adenylyl cyclase being the most sensitive (Yoshimura et al. 1995). This differential sensitivity means that various neurons and/or brain areas will differ in their response to perturbation of the cAMP signalling system by ethanol.

Cyclic AMP signalling has been shown to be one of the controlling elements in the modulation of ethanol sensitivity of ionotropic $GABA_A$ receptors on cerebellar Purkinje cells, which are the output neurons of the cerebellum. Ethanol had little effect on $GABA_A$ receptor function in the Purkinje cells in the absence of simultaneous activation of the cAMP/protein kinase A system (Lin et al. 1993; Freund et al. 1996). It is of interest to note that the ethanol-sensitive Type VII adenylyl cyclase is also localized to cerebellar neurons (Mons et al. 1998). It can, thus, be proposed that ethanol-induced stimulation of cAMP production would, in turn, lead to sensitization of the $GABA_A$ receptor in the cerebellar Purkinje cells to ethanol. This feed-forward mechanism may contribute to the incoordination and postural abnormalities seen in intoxicated individuals.

Metabotropic Receptors and Protein Kinase C

Another second messenger-related signalling system in neurons is the calcium- and phospholipid-dependent protein kinase, protein kinase C (PKC). Ethanol appears to have little effect on the activity of the isolated PKC enzyme in cell-free assay systems (Machu et al. 1992), but there is evidence that the actions of certain isoforms of PKC can be accentuated by ethanol in intact cells (e.g. Hundle et al. 1997). PKC has also been implicated in modulating the sensitivity of $GABA_A$ receptors to ethanol, since only receptors containing a subunit that could be phosphorylated by PKC (i.e., the γ2L subunit described earlier) were reported to be sensitive to ethanol (Wafford et al. 1991, 1992, Weiner et al. 1994). In addition, mice that lack a brain-specific isoform of PKC were found to be resistant to the sedative effect of ethanol and the ethanol potentiation of $GABA_A$ receptor function (Harris et al. 1995).

PKC may also modulate the response of the NMDA receptor to ethanol. In cultures of cerebellar granule neurons, activation of PKC, like ethanol, inhibited NMDA receptor function, and the actions of both ethanol and PKC could be blocked by PKC inhibitors (Snell et al. 1994). This mechanism appears to be specific to certain neurons and brain regions: PKC activation appears to to enhance rather than inhibit the response to NMDA in other brain areas (e.g. the hippocampus).

Tyrosine Kinases

Another protein kinase that may influence the ability of ethanol to inhibit NMDA receptor function is the tyrosine kinase Fyn (a tyrosine kinase phosphorylates tyrosine residues within a protein). Ethanol-induced inhibition of NMDA receptor function was altered in hippocampal tissue of mice deficient in Fyn, and these Fyn "knock-out" mice were more sensitive to the hypnotic action of alcohol than normal mice (Miyakawa et al. 1997). In this study, ethanol was shown to stimulate the phosphorylation of the hippocampal NMDA receptor in the normal mice, but not in the Fyn-deficient mice.

Integrated Effects of Ethanol as Measured by EEG Recording, including Evoked Potentials

The preceding sections have focused on the effects of ethanol on specific neurotransmitter systems, and have indicated that some of these systems are particularly sensitive to perturbation by ethanol. Some attempt has been made to describe interactions among these systems that are relevant to ethanol's effects. However, on a more global level, efforts have been made to elucidate the effects of alcohol on brain activity by examining electroencephalograms (EEGs) in human subjects and animals. The EEG measures the general activity of the cerebral cortex; electrodes attached to the scalp pick up the average electrical activity of large numbers of neurons at once. The largest electrical potentials are observed when the brain is at rest. Under these conditions, the activity of the cortical neurons tends to lock into a synchronized rhythmic oscillation. If the brain is aroused as a result of an environmental stimulus, the "idling" pattern is broken, resulting in a "desynchronized" EEG pattern. In conscious animals and human beings, low to moderate doses of alcohol, those that cause behavioural arousal and euphoria, desynchronize the EEG (Djik et al. 1992, Stenberg et al. 1994), while behaviourally depressant doses of alcohol increase EEG synchronization (Kalant et al. 1981, Lucas et al. 1986, Ehlers et al. 1989, Cohen et al. 1993). Both in rodents (Young et al. 1982) and in man (Lehtinen et al. 1981, Landolt et al. 1996), EEG changes outlasted measurable levels of ethanol in the blood, indicating that neuroadaptive events occur within a single session of intoxication.

The sensory evoked potential is a specific change in the EEG that reflects stimulation of a sensory pathway. These potentials are related to the processing of the characteristics of the stimulus, and are therefore useful for assessing the function of the sensory system. The components of the auditory evoked potential have been studied in most detail with regard to ethanol's actions. This potential consists of two sets of deflections, which reflect the different components of the auditory system. The later deflections are generated by neurons in the thalamus and auditory cortex, and have a number of components, labelled N (negative) and P (positive). Similar early and late components have been defined for visual evoked potentials.

The P3 component of visual and auditory evoked potentials in humans is particularly sensitive to ethanol, showing increases in latency and decreases in amplitude in response to ethanol, which suggests a selective effect on conscious processing of responses to novel or important stimuli (Rohrbaugh et al. 1987, Colrain et al. 1993, Wall et al. 1995). Ethanol-induced deficits in automatic processing of unattended stimuli have also been suggested (Jääskeläinen et al. 1995). In the latter case, the authors suggested that this phenomenon could result in improper orienting of attention to auditory stimuli in the environment. Such effects of ethanol on attentional processes may have a significant negative impact on one's ability to operate vehicles or attend to various important stimuli in one's environment.

EEG changes can also be seen in the absence of alcohol, in individuals who have previously drunk relatively large amounts of alcohol. For example, heavy social drinkers, in a sober condition, exhibited shorter P2 and longer P3 latencies, and decreased P3 amplitude in word identification (Nichols et al. 1996) and simulated driving tasks (Nichols et al. 1993) compared to controls. The latencies of several components of the auditory evoked potentials were also larger in abstinent chronic alcoholics than in controls (Begleiter et al. 1981, Realmuto et al. 1993). Begleiter and his colleagues have also presented data that the P3 characteristics are inherently different in many children of alcoholic fathers, compared to children of non-alcoholic fathers, and have proposed that particular P3 potential characteristics may reflect a genetic propensity to develop alcoholism (Begleiter et al. 1998, Porjesz et al. 1990, 1991) (see also Chapter 3).

Chronic Biochemical and Electrophysiological Effects of Ethanol

The central nervous system adapts to the chronic presence of ethanol, leading to the phenomena of tolerance and dependence (Tabakoff et al. 1983). Chronic exposure to ethanol is also associated with neuronal damage and loss (Charness 1993). In assessing the neuronal systems that are modified during neuroadaptive responses to ethanol, attention has focused to a great extent on the systems which are initially most sensitive to ethanol.

Tolerance

Tolerance to ethanol is defined as an acquired resistance to the effects of ethanol. However, tolerance is a complex phenomenon, which is manifest in a number of forms (Kalant 1998). The tolerance discussed here is functional tolerance, which is defined as a change at the cellular (neuronal) level that produces resistance to ethanol's effects (as opposed to metabolic tolerance, which depends on accelerated ethanol metabolism).

Functional tolerance can occur within a single alcohol exposure (acute tolerance), or can develop over longer periods of alcohol exposure (chronic tolerance). In addition, tolerance can have a learned or conditioned component. In this "conditioned" form of tolerance, the individual learns to associate environmental cues with the effects of alcohol and develops a conditioned response which counteracts the effects of alcohol. This conditioned response, which is opposite in direction to alcohol's effect, is manifest as tolerance, but only occurs in an environment associated with alcohol administration (environment-dependent tolerance). In a different environment, no conditioned response is elicited and no tolerance is displayed.

In trying to determine the neurochemical basis for tolerance, this complexity has often been overlooked, and researchers have simply administered alcohol for various time periods and then investigated changes in particular neurotransmitter systems. This approach has serious limitations, since any change in neuronal function is not isolated and can produce downstream effects, making it difficult to determine the primary event that is associated with tolerance to a particular behavioural effect of alcohol (Kalant 1998).

A more productive approach has been to alter a neuronal system prior to alcohol administration, and to determine the effect of this alteration on tolerance development. Early and more recent studies, in which chemical lesions of specific neurotransmitter systems were performed, have demonstrated the need for intact noradrenergic and serotonergic systems for the development of chronic alcohol tolerance (Tabakoff et al. 1977, Lê et al. 1981a, b, Campanelli et al. 1988, Trzaskowska et al. 1986, Kalant 1993, 1998). Interestingly, in the absence of an intact noradrenergic system, tolerance could be reinstated by treating the animals with an activator of adenylyl cyclase, suggesting that the adenylyl cyclase signal transduction pathway is necessary for tolerance development (Szabó et al. 1988a). The early work indicating the importance of cAMP signalling systems in determining sensitivity and tolerance to alcohol has been more recently substantiated with genetic studies with *Drosophila melanogaster* (fruit fly) mutants (Moore et al. 1998). Currently, it is thought that nor-adrenergic systems and cAMP signalling are components necessary for tolerance development while serotonergic systems modulate the rate and extent of tolerance development.

Studies with specific receptor antagonists have also suggested a role for voltage-sensitive calcium channels (Wu et al. 1987, Dolin et al. 1987), as well as the NMDA receptor (Khanna et al. 1992, Wu et al. 1993), in the development of alcohol tolerance. Interestingly, blockade of the NMDA receptor only attenuated the environment-dependent form of tolerance, suggesting that antagonism of the NMDA receptor interfered with the learning required for the acquisition of this form of tolerance (Khanna et al. 1994, Szabó et al. 1994).

The systems responsible for the decay of functional alcohol tolerance have also been investigated. Neuropeptides, including arginine vasopressin and neurotrophins, can reduce the rate of loss of tolerance (Szabó et al. 1988b, 1995). These actions appear to be dependent on gene expression, suggesting that processes dependent on gene expression are involved not only in tolerance development, but also in its loss (Giri et al. 1990, Szabó et al. 1996). Given that vasopressin and a number of pharmacological agents that modulate tolerance have little effect in animals whose noradrenergic or serotonergic systems have been destroyed (e.g. Hoffman et al. 1983, Speisky et al. 1985), a reasonable current assumption would be that a number of agents can modulate tolerance development and loss of tolerance by acting through noradrenergic and serotonergic neurons in mammalian brain.

Although the noradrenergic and serotonergic neuronal systems are important in modulating the development and maintenance of alcohol tolerance, the molecular changes that define (encode) the presence of functional tolerance are still under intense investigation. Currently, adaptive changes in subunit composition and function of the $GABA_A$ receptor hold promise for explaining some of the manifestations of chronic functional tolerance to certain effects of ethanol. For example, changes in the level of a number of subunits of the $GABA_A$ receptor, in various brain areas, have been noted in animals treated chronically with alcohol (Morrow et al. 1990, 1992, Montpied et al. 1991, Mhatre et al. 1992, 1993, Devaud et al. 1995, 1998, Ticku et al. 1994). Investigations of brain preparations from chronically alcohol-treated animals have also demonstrated a reduced ability of ethanol to potentiate GABA-mediated chloride ion flux through the $GABA_A$ receptor, suggesting that the system had become resistant (tolerant) to the effect of ethanol (Allan et al. 1987, Morrow et al. 1988). Since it has been suggested that the subunit composition of the GABA$_A$ receptor influences this receptor's sensitivity to ethanol, one can speculate that changes in subunit composition could lead to the decreased response of the receptor to ethanol. Another possible mechanism for resistance of the GABA$_A$ receptor to ethanol stimulation upon chronic alcohol exposure is a change in the adenylyl cyclase signalling system. As discussed earlier, ethanol enhancement of GABA$_A$ receptor function in cerebellar Purkinje cells depends on the simultaneous activation of adenylyl cyclase (Lin et al. 1993). After chronic alcohol exposure, decreased adenylyl cyclase activity has been found in many brain areas (see Tabakoff et al. 1998). This decrease in the activity of the cAMP-generating systems would be expected to blunt the response of the GABA$_A$ receptor to ethanol-induced stimulation (i.e. produce resistance to ethanol), at least in cerebellar Purkinje neurons.

Physical Dependence

The alcohol withdrawal syndrome involves anxiety, tremor, autonomic and CNS hyperexcitability, hallucinations, aberrations in body temperature, sleep disturbances and potentially fatal convulsions. The time course of appearance of symptoms after cessation of drinking is different, with the confusional state of "delirium tremens" occurring later than the other signs and symptoms in man (Victor et al. 1953).

EEG recordings during the earlier stages of alcholol withdrawal demonstrate epileptiform activity, with desynchronized activity and spiking in brain cortex. Recordings from rats suggest that this activity originates in subcortical regions, and spreads later to the cerebral cortex (Walker et al. 1974, Hunter et al. 1978, Veatch et al. 1996).

Increases in excitatory amino acid (glutamate) transmission and increases in calcium currents are now known to play a major role in the neuronal hyperexcitability seen during alcohol withdrawal, although almost all studies in this regard have used hippocampal neurons. Both AMPA/kainate and NMDA receptor-mediated transmission increased after withdrawal from chronic alcohol use (Shindou et al. 1994, Molleman et al. 1995a, Whittington et al. 1995). Consistent evidence has also been found of increased voltage-sensitive calcium channel activity (Shindou et al. 1994, Whittington et al. 1995, Perez-Velazquez et al. 1994, Huang et al. 1993). A progressive series of changes in the activity of hippocampal pyramidal cells *in vitro* during alcohol withdrawal may reflect the progression of the behavioural signs of withdrawal (Whittington et al. 1990, 1992, 1995, Bailey et al. 1998). Neurochemical studies have also implicated both voltage-sensitive calcium channels and NMDA receptors in the manifestation of the neuronal hyperexcitability of ethanol withdrawal. Increased numbers of voltage-sensitive calcium channels and NMDA receptors have been demonstrated in brains of animals exposed chronically to ethanol to induce physical dependence, as well as in cultured neurons treated *in vitro* with ethanol (Dolin et al. 1987, Lucchi et al. 1985, see Tabakoff et al. 1996b). The administration of calcium channel antagonists or NMDA receptor antagonists reduced alcohol withdrawal seizures, and treatments that prevented the increase in voltage-sensitive calcium channels or in NMDA receptors during the chronic administration of alcohol also attenuated withdrawal seizures (Little et al. 1986, Whittington et al. 1991, Grant et al. 1990b, Morrisett et al. 1990, Kotlinska et al. 1996, Snell et al. 1996). This body of evidence supports the contention that increases in NMDA receptors and in voltage-sensitive calcium channels may underlie the occurrence of a number of withdrawal signs and symptoms that define the presence of physical dependence on alcohol.

Although withdrawal anxiety, hyperexcitability and convulsions have been suggested by some to be due to decreases in GABA transmission during alcohol withdrawal, electrophysiological studies have not consistently supported this hypothesis. Hippocampal and medial septum/diagonal neurons showed no changes in any aspect of $GABA_A$ receptor-mediated transmission during alcohol withdrawal (Whittington et al. 1995, Frye et al. 1996), although Ibbotson et al. (1997) have found reduced inhibitory transmission in cerebral cortical cells. On the other hand, repeated alcohol withdrawals have been postulated to result in kindling of the CNS (Becker et al. 1989), which produces a prolonged, possibly permanent hyperexcitability that may depend more on changes in GABA transmission than do the overt signs seen during a single withdrawal episode. Kang et al. (1996) have reported a prolonged decrease in GABA-mediated inhibition in hippocampal slices after intermittent chronic alcohol exposure that may manifest a CNS kindling phenomenon.

Another manifestation of alcohol withdrawal is that the firing of dopaminergic neurons in the ventral tegmental area is considerably depressed, with decreases in spontaneous firing rates seen *in vivo* (Diana et al. 1992, 1995, Shen et al. 1993) and *in vitro* (Molleman et al. 1995b). Alcohol withdrawal also generates a decrease in the release of dopamine from neurons in mesolimbic regions of the brain (the ventral tegmental area) (Diana et al. 1993). Since glutamate released from glutamate-containing neurons acts through NMDA receptors to inhibit the activity of the dopamine-containing neurons (Imperato et al. 1990), the increase in NMDA receptor sensitivity to glutamate, along with increased glutamate release after chronic alcohol treatment, could contribute to the decreased activity of the dopamine-containing neurons during alcohol withdrawal. In fact, it has been observed that the administration of an NMDA receptor antagonist reverses the decreased release of dopamine in the nucleus accumbens of alcohol-withdrawn animals (Rossetti et al. 1991). Systemic administration of alcohol also reversed this change in dopamine release (Rossetti et al. 1992). These findings suggest that the increase in NMDA receptor function that occurs during alcohol withdrawal could contribute not only to the occurrence of the CNS hyperexcitability manifested as seizures (convulsions), but could also contribute to decreased function of dopamine neurons, which may result in the negative affect (dysphoria) that is associated with alcohol withdrawal and could contribute to the compulsion to drink alcohol and to relapse.

Neurotoxicity

The interaction of glutamate with the NMDA receptor can also, when the system is overstimulated, lead to neuronal death (excitotoxicity) (Choi 1992). It has been shown that the increase in NMDA receptor function produced by chronic ethanol exposure leads to greater susceptibility to glutamate-induced toxicity of neurons in culture (Iorio et al. 1993, Chandler et al. 1993, Ahern et al. 1994). In addition, animals treated chronically with alcohol were more susceptible to toxicity induced by injection of NMDA into the hippocampus (Davidson et al. 1993). These results suggest that the neuronal damage and loss observed in chronic alcoholics (Charness 1993) may be a result of the increase in NMDA receptor function that occurs during alcohol withdrawal.

Withdrawal-Induced "Craving", Anxiety, Anhedonia or Relapse

Recently, studies have begun to concentrate on neuronal changes that outlast the initial phase of withdrawal hyperexcitability after chronic alcohol exposure. This work is aimed at elucidating functional changes that remain for long periods after cessation of drinking, because such changes may be involved in the persistent desire to drink excessively, in the anxiety and anhedonia that persist beyond the acute withdrawal phase, and in the craving for alcohol seen in alcoholics.

Decreased activity of dopaminergic neurons in the ventral tegmentum has been found to outlast the acute phase of ethanol withdrawal. Diana et al. (1996) found decreases in neuronal firing *in vivo* twenty-four hours after cessation of behavioural withdrawal signs, and firing rates *in vitro* were still depressed at six days, but not two months, after alcohol withdrawal in the mouse (Bailey et al. 1997a, b). Persistent changes in neuronal function after withdrawal from chronic alcohol treatment (Durand et al. 1984a, Abraham et al. 1984) may be involved in long-term anxiety in alcohol-withdrawn subjects, and prolonged decreases in LTP in hippocampal neurons have also been found after withdrawal of rats from chronic alcohol treatment (Durand et al. 1984b, Tremwell et al. 1994). Such changes may be of considerable importance in the chronic actions of alcohol on cognition in humans (see above).

Conclusions

Although ethanol seems to produce a myriad of actions in the CNS of mammals, a closer examination reveals that a significant number of manifestations of ethanol's effects are secondary to its actions on a limited number of brain proteins. The primary sites of ethanol's actions seem to be the receptor/ligand-gated ion channels (including the $GABA_A$, NMDA, 5-HT_3, and possibly nicotinic cholinergic receptors). These receptor-gated ion channels are significant in their ability to control neuronal excitability, and one can postulate that ethanol's actions at these receptor-gated channels would result in many of the observed effects of ethanol on neuronal firing patterns and the release of particular transmitter substances (for example, ethanol seems to have little direct action on the release of dopamine from neuron terminals, but enhances dopamine release in conjunction with enhanced firing of the dopaminergic neurons in certain brain areas). It is of interest to note that ethanol can have a biphasic effect on the activity of certain receptors and ion channels. At low doses ethanol can potentiate the activity of NMDA and muscarinic and nicotinic cholinergic receptors, and these low dose actions of ethanol may be responsible for some of the behavioural activation seen with alcohol. The selectivity of ethanol's actions for particular neuronal systems may reside in the presence of the ethanol-sensitive, receptor-gated ion channels on particular neurons and the character of these ion channels in terms of their subunit composition. A number of findings described above indicate that receptor-gated ion channels of different subunit composition differ significantly in their response to ethanol. The sensitivity of the receptor-gated ion channels to ethanol's actions can also be significantly modulated by the action of protein kinases (i.e. by the phosphorylation state of ethanol's target proteins). One can consider the protein kinases (PKA, PKC, Fyn, etc.) as entities for setting the tone (responsivity) of the CNS to ethanol's actions. One can also postulate that environmental signals acting through the protein kinases can, in a moment-to-moment fashion, influence the magnitude and character of an individual's response to alcohol. The actions of ethanol on second messenger systems (e.g. the systems that generate cAMP), and indirectly on protein kinases, not only produce a rather immediate effect on the responsivity of neurons to ethanol, but also set in motion neuroadaptive events that can produce long-term changes in neuronal excitability that manifest themselves as tolerance to and physical dependence on alcohol. The chronic effects of ethanol on the CNS are generally viewed as a result of adaptations to the acute perturbations produced by ethanol. These adaptations may counter the effects of ethanol on the organism (e.g. tolerance) or may themselves generate negative consequences (physical dependence, neurotoxicity, "craving"). To date, several neurotransmitter systems have been implicated in the development, expression and loss of tolerance. The noradrenergic, serotonergic and vasopressin systems seem intimately involved in this adaptive process.

Similarly, inroads have been made in identifying neurotransmitter systems that are involved in the generation of physical dependence on alcohol and certain signs of withdrawal. Changes in voltage-sensitive calcium channels and glutamate-mediated transmission may underlie not only withdrawal signs, but also ethanol withdrawal-induced neurotoxicity. The demonstration that NMDA receptor antagonists reduce the intensity of withdrawal signs, reduce withdrawal-induced neuronal damage, and normalize the activity of dopaminergic neurons whose malfunction may lead to the dysphoria associated with withdrawal, represents an important advance. The molecular/neuro-chemical/neurophysiological mechanisms that underlie pathological alcohol-seeking behaviour and "craving" for alcohol seem to also involve, in part, a malfunctioning mesolimbic dopaminergic system. However, the current evidence suggests that interactions among various ethanol-"adapted" neurotransmitter systems (GABA, NMDA, 5-HT, dopamine and opioids) are of substantial importance in determining the components of alcohol dependence and relapse phenomena.

Some Recommendations for Further Research

1. Further studies on the biphasic actions of ethanol on certain receptor systems (e.g. NMDA, cholinergic and opioid systems) should be pursued. These studies could uncover determinants of the lower-dose, behaviour-activating effects of alcohol which have been an enigmatic but integral component of the behavioural manifestations of alcohol ingestion by human beings.

2. Studies on the determinants of the brain region-specific effects of ethanol need to continue to be pursued. Knowledge of these determinants will provide insight into the factors responsible for the characteristic spectrum of ethanol's actions and may indicate the brain sites that determine differences in individual responses to alcohol (including the aversive and the pleasurable actions of alcohol).

3. Genetic studies involving selectively bred and genetically engineered animals (transgenics, knock-outs) need to be expanded to test hypotheses on involvement of particular neuronal systems in some of the more critical actions of ethanol, including the anxiolytic and other reinforcing effects of ethanol.

4. Epidemiological and mechanistic studies of long-term moderate alcohol use on brain function need to be expanded to complement studies on the effects of chronic high levels of alcohol intake.

5. The neuroadaptive events that significantly impact an individual's ability to moderate alcohol intake need to be defined and characterized (i.e. the neuroadaptations that generate dependence, craving and tolerance).

6. The knowledge already gathered and the results of future studies of the dependence-producing and neuronal damaging effects of ethanol need to be utilized to develop more efficacious medications to treat alcohol dependence and alcohol-induced brain damage.

Acknowledgement

We wish to thank Donna Moye and Marj Becker for their assistance in preparing this manuscript.

References

Abraham WC, Rogers CJ, Hunter BE (1984) Chronic ethanol-induced decreases in the responses of dentate granule cells to perforant path input in the rat. Exp Brain Res 54: 406–14

Abrams DG, Wilson GT (1979) Effects of alcohol on social anxiety in women: cognitive versus physiological processes. J Abnorm Psychol 88: 161–73

Acquas E, Meloni M, Di Chiara G (1993) Blockade of δ-opioid receptors in the nucleus accumbens prevents ethanol-induced stimulation of dopamine release. Eur J Pharmacol 230: 239–41

Ahern KvB, Lustig HS, Greenberg DA (1994) Enhancement of NMDA toxicity and calcium responses by chronic exposure of cultured cortical neurons to ethanol. Neurosci Lett 165: 211–14

Alkana RL, Parker ES (1979) Memory facilitation by post-training injection of ethanol. Psychopharmacology (Berlin) 66: 117–19

Allan AM , Harris RA (1986) Gamma-aminobutyric acid and alcohol actions: neurochemical studies of long sleep and short sleep mice. Life Sci 39: 2005–15

Allan AM, Harris RA (1987) Acute and chronic ethanol treatments alter GABA receptor-operated chloride channels. Pharmacol Biochem Behav 27: 665–70.

Anantharam V, Bayley H, Wilson A, et al. (1992) Differential effects of ethanol on electrical properties of various potassium channels expressed in oocytes. Mol Pharmacol 42: 499–505

Aston-Jones G, Foote SL, Bloom FE (1982) Low doses of ethanol disrupt sensory responses of brain noradrenergic neurons. Nature 296: 857–60

Babor TF, Berglas S, Mendelson JH, et al. (1983) Alcohol, affect, and the disinhibition of verbal behavior. Psychopharmacology (Berlin) 80: 53–60

Bailey CP, Little HJ (1997a) Prolonged alterations in VTA neuronal function after chronic ethanol intake. Pharmacologist 39: 379

Bailey CP, Molleman A, Little HJ (1997b) Prolonged changes in activity of ventral tegmental neurones after chronic ethanol treatment. Br J Pharmacol 120: 136P

Bailey CP, Molleman A, Little HJ (1998) Comparison of the effects of drugs on hyperexcitability induced in hippocampal slices by withdrawal from chronic ethanol administration. Br J Pharmacol 123: 215–22

Barrett JE, Brady LS, Witkin JM (1985) Behavioral studies with anxiolytic drugs. I. Interactions of the benzodiazepine antagonist Ro15-1788 with chlordiazepoxide, pentobarbital and ethanol. J Pharmacol Exp Ther 233: 554–59

Barrett JE, Vanover K (1993) 5-HT receptors as targets for the development of novel anxiolytic drugs: models, mechanisms and future directions. Psychopharmacology (Berlin) 112: 1–12

Becker HC , Hale RL (1989) Ethanol-induced locomotor stimulation in C57BL/6 mice following RO15-4513 administration. Psychopharmacology (Berlin) 99: 333–36

Begleiter H, Porjesz B and Chou CL (1981) Auditory brainstem potentials in chronic alcoholics. Science 211: 1064–66

Begleiter H, Porjesz B, Reich T, et al. (1998) Quantitative trait loci analysis of human event-related brain potentials: P3 voltage. Electroencephalogr Clin Neurophysiol 108: 244–50

Benjamin D, Grant ER, Pohorecky LA (1993) Naltrexone reverses the ethanol-induced dopamine release in the nucleus accumbens in awake, freely moving rats. Brain Res 621: 137–40

Birnbaum IM, Taylor TH, Parker ES (1983) Alcohol and sober mood state in female social drinkers. Alcohol Clin Exp Res 7: 362–68

Blanchard BA, Steindorf S, Wang S, et al. (1993) Sex differences in ethanol-induced dopamine release in nucleus accumbens and in ethanol consumption in rats. Alcohol Clin Exp Res 17: 968–73

Blanchard RJ, Hori K, Blanchard DC, et al. (1987) Ethanol effects on aggression of rats selected for different levels of agressiveness. Pharmacol Biochem Behav 27: 641–44

Blitzer RD, Gil O, Landau EM (1990) Long-term potentiation in rat hippocampus is inhibited by low concentrations of ethanol. Brain Res 537:203–08

Brandao ML, Fontes JCS, Graeff FG (1980) Facilitatory effect of ketamine on punished behavior. Pharmacol Biochem Behav 13: 1–4

Brewers Association of Canada (1995) The changing pattern of alcohol use, drinking problems and public policy. Bottom Line 16: 5–28.

Brodie MS, Shefner SA, Dunwiddie TV (1990) Ethanol increases the firing rate of dopamine neurons of the rat ventral tegmental area in vitro. Brain Res 508: 65–69

Brodie MS, Trifunovic RD, Shefner SA (1995) Serotonin potentiates ethanol-induced excitation of ventral tegmental area neurons in brain slices from three different rat strains. J Pharmacol Exp Ther 273: 1139–46

Brodie MS, Appel SB (1998) The effects of ethanol on dopaminergic neurons of the ventral tegmental area studied with intracellular recording in brain slices. Alcohol Clin Exp Res 22: 236–44

Buchholtz NS, Zhou DF, Tabakoff B (1989) Ethanol does not affect serotonin receptor binding in rodent brain. Alcohol 6: 277–80

Buller AL, Larson HC, Morrisett RA, et al. (1995) Glycine modulates inhibition of heteromeric N-methyl-D-aspartate receptors expressed in Xenopus oocytes. Mol Pharmacol 48: 717–23

Cala LA (1985) CT demonstration of the early effects of alcohol on the brain. In: Galanter M (ed.), Recent Developments in Alcoholism Vol. 3. Plenum Press, New York, pp. 253–64

Campanelli C, Lê AD, Khanna JM, et al. (1988) Effect of raphe lesions on the development of acute tolerance to ethanol and pentobarbital. Psychopharmacology (Berlin) 96: 454–57

Carboni E, Acquas E, Frau R, et al. (1989) Differential inhibitory effects of a 5-HT3 antagonist on drug-induced stimulation of dopamine release. Eur J Pharmacol 164: 515–19

Carey KB, Maisto SA (1987) Effect of a change in drinking pattern on the cognitive function of female social drinkers. J Stud Alcohol 48: 236–42

Carlen PL, Gurevich N., Durand D (1982) Ethanol in low doses augments calcium-mediated mechanisms measured intracellularly in hippocampal neurones. Science 215: 306–09

Celentano JJ, Gibbs TT, Farb DH (1988) Ethanol potentiates GABA- and glycine-induced chloride currents in chick spinal cord neurons. Brain Res 455: 377–80

Chait LD, Wenger GR, McMillan DE (1981) Effects of phencyclidine and ketamine on punished and unpunished responding by pigeons. Pharmacol Biochem Behav 15: 145–48

Chandler LJ, Sumners C, Crews FT (1991) Ethanol inhibits NMDA-mediated excitoxicity in rat primary neuronal cultures. Alcohol Clin Exp Res 17: 54–60

Chandler LJ, Newsom H, Sumners C, et al. (1993) Chronic ethanol exposure potentiates NMDA excitotoxicity in cerebral cortical neurons. J Neurochem 60: 1578–81

Charness ME (1993) Brain lesions in alcoholics. Alcohol Clin Exp Res 17: 2–11

Choi DW (1992) Excitotoxic cell death. J Neurobiol 23: 1261–76

Chu B, Anantharam V, Treistman SN (1995) Ethanol inhibition of recombinant heteromeric NMDA channels in the presence and absence of modulators. J Neurochem 65: 140–48

Chutuape MAD, de Wit H (1995) Preferences for ethanol and diazepam in anxious individuals: an evaluation of the self-medication hypothesis. Psychopharmacology (Berlin) 121: 91–103.

Cloninger CR (1988) Etiologic factors in substance abuse: an adoption study perspective. In: Pickens RW, Svikis DS (eds.), Biological vulnerability to drug abuse. National Institute on Drug Abuse, DHSS Pub. No. (ADM) 88-1590 U.S., pp. 52–71

Cohen HL, Porjesz B, Begleiter H (1993) Ethanol-induced alterations in electroencephalographic activity. Neuropsychopharmacology 8: 365–70

Collingridge GL, Lester RAJ (1989) Excitatory amino acid receptors in the vertebrate central nervous system. Pharmacol Rev 40: 143–210

Collins AC (1996) The nicotinic cholinergic receptor as a potential site of ethanol action. In: Deitrich RA, Erwin VG (eds.), Pharmacological effects of ethanol on the nervous system. CRC Press, Boca Raton, FL, pp. 95–115

Colombo G, Agabio R, Lobina C, et al. (1995) Sardinian alcohol-preferring rats: a genetic animal model of anxiety. Physiol Behav 57: 1181–85

Colrain IM, Taylor KJ, McLean S, et al. (1993) Dose dependent effects of alcohol on visual evoked potentials. Psychopharmacology (Berlin) 112: 383–88

Costall B, Naylor RJ, Tyers MB (1990) The psychopharmacology of 5-HT$_3$ receptors. Pharmacol Ther 47: 181–202

Covernton PJO, Connelly JG (1997) Differential modification of rat neuronal nicotinic receptor subtypes by acute application of ethanol. Br J Pharmacol 122: 1661–68

Crabbe JC, Phillips TJ, Feller DJ, et al. (1996) Elevated alcohol consumption in null mutant mice lacking 5-HT1B serotonin receptors. Nature Genet 14: 98–101

Criswell HE, Simson PE, Knapp DJ, et al. (1995) Effect of zolpidem on gamma-aminobutyric acid (GABA)-induced inhibition predicts the interaction of ethanol with GABA on individual neurons in several rat brain regions. J Pharmacol Exp Ther 273: 526–36

Crum RM, Muntraner C, Eaton WW, et al. (1995) Occupational stress and the risk of alcohol abuse and dependence. Alcohol Clin Exp Res 19: 647–55

Cunningham CL, Henderson CM, Bormann NM (1998) Extinction of ethanol-induced conditioned place preference and conditioned place aversion: effects of naloxone. Psychopharmacology (Berlin) 139: 62–70

Daniell LC, Brass EP, Harris RA (1987) Effect of ethanol on intracellular ionized calcium concentrations in synaptosomes and hepatocytes. Mol Pharmacol 32: 831–37

Dar MS (1990) Central adenosinergic system involvement in ethanol-induced motor incoordination in mice. J Pharmacol Exp Ther 255: 1202–09

Dar MS, Mustafa SJ, Wooles WR (1983) Possible role of adenosine in the CNS effects of ethanol. Life Sci 33: 1363–74

Davidson MD, Wilce P, Shanley BC (1993) Increased sensitivity of the hippocampus in ethanol-dependent rats to toxic effect of N-methyl-D-aspartic acid $in vivo$. Brain Res 606: 5–9

Devaud LL, Morrow AL (1998) Gender influences the effects of ethanol dependence on $GABA_A$ and NMDA receptor subunit peptide expression in rat cortex and hypothalamus. Alcohol Clin Exp Res 21: 88A

Devaud LL, Smith FD, Grayson DR, et al. (1995) Chronic ethanol consumption differentially alters the expression of γ-aminobutyric acid$_A$ receptor subunit mRNAs in rat cerebral cortex: competitive quantitative reverse transcriptase-polymerase chain reaction analysis. Mol Pharmacol 48: 861–68

De Vry J (1995) 5-HT$_{1A}$ receptor agonists: recent developments and controversial issues. Psychopharmacology (Berlin) 121: 1–26

Diana M, Pistis M, Muntoni A, et al. (1992) Marked decrease of A10 dopamine neuronal firing during ethanol withdrawal syndrome in rats. Eur J Pharmacol 221: 403–04

Diana M, Pistis M, Carboni S, et al. (1993) Profound decrement of mesolimbic dopaminergic neuronal activity during ethanol withdrawal syndrome in rats: electrophysiological and biochemical evidence. Proc Natl Acad Sci USA 90: 7966–69

Diana M, Pistis M, Muntoni AL, et al. (1995) Ethanol withdrawal does not induce a reduction in the number of spontaneously active dopaminergic neurons in the mesolimbic system. Brain Res 682: 29–34

Diana M, Pistis M, Muntoni A, et al. (1996) Mesolimbic dopaminergic reduction outlasts ethanol withdrawal syndrome. Neuroscience 71: 411–15

Diao L, Dunwiddie TV (1996) Interactions between ethanol, endogenous adenosine and adenosine uptake in hippocampal brain slices. J Pharmacol Exp Ther 278: 542–46

Di Chiara G, Morelli M, Consolo S (1994) Modulatory functions of neurotransmitters in the striatum: ACh/dopamine/NMDA interactions. Trends Neurosci 17: 228–33

Dijk DJ, Brunner DP, Aeschbach D, et al. (1992) The effects of ethanol on human sleep EEG power spectra differ from those of benzodiazepine agonists. Neuropsychopharmacology 7: 225–32

Dildy-Mayfield JE, Harris RA (1992a) Comparison of ethanol sensitivity of rat brain kainate, DL-ᵡ-amino-3-hydroxy-5-methyl-4-isoxalone propionic acid and N-methyl-D-aspartate receptors expressed in *Xenopus* oocytes. J Pharmacol Exp Ther 262: 487–94

Dildy-Mayfield JE, Harris RA (1992b) Acute and chronic ethanol exposure alters the function of hippocampal kainate receptors expressed in *Xenopus* oocytes. J Neurochem 58: 1569–72

Dolin S, Hudspith M, Pagonis C, et al. (1987) Increased dihydropyridine-sensitive calcium channels in rat brain may underlie ethanol physical dependence. Neuropharmacology 26: 275–79

Durand D, Carlen PL (1984a) Decreased neuronal inhibition in vitro after long term administration of ethanol. Science 224: 1359–61

Durand D, Carlen PL (1984b) Impairement of long term potentiation in rat hippocampus following chronic ethanol treatment. Brain Res 308: 325–32

Eckardt MJ, File SE, Gessa LG, et al. (1998) Effects of moderate alcohol consumption on the central nervous system. Alcohol Clin Exp Res 22: 998–1040

Ehlers CL, Wall TL, Shuckit MA (1989) EEG spectral characteristics following ethanol administration in young men. Electroencephalogr Clin Neurophysiol 73: 179–87

Emmett-Oglesby MW, Mathis DA, Moon RTY, et al. (1990) Animal models of drug withdrawal symptoms. Psychopharmacology (Berlin) 101: 292–309

Fadda F, Garau B, Marchei F, et al. (1991) MDL 72222, a selective 5-HT$_3$ receptor antagonist, suppresses voluntary ethanol consumption in alcohol-preferring rats. Alcohol Alcoholism 26: 107–10

Faiman CP, Viu E, Skolnick P, et al. (1994) Differential effects of compounds that act at strychnine-insensitive glycine receptors in a punishment procedure. J Pharmacol Exp Ther 270: 528–33

Frenkel C, Wartenberg HC, Rehberg B (1997) Interactions of ethanol with single human brain sodium channels. Neurosci Res Comm 20: 113–20

Freund RK, Palmer MR (1996) 8-Bromo-cAMP mimics β-adrenergic sensitization of GABA responses to ethanol in cerebellar Purkinje neurons *in vivo*. Alcohol Clin Exp Res 20: 408–12

Freund RK, Palmer MR (1997) Ethanol depression of cerebellar Purkinje neuron firing involves nicotinic acetylcholine receptors. Exp Neurol 143: 319–22

Froehlich JC, Harts J, Lumeng L, et al. (1988) Differences in response to the aversive properties of ethanol in rats selectively bred for oral ethanol preference. Pharmacol Biochem Behav 31: 215–22

Froehlich JC, Li T-K (1993) Recent developments in alcoholism: opioid peptides. Recent Dev Alcohol 11: 187–205

Froehlich JC, Li TK (1994) Opioid involvement in alcohol drinking. Ann NY Acad Sci 739: 156–67

Froehlich JC, Badia-Elder NE, Zink RW, et al. (1998) Contribution of the opioid system to alcohol aversion and alcohol drinking behavior. J Pharmacol Exp Ther

Frohlich R, Patzelt C, Illes P (1994) Inhibition by ethanol of excitatory amino acid receptors and nicotinic acetylcholine receptors at rat locus coeruleus neurons. N-S Arch Pharmacol 350: 626–31

Frye GD, Fincher AS (1996) Sensitivity of postsynaptic GABAB receptors on hippocampal CA1 and CA3 pyramidal neurons to ethanol. Brain Res 735: 239–48

Gatto GJ, McBride WJ, Murphy JM, et al. (1994) Ethanol self-infusion into the ventral tegmental area by alcohol-preferring rats. Alcohol 11: 557–64

Gauvin DV, Harland RD, Criado JR, et al. (1989) The discriminative stimulus properties of ethanol and acute ethanol withdrawal states in rats. Drug Alcohol Depend 24: 103–13

Gauvin DV, Youngblood BD, Holloway FA (1992) The discriminative stimulus properties of acute ethanol withdrawal (hangover) in rats. Alcohol Clin Exp Res 16: 336–41

Giri PR, Dave JR, Tabakoff B, et al. (1990) Arginine vasopressin induces the expression of c-fos in the mouse septum and hippocampus. Mol Brain Res 7: 131–37

Goldstein DB, Chin JH (1981) Interaction of ethanol with biological membranes. Fed Proc 40: 2073–76

Gonzales RA, Weiss F (1998) Suppression of ethanol-reinforced behavior by naltrexone is associated with attenuation of the ethanol-induced increase in dialysate dopamine levels in the nucleus accumbens. J Neurosci 18: 10663–71

Grant KA (1995) Animal models of alcohol abuse. In: Kranzeler H (ed.), Handbook of Experimental Pharmacology, Vol. 114: The Pharmacology of Alcohol Abuse. Springer-Verlag, Berlin, pp. 186–229

Grant KA, Hoffman PL, Tabakoff B (1990a) Neurobiological and behavioral approaches to tolerance and dependence. In: Edwards G, Lader M (eds.), The nature of drug dependence. Oxford University Press, Oxford, pp. 135–69

Grant KA, Valverius P, Hudspith M, et al. (1990b) Ethanol withdrawal seizures and the NMDA receptor complex. Eur J Pharmacol 176: 289–96

Grant KA, Colombo G, Gatto GJ (1997) Characterization of the ethanol-like discriminative stimulus effects of 5-HT$_1$ receptor agonists as a function of ethanol training dose. Psychopharmacology (Berlin) 133: 133–41

Gustafson R (1993) What do experimental paradigms tell us about alcohol-related aggressive responding? J Stud Alcohol 11: 19–29

Hannon R, Butler CP, Day CL, et al. (1987) Social drinking and cognitive functioning in college students: a replication and reversibility study. J Stud Alcohol 48: 502–06

Harris RA, McQuilkin SJ, Paylor R, et al. (1995) Mutant mice lacking the γ isoform of protein kinase C show decreased behavioral actions of ethanol and altered function of γ-amino-butyrate type A receptors. Proc Natl Acad Sci USA 92: 3633–35

Heidbreder C, De Witte P (1993) Ethanol differentially affects extracellular monoamines and GABA in the nucleus accumbens. Pharmacol Biochem Behav 46: 477–81

Hellevuo K, Hoffman PL, Tabakoff B (1991) Ethanol fails to modify [^{3}H]GR65630 binding to 5-HT$_3$ receptors in NCB-20 cells and in rat cerebellar membranes. Alcohol Clin Exp Res 15: 775–78

Henn C, Löffelholz K, Klein J (1998) Stimulatory and inhibitory effects of ethanol on hippocampal acetylcholine release. N-S Arch Pharmacol 357: 640–47

Higgins ST, Stitzer ML (1988) Effects of alcohol on speaking in isolated humans. Psychopharmacology (Berlin) 95: 189–94

Hindmarch I, Kerr JS, Sherwood N (1991) The effects of alcohol and other drugs on psychomotor performance and cognitive function. Alcohol Alcoholism 26: 71–79

Hitchcott PK, Bonardi CMT, Phillips GD (1997a) Enhanced stimulus-reward learning by intra-amygdala administration of a D3 dopamine receptor agonist. Psychopharmacology (Berlin) 133: 240–48

Hitchcott PK, Harmer CJ, Phillips GD (1997b) Enhanced acquisition of discriminative approach following intra-amygdala d-amphetamine. Psychopharmacology (Berlin) 132: 237–46

Hodge C, Chappelle A, Samson H (1996) Dopamine receptors in the medial prefrontal cortex influence ethanol and sucrose-reinforced responding. Alcohol Clin Exp Res 20: 1631–38

Hoffman PL, Melchior CL, Tabakoff B (1983) Vasopressin maintenance of ethanol tolerance requires intact brain noradrenergic systems. Life Sci 32: 1065–71

Hoffman PL, Tabakoff B (1985) Ethanol's action on brain biochemistry. In: Tarter RE, Van Thiel DH (eds), Alcohol and the brain: chronic effects. Plenum, New York, pp. 19–68

Huang GJ, McArdle JJ (1993) Chronic ingestion of ethanol increases the number of calcium channels of hippocampal neurones of long sleep but not short sleep mice. Brain Res 615: 328–30

Hundle B, McMahon T, Dadgar J, et al. (1997) An inhibitory fragment derived from protein kinase Cε prevents enhancement of nerve growth factor responses by ethanol and phorbol esters. J Biol Chem 272: 15028–35

Hunter BE, Walker DW (1978) Ethanol dependence in the rat: role of extrapyramidal motor systems in the withdrawal reaction. Exp Neurol 62: 374–92

Hupkens CLH, Knibbe RA, Drop MJ (1993) Alcohol consumption in the European community: uniformity and diversity in drinking patterns. Addiction 88: 1391–1404

Ibbotson T, Field MJ, Boden PR (1997) Effect of chronic ethanol treatment in vivo on excitability in mouse cortical neurones in vitro. Br J Pharmacol 122: 956–62

Imperato A, Di Chiara G (1986) Preferential stimulation of dopamine release in the nucleus accumbens of freely moving rats by ethanol. J Pharmacol Exp Ther 239: 219–28

Imperato A, Scrocco MG, Bacchi S, et al. (1990) NMDA receptors and in vivo dopamine release in the nucleus accumbens and caudatus. Eur J Pharmacol 187: 555–56

Iorio KR, Tabakoff B, Hoffman PL (1993) Glutamate-induced neurotoxicity is increased in cerebellar granule cells exposed chronically to ethanol. Eur J Pharmacol 248: 209–12

Jääskeläinen IP, Lehtokoski A, Alho K, et al. (1995) Low dose of ethanol suppresses mismatch negativity of auditory event-related potentials. Alcohol Clin Exp Res 19: 607–10

Jerusalinsky D, Kornisiuk E, Izquierdo I (1997) Cholinergic neurotransmission and synaptic plasticity concerning memory processing. Neurochem Res 22: 507–15

Jessor R, Collins MI, Jessor SL (1972) On becoming a drinker: social-psychological aspects of an adolescent transition. Ann N Y Acad Sci 197: 199–213

Jessor R, Jessor SL (1975) Adolescent development and the onset of drinking: a longitudinal study. J Stud Alcohol 36: 27–51

Kalant H (1993) Problems in the search for mechanisms of tolerance. Alcohol Alcoholism Suppl. 2: 1–8

Kalant H (1998) Research on tolerance: what can we learn from history? Alcohol Clin Exp Res 22: 67–76

Kalant H, Woo N (1981) Electrophysiological effects of ethanol on the nervous system. Pharmacol Ther 14: 431–57

Kandel DB, Kessler RC, Margulies RZ (1978) Antecedents of adolescent initiation into stages of drug use: a developmental analysis. In: Kandel DB (ed.), Longitudinal research in drug use. Halsted Press, New York, pp. 73–99

Kang MH, Spigelman I, Sapp DW, et al. (1996) Persistent reduction of GABA(A) receptor-mediated inhibition in the rat hippocampus after chronic intermittent ethanol treatment. Brain Res 709: 221–28

Khanna JM, Kalant H, Shah G, et al. (1992) Effect of (+)MK-801 and ketamine on rapid tolerance to ethanol. Brain Res Bull 28: 311–14

Khanna JM, Morato GS, Chau A, et al. (1994) Effect of NMDA antagonists on rapid and chronic tolerance to ethanol: importance of intoxicated practice. Pharmacol Biochem Behav 48: 755–63

Koltchine V, Anantharam V, Wilson A, et al. (1993) Homomeric assemblies of NMDAR1 splice variants are sensitive to ethanol. Neurosci Lett 152: 13–16

Kotlinska J, Liljequist S (1996) Oral administration of glycine and polyamine receptor antagonists blocks ethanol withdrawal seizures. Psychopharmacology (Berlin) 127: 238–44

Kuner T, Schoepfer R, Korpi ER (1993) Ethanol inhibits glutamate-induced currents in heteromeric NMDA receptor subtypes. Neuroreport 5: 297–300

Lal H, Harris CM, Benjamin D, et al. (1988) Characterization of a pentylenetetrazol-like interoceptive stimulus produced by ethanol withdrawal. J Pharmacol Exp Ther 247: 508–18

Landolt HP, Roth C, Dijk DJ, et al. (1996) Late afternoon ethanol intake affects nocturnal sleep and the sleep EEG in middle-aged men. J Clin Psychopharmacol 16: 428–36

Langenbucher JE, Nathan PE (1990) The tension-reduction hypothesis: a reanalysis of some early crucial data. In: Cox WM (ed.), Why people drink: parameters of alcohol as a reinforcer. Gardner Press, New York, pp. 131–68

Lau AHL, Frye GD (1996) Acute and chronic actions of ethanol on CA1 hippocampal responses to serotonin. Brain Res 731: 12–20

Lê AD, Khanna JM, Kalant H, et al. (1981a) Effect of modification of brain serotonin (5-HT), norepinephrine (NE) and dopamine (DA) on ethanol tolerance. Psychopharmacology (Berlin) 75: 231–35

Lê AD, Khanna JM, Kalant H, et al. (1981b) The effect of lesions in the dorsal, median and magnus raphe nuclei on the development of tolerance to ethanol. J Pharmacol Exp Ther 218: 525–29

Le Marquand D, Pihl RO, Benkelfat C (1994a) Serotonin and alcohol intake, abuse, and dependence: clinical evidence. Biol Psychiatry 36: 326–37

Le Marquand D, Pihl RO, Benkelfat C (1994b) Serotonin and alcohol intake, abuse, and dependence: findings of animal studies. Biol Psychiatry 36: 395–421

Lehtinen I, Lang AH, Jantti V, et al. (1981) Ethanol-induced disturbance in human arousal mechanism. Psychopharmacology (Berlin) 73: 223–29

Leonard BE (1996) Serotonin receptors and their function in sleep, anxiety disorders and depression. Psychother Psychosom 65: 66–75

Li CY, Peoples RW, Weight FF (1994) Alcohol action on a neuronal membrane receptor: evidence for a direct interaction with the receptor protein. Proc Natl Acad Sci USA 91: 8200–04

Lima-Landman MT, Albuquerque EX (1989) Ethanol potentiates and blocks NMDA-activated single-channel currents in rat hippocampal pyramidal cells. FEBS Lett 247: 61–67

Lin AMY, Freund RK, Palmer MR (1993) Sensitization of γ–aminobutyric acid-induced depressions of cerebellar Purkinje neurons to the potentiative effects of ethanol by 2 adrenergic mechanisms in rat brain. J Pharmacol Exp Ther 265: 426–32

Lister RG, Gorenstein C, Risher-Flowers D, et al. (1991) Dissociation of the acute effects of alcohol on implicit and explicit memory processes. Neuropsychologia 29: 1205–12

Little HJ, Dolin SJ, Halsey MJ (1986) Calcium channel antagonists decrease the ethanol withdrawal syndrome. Ann NY Acad Sci 560: 465–66

Lovinger DM (1991) Ethanol potentiation of 5-HT$_3$ receptor-mediated ion current in NCB-20 neuroblastoma cells. Neurosci Lett 122: 57–60

Lovinger DM, White G (1991) Ethanol potentiation of 5-hydroxytryptamine$_3$ receptor-mediated ion current in neuroblastoma cells and isolated adult mammalian neurons. Mol Pharmacol 40: 263–70

Lovinger DM, Zhou Q (1994) Alcohols potentiate ion current mediated by recombinant 5-HT$_3$RA receptors expressed in a mammalian cell line. Neuropharmacology 33: 1567–72

Lucas SE, Mendelson JH, Benedikt RA, et al. (1986) EEG, physiologic and behavioral effects of ethanol administration. NIDA Res Monogr 67: 209–14

Lucchi L, Govoni S, Battaini F, et al. (1985) Ethanol administration in vivo alters calcium ions control in rat striatum. Brain Res 332: 376–79

Lustig HS, Chan J, Greenberg DA (1992) Ethanol inhibits excitotoxicity in cerebral cortical cultures. Neurosci Lett 135: 259–61

Macdonald RL, Olsen RW (1994) GABA$_A$ receptor channels. Annu Rev Neurosci 17: 569–602

Machu TK, Olsen RW, Browning MD (1992) Ethanol has no effect on cAMP-dependent protein kinase-, protein kinase C-, or Ca(2+)-calmodulin-dependent protein kinase II-stimulated phosphorylation of highly purified substances in vitro. Alcohol Clin Exp Res 16: 290–94

Madamba SG, Hsu M, Schweitzer P, et al. (1995) Ethanol enhances muscarinic cholinergic neurotransmission in rat hippocampus in vitro. Brain Res 685: 21–32

Mancillas JR, Siggins GR, Bloom FE (1986) Systemic ethanol: selective enhancement of responses to acetylcholine and somatostatin in hippocampus. Science 231: 161–63

Mann JJ (1995) Violence and aggression. In: Bloom FE, Kupfer DJ (eds), Psychopharmacology: the fourth generation of progress. Raven Press, New York, pp. 1919–28

Marlatt GA, Baer J, Donovan DM, et al. (1988) Addictive behaviors: etiology and treatment. Annu Rev Psychol 39: 223–52

Marszala W, Kurata Y, Hamilton BJ, et al. (1994) Selective effects of alcohols on γ-aminobutyric acid A receptor subunits expressed in human embryonic kidney cells. J Pharmacol Exp Ther 269: 157–63

Martin D, Tayyeb MI, Swartzwelder HS (1995) Ethanol inhibition of AMPA and kainate receptor-mediated depolarisations of hippocampal area CA1. Alcohol Clin Exp Res 19: 1312–16

Masood K, Wu CP, Brauneis U, et al. (1994) Differential ethanol sensitivity of recombinant N-methyl-D-aspartate receptor subunits. Mol Pharmacol 45: 324–29

McBain CJ, Mayer ML (1994) N-methyl-D-aspartic acid receptor structure and function. Physiol Rev 74: 723–60

Mehta AK, Ticku MK (1988) Ethanol potentiation of GABAergic transmission in cultured spinal cord neurons involves γ-aminobutyric acid$_A$-gated chloride channels. J Pharmacol Exp Ther 246: 558–64

Mendelson WB (1979) Pharmacologic and electrophysiologic effects of ethanol in relation to sleep. In: Majchrowicz E, Noble EP (eds.), Biochemistry and pharmacology of ethanol, Vol. 2. Plenum Press, New York, pp. 467–84

Mereu G, Fadda F, Gessa GL (1984) Ethanol stimulates the firing rate of nigral dopaminergic neurons in unanesthetized rats. Brain Res 292: 63–69

Mhatre MC, Ticku MK (1992) Chronic ethanol administration alters γ-aminobutyric acid$_A$ receptor gene expression. Mol Pharmacol 42: 415-22

Mhatre MC, Pena G, Sieghart W, et al. (1993) Antibodies specific for GABA$_A$ receptor α subunits reveal that chronic alcohol treatment down-regulates α–subunit expression in rat brain. J Neurochem 61: 1620–25.

Miczek KA, Weertz EM, DeBold JF (1993) Alcohol, benzodiazepine-GABA$_A$ receptor complex and aggression: ethological analysis of individual differences in rodents and primates. J Stud Alcohol Suppl 11: 170–78

Mihic SJ, Ye Q, Wick MJ, et al. (1997) Sites of alcohol and volatile anaesthetic action on GABA$_A$ and glycine receptors. Nature 389: 385–89

Minami K, Minami M, Harris RA (1997a) Inhibition of 5-hydroxytryptamine type 2A receptor-induced currents by n-alcohols and anesthetics. J Pharmacol Exp Ther 281: 1136–43

Minami K, Vanderah TW, Minami M, et al. (1997b) Inhibitory effects of anesthetics and ethanol on muscarinic receptors expressed in *Xenopus* oocytes. Eur J Pharmacol 339: 237–44

Miyakawa T, Yagi T, Kitazawa H, et al. (1997) Fyn-kinase as a determinant of ethanol sensitivity: relation to NMDA-receptor function. Science 278: 698–701

Molleman A, Little HJ (1995a) Increases in non-NMDA glutaminergic transmission, but no change in GABA$_B$ transmission, in CA1 neurons during withdrawal from in vivo chronic ethanol treatment. J Pharmacol Exp Ther 274: 1035–41

Molleman A, Little HJ (1995b) Effects of withdrawal from chronic ethanol treatment on spontaneous firing in rat ventral tegmental area slices. Br J Pharmacol 116: 394P

Mons N, Yoshimura M, Ikeda H, et al. (1998) Immunological assessment of the distribution of Type VII adenylyl cyclase in brain. Brain Res 788: 251–61

Montpied P, Morrow AL, Karanian JW, *et al.* (1991) Prolonged ethanol inhibition decreases gamma-aminobutyric acid $_A$ receptor α subunit mRNAs in the rat cerebral cortex. Mol Pharmacol 39: 157–63

Moore MS, DeZazzo J, Luk AY, et al. (1998) Ethanol intoxication in *Drosophila*: genetic and pharmacological evidence for regulation by the cAMP signaling pathway. Cell 93: 997–1007

Morrisett RA, Rezvani AH, Overstreet D, et al. (1990) MK-801 potently inhibits alcohol withdrawal seizures in rats. Eur J Pharmacol 176: 103–05

Morrisett RA, Swartzwelder HS (1993) Attenuation of hippocampal long term potentiation by ethanol: a patch clamp analysis of glutamatergic and GABAergic mechanisms. J Neurosci 13: 2264–72

Morrow AL, Suzdak PD, Karanian JW, et al. (1988) Chronic ethanol administration alters γ-aminobutyric acid, pentobarbital and ethanol-mediated $^{36}Cl^-$ uptake in cerebral cortical synaptoneurosomes. J Pharmacol Exp Ther 246: 158–64

Morrow AL, Montpied P, Lingford-Hughes A, et al. (1990) Chronic ethanol and pentobarbital administration in the rat: effects on $GABA_A$ receptor function and expression in brain. Alcohol 7: 237–44

Morrow AL, Herbert JS, Montpied P (1992) Differential effects of chronic ethanol administration on $GABA_A$ receptor $\alpha 1$ and $\alpha 6$ subunit mRNA levels in rat cerebellum. Mol Cell Neurosci 3: 251–58

Mulvihill LE, Skilling TA, Vogel-Sprott M (1997) Alcohol and the ability to inhibit behavior in men and women. J Stud Alcohol 58: 600–05

Nagy LE, Diamond I, Collier K, et al. (1989) Adenosine is required for ethanol-induced heterologous desensitization. Mol Pharmacol 36: 744–48

Nagy LE, Diamond I, Casso DJ, et al. (1990) Ethanol increases extracellular adenosine by inhibiting adenosine uptake via the nucleoside transporter. J Biol Chem 265: 1946–51

Nagy LE, Diamond I, Gordon AS (1991) cAMP-dependent protein kinase regulates inhibiton of adenosine transport by ethanol. Mol Pharmacol 40: 812–17

Nestoros JN (1980) Ethanol specifically potentiates GABA-mediated neuro-transmission in feline cerebral cortex. Science 209: 708–10

NIAAA (National Institute on Alcohol Abuse and Alcoholism) (1994) Eighth Special Report to the U.S. Congress on Alcohol and Health, NIH Publication 94-3699, U.S. Dept. of Health and Human Services

Nichols JM, Martin F (1993) P300 in heavy social drinkers: the effect of lorazepam. Alcohol 10: 269–74

Nichols JM, Martin F (1996) The effect of heavy social drinking on recall and event-related potentials. J Stud Alcohol 57: 125–35

Nie Z, Yuan X, Madamba SG, et al. (1993) Ethanol decreases glutamatergic synaptic transmission in rat nucleus accumbens in vitro: naloxone reversal. J Pharmacol Exp Ther 266: 1705–12

Nie Z, Madamba SG, Siggins GR (1994) Ethanol inhibits glutamatergic neurotransmission in nucleus accumbens neurons by multiple mechanisms. J Pharmacol Exp Ther 271: 1566–73

Nixon SJ (1995) Alcohol's effect on cognition. Alcohol Health Res World 19: 97–103

Oakes SG, Pozos RS (1982) Electrophysiological effects of acute ethanol exposure. I. Alterations in the action potentials of dorsal root ganglia neurons in dissociated culture. Dev Brain Res 5: 243–49

Olivier B, Mos J, Tulp M, et al. (1990) Serotonergic involvement in aggressive behavior in animals. In: van Praag HM, Plutchik R, Apter A (eds.), Violence and suicidality. Brunner/Mazel Publishers, New York, pp. 79–137

O'Malley SS, Jaffe A, Chang G, et al. (1992) Naltrexone and coping skills therapy for alcohol dependence: a controlled study. Arch Gen Psych 49: 881–87

Orgogozo J-M, Dartigues J-F, Lafont S, et al. (1997) Wine consumption and dementia in the elderly: a prospective community study in the Bordeaux area. Rev Neurol (Paris) 153: 185–92

Oscar-Berman M, Hunter N (1996) Visual laterality patterns for the perception of emotional words in alcoholic and aging individuals. J Stud Alcohol 57: 144–54

Peoples RW, Weight FF (1995) Cut-off in potency implicates alcohol inhibition of N-methyl-D-aspartate receptors in alcohol intoxication. Proc Natl Acad Sci USA 92: 2825–29

Perez-Velazquez JL, Valiante TA, Carlen PL (1994) Changes in calcium currents during ethanol withdrawal in a genetic mouse model. Brain Res 649: 305–09

Phillips TJ, Crabbe JC (1991) Behavioral studies of genetic differences in alcohol action. In: Crabbe JC, Harris RA (eds.), The genetic basis of alcohol and drug actions. Plenum Press, New York, pp. 25–104

Pickens RW, Svikis DS, McGue M, et al. (1991) Heterogeneity in the inheritance of alcoholism. Arch Gen Psych 48: 19–28

Pohorecky LA (1981) The interaction of alcohol and stress. Neurosci Biobehav Rev 5: 209–29

Porjesz B, Begleiter H (1990) Event-related potentials in individuals at risk for alcoholism. Alcohol 7: 465–69

Porjesz B, Begleiter H (1991) Neurophysiological factors in individuals at risk for alcoholism. Recent Dev Alcohol 9: 53–67

Procter WR, Allan AM, Dunwiddie TV (1992) Brain region-dependent sensitivity of $GABA_A$ receptor mediated responses to modulation by ethanol. Alcohol Clin Exp Res 16: 480–89

Realmuto G, Begleiter H, Odencrantz J, et al. (1993) Event-related potential evidence of dysfunction in automatic processing in abstinent alcoholics. Biol Psychiatry 33: 594–601

Risinger FO (1997) Fluoxetine's effects on ethanol's rewarding, aversive and stimulus properties. Life Sci 61: 235–42

Risinger FO, Dickinson SD, Cunningham CL (1992) Haloperidol reduces ethanol-induced motor activity stimulation but not conditioned place preference. Psychopharmacology (Berlin) 107: 453–56

Risinger FO, Malott DH, Prather LK, et al. (1994) Motivational properties of ethanol in mice selectively bred for ethanol-induced locomotor differences. Psychopharmacology (Berlin) 116: 207–16

Rohrbaugh JW, Stapleton JM, Parasuraman R, et al. (1987) Dose-related effect of ethanol on visual sustained attention and event-related potentials. Alcohol 4: 293–300

Rossetti ZL, Melis F, Carboni S, et al. (1991) Marked decrease of extraneuronal dopamine after alcohol withdrawal in rats: reversal by MK-801. Eur J Pharmacol 200: 371–72

Rossetti ZL, Melis F, Carboni S, et al. (1992) Alcohol withdrawal in rats is associated with a marked fall in extraneuronal dopamine. Alcohol Clin Exp Res 16: 529–32

Salamone JD (1994) The involvement of nucleus accumbens dopamine in appetitive and aversive motion. Behav Brain Res 61: 117–33

Samson HH, Fromme K (1984) Social drinking in a simulated tavern: an experimental analysis. Drug Alcohol Depend 14: 141–63

Samson HH, Hodge CW, Erickson HL, et al. (1997) The effects of local application of ethanol in the n. accumbens on dopamine overflow and clearance. Alcohol 14: 485–92

Sanna E, Dildy-Mayfield JE, Harris RA (1994) Ethanol inhibits the function of 5-hydroxytryptamine type-1C and muscarinic-M1, G-protein linked receptors in Xenopus oocytes expressing brain messenger RNA: role of protein kinase. Mol Pharmacol 45: 1004–12

Saudou F, Amara DA, Deirich A, et al. (1994) Enhanced aggressive behavior in mice lacking 5-HT$_{1b}$ receptor. Science 265: 1875–78

Schandler SL, Cohen MJ, McArther DL (1988) Event-related brain potentials in intoxicated and detoxified alcoholics during visuospatial learning. Psychopharmacology (Berlin) 94: 275–83

Schechter MD, Krimmer EC (1992) Differences in response to the aversive properties and activity effects of low dose ethanol in LAS and HAS selectively bred rats. Psychopharmacology (Berlin) 107: 564–68

Shah J, Pant HC (1988) Spontaneous calcium release induced by ethanol in the isolated rat brain microsomes. Brain Res 474: 94–99

Shefner SA, Proctor WR, Brodie MS, et al. (1986) Locus coeruleus neurons from short-sleep and long-sleep mice differ in their responses to ethanol in vivo. Soc Neurosci Abstr 12: 281

Shefner SA, Tabakoff B (1985) Basal firing of rat locus coeruleus neurons affects sensitivity to ethanol. Alcohol 2: 239–43

Shen RY, Chiodo LA (1993) Acute withdrawal after repeated ethanol treatment reduces the number of spontaneously active dopaminergic neurons in the ventral tegmental area. Brain Res 622: 289–93

Shindou T, Watanabe S, Kamata O, et al. (1994) Calcium-dependent hyperexcitability of hippocampal CA1 pyramidal cells in an in vitro slice after ethanol withdrawal of the rat. Brain Res 656: 432–36

Sigel E, Baur R, Malherbe P (1993) Recombinant GABA$_A$ receptor function and ethanol. FEBS Lett 324: 140–42

Siggins GR, Pittman QJ, French ED (1987) Effects of ethanol on CA1 and CA3 pyramidal cells in the hippocampal slice preparation: an intracellular study. Brain Res 414: 22–34

Siggins GR, Nie Z, Madamba S (1998) A metabotropic hypothesis for ethanol sensivity of GABAergic glutamatergic central synapses. In: Liu Y (ed.), The "Drunken" Synapse: Studies of Alcohol Related Disorders.

Sinclair JG, Lo GF (1986) Ethanol blocks tetanic and calcium-induced long-term potentiation in the hippocampal slice. Gen Pharmacol 17: 231–33

Snell LD, Iorio KR, Tabakoff B, et al. (1994) Protein kinase C activation attenuates N-methyl-D-aspartate-induced increases in intracellular calcium in cerebellar granule cells. J Neurochem 62: 1783–89

Snell LD, Szabó G, Tabakoff B, et al. (1996) Gangliosides reduce the development of ethanol dependence without affecting ethanol tolerance. J Pharmacol Exp Ther 279: 128–36

Solem M, McMahon T, Messing RO (1997) Protein kinase A regulates inhibition of N- and P/Q-type calcium channels by ethanol in PC12 cells. J Pharmacol Exp Ther 282: 1487–95

Speisky MB, Kalant H (1985) Site of interaction of serotonin and desglycinamide-arginine-vasopressin in maintenance of ethanol tolerance. Brain Res 326: 281–90

Stenberg G, Sano M, Rosen I, et al. (1994) EEG topography of acute ethanol effects in resting and activated normals. J Stud Alcohol 55: 645–56

Stewart RB, Gatto GJ, Lumeng L, et al. (1993) Comparison of alcohol-preferring (P) and non-preferring (NP) rats on tests of anxiety and for the anxiolytic effects of ethanol. Alcohol 10: 1–10

Stitzer ML, Griffiths RR, Bigelow GE, et al. (1981) Human social conversation: effects of ethanol, secobarbital and chlorpromazine. Pharmacol Biochem Behav 14: 353–60

Stritzke WGK, Lang AR, Patrick CJ (1996) Beyond stress and arousal: a reconceptualization of alcohol-emotion relations with reference to psycho-physiological methods. Psychol Bull 120: 376–95

Suzdak PD, Glowa JR, Crawley JN, et al. (1986) A selective imidazo-benzodiazepine antagonist of ethanol in the rat. Science 234: 1243–47

Swartzwelder HS, Wilson WA, Tayyeb MI (1995) Differential sensitivity of NMDA receptor-mediated synaptic potentials in immature versus mature hippocampus. Alcohol Clin Exp Res 19: 320–23

Szabó G, Hoffman PL, Tabakoff B (1988a) Forskolin promotes the development of ethanol tolerance in 6-hydroxydopamine-treated mice. Life Sci 42: 615–21

Szabó G, Tabakoff B, Hoffman PL (1988b) Receptors with V1 characteristics mediate the maintenance of ethanol tolerance by vasopressin. J Pharmacol Exp Ther 247: 536–41

Szabó G, Tabakoff B, Hoffman PL (1994) The NMDA receptor antagonist dizocilpine differentially affects environment-dependent and environ-ment-independent ethanol tolerance. Psychopharmacology (Berlin) 113: 511–17

Szabó G, Hoffman PL (1995) Brain-derived neurotrophic factor, neurotrophin-3 and neurotrophin-4/5 maintain functional tolerance to ethanol. Eur J Pharmacol 287: 35–41

Szabó G, Nunley KR, Hoffman PL (1996) Antisense oligonucleotide to c-*fos* blocks the ability of arginine vasopressin to maintain ethanol tolerance. Eur J Pharmacol 306: 67–72

Tabakoff B, Ritzmann RF (1977) The effects of 6-hydroxydopamine on tolerance to and dependence on ethanol. J Pharmacol Exp Ther 203: 319–32

Tabakoff B, Hoffman PL (1983a) Alcohol interactions with brain opiate receptors. Life Sci 32: 197–204

Tabakoff B and Rothstein JD (1983b) Biology of tolerance and dependence. In: Tabakoff B, Sutker PB, Randall CL (eds), Medical and social aspects of alcohol abuse. Plenum Press, New York, pp. 187–220

Tabakoff B, Hoffman PL (1996a) Effect of alcohol on neurotransmitters and their receptors and enzymes. In: Begleiter H, Kissin B (eds.), The pharmacology of alcohol and alcohol dependence. Oxford University Press, New York, pp. 356–430

Tabakoff B, Hoffman PL (1996b) Ethanol and glutamate receptors. In: Deitrich RA, Erwin VG (eds), Pharmacological effects of ethanol on the nervous system. CRC Press, Boca Raton, FL, pp. 73–93

Tabakoff B, Hoffman PL (1998) Adenylyl cyclases and alcohol. In: Cooper DMF (ed.), Advances in second messenger and phosphoprotein research, Vol. 32. Lippincott-Raven, Philadelphia, PA, pp. 173–93

Takada R, Saito K, Matsuura H, et al. (1989) Effect of ethanol on hippocampal GABA receptors in the rat brain. Alcohol 6: 115–19

Takadera T, Suzuki R, Mohri T (1990) Protection by ethanol of cortical neurons from N-methyl-D-aspartate-induced neurotoxicity is associated with blocking calcium influx. Brain Res 537: 109–15

Tarter RE (1988) The high risk paradigm in alcohol and drug abuse research. In: Pickens RW, Svikis DS (eds.), Biological vulnerability to drug abuse. US Government Printing Office, Washington, DC, pp. 73–86

Ticku MK, Lowrimore P, Lehoullier P (1986) Ethanol enhances GABA-induced ^{36}Cl-influx in primary spinal cord cultured neurons. Brain Res Bull 17: 123–26

Ticku MK, Mhatre M (1994) Chronic ethanol treatment produces bidirectional changes in GABA$_A$ receptor gene and polypeptide expression. Alcohol Clin Exp Res 18: 447

Tomkins DM, Lê AD, Sellers EM (1995) Effect of the 5-HT$_3$ antagonist ondansentron on voluntary ethanol intake in rats and mice maintained on a limited access procedure. Psychopharmacology (Berlin) 117: 479–85

Tornatzky W, Miczek KA (1995) Alcohol, anxiolytics and social stress in rats. Psychopharmacology (Berlin) 121: 135--44

Tremwell MF, Hunter BE (1994) Effects of chronic ethanol ingestion on long term potentiation remain even after a prolonged recovery from ethanol exposure. Synapse 17: 141–48

Trzaskowska E, Pucilowski O, Dyr W, et al. (1986) Suppression of ethanol tolerance and dependence in rats treated with DSP-4, a noradrenergic neurotoxin. Drug Alcohol Depend 18: 349–53

Veatch LM, Gonzalez LP (1996) Repeated ethanol withdrawal produces site-dependent increases in EEG spiking. Alcohol Clin Exp Res 20: 262–67

Victor M, Adams KD (1953) The effect of alcohol on the nervous system. Res Publ Ass Res Nerv Ment Dis 32: 526–73

Volkow ND, Wang GJ, Hitzemann R, et al. (1994) Recovery of brain glucose metabolism in detoxified alcoholics. Am J Psychiatry 151: 178–83

Volpicelli JR, Alterman AI, Hayashida M, et al. (1992) Naltrexone in the treatment of alcohol dependence. Arch Gen Psychiatry 49: 876–80

Wafford KA, Burnett DM, Leidenheimer NJ, et al. (1991) Ethanol sensitivity of the GABA$_A$ receptor expressed in *Xenopus* oocytes requires eight amino acids contained in the γ 2L subunit of the receptor complex. Neuron 7: 27–33

Wafford KA, Whiting PJ (1992) Ethanol potentiation of GABA$_A$ receptors requires phosphorylation of the alternatively spliced variant of the gamma 2 subunit. FEBS Lett 313: 113–17

Walker DW, Zornetzer SF (1974) Alcohol withdrawal in mice: electro-encephalographic and behavioural correlates. Electroencephalogr Clin Neurophysiol 36: 233–43

Wall TL, Ehlers CL (1995) Acute effects of alcohol on P300 in Asians with different ALDH2 genotypes. Alcohol Clin Exp Res 19: 617–22

Wang XM, Lemos JR, Dayanithi G, et al. (1991a) Ethanol reduces vasopressin release by inhibiting calcium currents in nerve terminals. Brain Res 551: 338–41

Wang XM, Dayanithi G, Lemos JR, et al. (1991b) Calcium currents and peptide release from neurohypophyseal terminals are inhibited by ethanol. J Pharmacol Exp Ther 259: 705–11

Wang Y, Palmer MR, Cline EJ, et al. (1997) Effects of ethanol on striatal dopamine overflow and clearance: an in vivo electrochemical study. Alcohol 14: 593–601

Weertz EM, Miczek KA (1996) Primate vocalizations during social separation and aggression: effects of alcohol and benzodiazepines. Psychopharmacology (Berlin) 127: 255–64.

Weiner JL, Zhang L, Carlen PL (1994) Potentiation of GABA$_A$-mediated synaptic current by ethanol in hippocampal CA1 neurons: possible role of protein kinase C. J Pharmacol Exp Ther 268: 1388–95

Weiss F, Lorang MT, Bloom FE, et al. (1993) Oral alcohol self-administration stimulates dopamine release in the rat nucleus accumbens: genetic and motivational determinants. J Pharmacol Exp Ther 267: 250–58

White HR, Brick J, Hansell S (1993) A longitudinal investigation of alcohol use and aggression in adolescence. J Stud Alcohol Suppl 11: 62–77

Whittington MA, Little HJ (1990) Patterns of changes in field potentials in the isolated hippocampal slice on withdrawal from chronic ethanol treatment of mice in vivo. Brain Res 523: 237–44

Whittington MA, Dolin SJ, Patch TL, et al. (1991) Chronic dihydropyridine treatment can reverse the behavioural consequences of, and prevent the adaptations to, chronic ethanol treatment. Br J Pharmacol 103: 1669–76

Whittington MA, Little HJ, Lambert JDC (1992) Changes in intrinsic inhibition in isolated hippocampal slices during ethanol withdrawal; lack of correlation with withdrawal hyperexcitability. Br J Pharmacol 107: 521–27

Whittington MA, Lambert JDC, Little HJ (1995) Increased NMDA-receptor and calcium channel activity during ethanol withdrawal hyperexcitability. Alcohol Alcoholism 30: 105–14

Whitton PS (1997) Glutamatergic control over brain dopamine release in vivo and in vitro. Neurosci Biobehav Rev 21: 481–88

Williams AF (1966) Social drinking, anxiety and depression. J Pers Soc Psychol 3: 689–93

Wise RA, Bozarth MA (1987) A psychomotor stimulant theory of addiction. Psychol Rev 94: 469–92.

Wood WG, Schroeder WG (1992) Membrane exofacial and cytofacial leaflets: a new approach to understanding how ethanol alters brain membranes. In: Watson RR (ed.), Alcohol and Neurobiology. Receptors, Membranes and Channels. CRC Press, Boca Raton, FL, pp. 161–84

WHO (World Health Organization) (1995) Profile of alcohol in the member states of the European region of the World Health Organization. WHO Regional Office for Europe, Copenhagen, 1–3 June 1995

Wozniak KM, Pert A, Linnoila M (1990) Antagonism of 5-HT$_3$ receptors attenuates the effects of ethanol on extracellular dopamine. Eur J Pharmacol 187: 287–89

Wozniak KM, Pert A, Mele A, et al. (1991) Focal application of alcohols elevates extracellular dopamine in rat brain: a microdialysis study. Brain Res 540: 31–40

Wu PH, Pham T, Naranjo CA (1987) Nifedipine delays the acquisition of ethanol tolerance. Eur J Pharmacol 139: 233–36

Wu PH, Mihic SJ, Liu JF, et al. (1993) Blockade of chronic tolerance to ethanol by the NMDA antagonist, (+)MK-801. Eur J Pharmacol 231: 157–64

Xie ZC, Buckner E, Commissaris RL (1995) Anticonflict effect of MK-801 in rats: time course and chronic treatment studies. Pharmacol Biochem Behav 51: 635–40

Yang X, Criswell HE, Breese GR (1996a) Nicotine-induced inhibition in medial septum involves activation of presynaptic nicotinic cholinergic receptors on gamma-aminobutyric acid-containing neurons. J Pharmacol Exp Ther 276: 482–89

Yang X, Criswell HE, Simson P, et al. (1996b) Evidence for a selective effect of ethanol on *N*-methyl-D-aspartate responses: ethanol affects a subtype of the ifenprodil-sensitive *N*-methyl-D-aspartate receptors. J Pharmacol Exp Ther 278: 114-4

Yoshimoto K, McBride WJ, Lumeng L, et al. (1992) Alcohol stimulates the release of dopamine and serotonin in the nucleus accumbens. Alcohol 9: 17–22

Yoshimura M, Tabakoff B (1995) Selective effects of ethanol on the generation of cAMP by particular members of the adenylyl cyclase family. Alcohol Clin Exp Res 19: 1435–40

Young GA, Wolf DL, Khazan N (1982) Relationship between blood EEG levels and ethanol-induced changes in cortical EEG power spectra in the rat. Neuropharmacology 21: 721–23

Yu D, Zhang L, Eisele JL, et al. (1996) Ethanol inhibition of nicotinic acetylcholine type alpha-7 receptors involves the amino-terminal domain of the receptor. Mol Pharmacol 50: 1010–16

Alcoholic Beverages and Cancers of the Digestive Tract and Larynx

R. Doll
Radcliffe Infirmary, Oxford, UK

D. Forman
Radcliffe Infirmary, Oxford, UK

C. La Vecchia
Institut Universitaire de Médicine Sociale et Préventive,
Lausanne, Switzerland,
and Istituto di Ricerche Farmacologiche "Mario Negri",
Milan, Italy

R. Woutersen
TNO Nutrition and Food Research Institute,
Zeist, The Netherlands

Abstract

Ethanol is not a carcinogen by standard laboratory tests. Animal experiments suggest, however, that, given by mouth, it may act as a co-carcinogen in the production of cancers in the oesophagus and possibly also in the non-glandular (fore)stomach, but not in the glandular stomach or pancreas. The evidence relating to the production of colorectal cancer is conflicting, and no conclusion can be drawn from it.

Epidemiological evidence shows that the use of alcoholic beverages increases the risk of developing cancers of the mouth (other than the salivary glands), pharynx (other than the nasopharynx) and larynx; that the risks are principally due to the presence of ethanol and increase with the quantity consumed; that the risks increase with increasing smoking level, each agent roughly multiplying the effect of the other; and that, in the absence of smoking, the risks in developed countries are small unless alcohol use is exceptionally heavy. The risks may be diminished by a diet rich in fruit and green vegetables, but the evidence is inconclusive. Whether the co-carcinogenic effects of different alcoholic beverages depend solely on the presence of ethanol and are unaffected by its concentration or by the presence of congeners is uncertain.

The epidemiological evidence also suggests that there may be some direct relationship between alcohol use and colorectal cancer. The apparent relationship is quantitatively moderate, and even with heavy drinking doubling of the normal risk can be excluded. No apparent difference in susceptibility exists between men and women or between the two sites (colon and rectum), or between the different types of alcoholic beverage. The nature of the observed relationship remains in doubt. The relationship may be causal; it may be due to confounding between the consumption of alcoholic beverages and some other dietary factor that increases the risk of the disease, and it may be due, at least in part, to the selective publication of positive results.

The balance of the evidence suggests that alcoholic beverages do not cause cancers of the stomach or pancreas, but it does not rule out the possibility altogether. Alcohol may contribute specifically to the production of cancer of the gastric cardia and, indirectly through the production of chronic (calcifying) pancreatitis, to cancer of the pancreas; but the evidence is insufficient for any conclusion to be reached.

Introduction

A relationship between heavy use of alcoholic beverages and the development of carcinoma of the oesophagus was recognized clinically before the First World War (Lamy 1910), but it was only with the publication of national occupational mortality statistics for England and Wales in the mid-1920s that evidence was obtained of a similar relationship with the development of cancers of the upper respiratory and digestive tracts as a group (Young et al. 1926). No useful evidence that these relationships were causal was obtained until after the Second World War, when epidemiological techniques for investigating the aetiology of non-infectious diseases were developed. The evidence that has subsequently accrued relating to these and other cancers of the digestive tract has enabled some definitive conclusions to be reached about the role of alcoholic beverages in their production, but several important aspects of the observed relationships remain to be resolved. These are set out separately after the sections on animal experiments and after the four epidemiological sections dealing with (1) cancers of the mouth, pharynx, oesophagus and larynx; (2) cancer of the stomach; (3) cancer of the pancreas; and (4) cancers of the large bowel.

For the purposes of this report, a carcinogen is defined as an agent that has initiating capacity and can induce tumours that rarely or never occur spontaneously; an agent that enhances the carcinogenic process without having initiating capacity is described as a co-carcinogen.

Evidence from Animal Experiments

Ethanol or alcoholic beverages have been tested for their carcinogenic potential in only a few adequately performed long-term studies with mice or rats. Most of the studies that have been described in the literature cannot be used for evaluation of the carcinogenicity of alcohol due to severe limitations in experimental design (IARC 1988).

In one adequate study, a group of 108 male and 42 female CF1 mice was given 43% ethanol in water for up to 1020 days (Horie et al. 1965). Another group of mice was given 14% ethanol, similarly, for up to 735 days, and a further group of 100 male mice was given 19.5% as the drinking fluid for a maximum of 664 days. No differences in incidence of tumours was found.

Based on these rather limited data, it may be concluded that there is no experimental evidence that alcohol is a carcinogen. However, over the past 25 years several studies have been published reporting a co-carcinogenic or promoting effect of ethanol when administered to animals in combination with well-known chemical carcinogens. The present review concentrates on the effects of alcohol on digestive tract carcinogenesis in experimental animals.

Modifying Effects of Ethanol on the Activity of Known Carcinogens

Oesophagus and Stomach

When polycyclic hydrocarbons such as benzo(a)pyrene or dimethylbenzanthracene were applied locally to the oesophagus of mice, their carcinogenic potential was significantly enhanced when ethanol was used as a solvent (Horie et al. 1965). In this experiment, ethanol most likely has acted as a tumour promoter by its irritating effects on the tissue.

Mufti et al. (1989) demonstrated that ethanol, when administered to rats after initiation by intraperitoneal injection with the oesophageal specific carcinogen N-nitrosomethylbenzylamine (NMBZA), increased the incidence of oesophageal tumours. When ethanol was administered before and during initiation with NMBZA, the incidence of oesophageal nodules and tumours was decreased as compared to control rats. These results indicate that the occurrence of oesophageal tumours is inhibited by simultaneous ethanol administration but enhanced when ethanol is administered after initiation, most probably by allowing extensive dysplastic proliferation of the carcinogen-induced lesions.

Griciuté et al. (1982, 1984) exposed C57B mice by gastric intubation to N-nitrosodiethylamine (NDEA) or N-nitrosodi-n-propylamine (NDPA), either in tap water or in a 40% ethanol solution, twice a week for 50 weeks. A significant increase in incidence of squamous cell carcinomas of the oesophagus/forestomach was observed in the group given the carcinogens in ethanol relative to the group given the nitrosamines in tap water.

Gibel (1967) exposed Sprague-Dawley rats by intragastric intubation to NDEA or N,N′-dinitrosopiperazine (DNPIP) in tap water or 30% (v/v) ethanol. The combination of NDEA plus ethanol increased the incidence of papillomas and carcinomas of the oesophagus/forestomach, whereas DNPIP plus ethanol increased the numbers of oesophageal/forestomach papillomas but not of carcinomas as compared with DNPIP alone.

Konishi et al. (1986) did not find a significant effect of ethanol on the incidence of oesophageal carcinomas induced by N-nitrosopiperidine (NPIP) in rats. In this study NPIP was given via the diet, and ethanol via a tube inserted into the pharynx, either followed or not by 10% ethanol in drinking water for 12 weeks.

Castonguay et al. (1984) did not find an effect of a liquid diet containing 66 g/l ethanol on the incidence of oesophageal tumours induced by subcutaneous injection of N′-nitrosonornicotine (NNN).

Takahashi et al. (1986) exposed rats via the drinking water to N-methyl-N′-nitro-N-nitrosoguanidine (MNNG) for 8 weeks followed by either tap water or 10% ethanol in water as drinking fluid. After 40 weeks, the incidence of adenocarcinomas in the glandular stomach of animals of the 10% ethanol group was similar to that in the controls.

PANCREAS

The results of a long-term study with azaserine-treated rats (model for acinar adenocarcinomas of exocrine pancreas) demonstrated that ethanol caused an increase in multiplicity but not in incidence of malignant pancreatic tumours, pointing to an enhancing effect on the development of acinar adenocarcinomas in carcinoma-bearing animals (Woutersen et al. 1989).

In N-nitrosobis(2-oxopropyl)amine (BOP)-treated hamsters (a model for ductular adenocarcinomas in exocrine pancreas), ethanol did not modulate pancreatic carcinogenesis (Woutersen et al. 1986b, 1989). These findings are in agreement with those of Pour et al. (1983), who found that ethanol given to outbred Syrian golden hamsters in drinking water at a 50 g/l concentration for life, beginning either before or after a single dose of BOP, had no effect on tumour induction. This observation was in contrast with the results of a previous study of this group (Tweedie et al. 1981) in which a higher concentration of ethanol (250 g/l) inhibited the development of BOP-induced pancreatic lesions. The observation of Pour et al. (1983) that hamsters treated with BOP and maintained on ethanol for life exhibited a few atypical acinar cell foci, might point to the pancreatic acinar cell as the main target cell for ethanol and not the centro-acinar or ductular cell. The results in the chronic studies performed by Woutersen et al. (1989) support this hypothesis, since ethanol influenced pancreatic carcinogenesis in azaserine-treated rats but not in BOP-treated hamsters.

The pancreatic tumours induced in the hamster pancreas by BOP are morphologically closely similar to pancreatic cancers occurring in human beings. The absence of an enhancing effect of ethanol on pancreatic carcinogenesis in hamsters may be more relevant to the human situation than the enhancing effects found in the rat studies.

Long-term ethanol ingestion in rats (14–53 weeks) produced changes in acinar, centroacinar and ductular cells. Microscopic changes comprised degeneration and atrophic changes of acinar cells, fibrosis and intraductal protein precipitates (Sarles et al. 1971). The pseudoductular cysts are lined by cuboidal epithelium of ductal type, which may represent dedifferentiation of acinar structures or hyper-plasia of centroacinar cells accompanied by atrophy of surrounding acini. A similar phenomenon has been observed in BOP-treated hamsters (Pour 1984, 1988, Meijers et al. 1989, Levitt et al. 1977, Takahashi et al. 1980, Flaks et al. 1980, 1981).

COLON AND RECTUM

Hamilton et al. (1987, 1988) studied the effects of chronic dietary alcohol use (Lieber-DeCarli-type liquid diet containing 33% of energy as ethanol) during the initiation phase in an azoxymethane (AOM)-treated rat model. They found a significantly lower incidence of tumours of the left colon when the liquid-ethanol diet was given prior to and during administration of carcinogen, whereas administration of the liquid-ethanol diet after injection of the carcinogen had no effect on the incidence of tumours of the colon. Thus, inhibition of tumorigenesis may result from suppression of metabolic activation of AOM and the consequent reduced formation of DNA damage during the initiation phase of the model.

Seitz et al. (1984) studied the effect of chronic ethanol administration on 1,2-dimethylhydrazine (DMH; subcutaneously injected) induced rectal carcinogenesis in male Sprague-Dawley rats fed a nutritionally adequate liquid diet containing 36% of total energy as ethanol or isocaloric carbohydrates. Chronic ethanol ingestion increased the total number of rectal tumours significantly (17 vs. 6; $P<0.02$), whereas no cocarcinogenic effect of ethanol was observed in other parts of the intestine. Alcohol did not influence the size or type of the tumours.

Howarth et al. (1985) injected male inbred D/A rats subcutaneously with DMH and maintained the animals on tap water, commercially available beer or 4.8% (v/v) ethanol in water as the drinking fluid. They found no significant difference in the incidence of intestinal cancer between the groups given ethanol or beer and the group given tap water. Nelson et al. (1985), who conducted a similar experiment with Sprague-Dawley rats exposed to DMH and maintained on either 5% (v/v) ethanol or tap water as the drinking fluid, also found no effect of ethanol on the development of colonic tumours.

Conclusions

It is generally accepted that alcohol per se is not a carcinogen. However, the available data on the effects of ethanol on digestive tract cancer induced in experimental animals by well-known chemical carcinogens suggest that chronic oral alcohol ingestion may have a co-carcinogenic effect on the oesophagus and possibly also the non-glandular (fore)stomach, but not on the glandular stomach or the pancreas. There has been very little work on the influence of ethanol on experimentally induced colorectal cancer, and the few results available are conflicting; it is not possible to draw from these findings any conclusions about a possible co-carcinogenic effect of ethanol on the colon/rectum.

While a number of studies indicate that ethanol increases the incidence of some specific chemically induced digestive tract tumours, other studies do not. One possible explanation for these contradictory results may be that ethanol has differential effects at various stages of the carcinogenic process. In fact, the controversial results obtained with various studies investigating the modifying effects of ethanol on the activity of known carcinogens can be explained by differences in experimental design, such as the method (in drinking water, as liquid diet, intragastrically; prior to, with or after carcinogen application), dose, concentration and duration of ethanol administration as well as type, dose, duration and method of carcinogen application.

Experimental work has so far failed to elucidate the underlying mechanism by which excessive consumption of alcoholic beverages, which are complex solutions containing many compounds in addition to alcohol, may act as a co-carcinogen under certain conditions.

Epidemiological Evidence

Epidemiological evidence of the role of alcoholic beverages in the production of cancers of the digestive tract and larynx has been obtained from a few ecological studies, many cohort studies and a very large number of case-control studies.

The best evidence has been obtained from cohort studies in which incidence or mortality rates for specific types of cancer have been observed in men and women who have previously been classified according to the amount of alcohol they habitually drink.[1] Even these studies, however, provide only imprecise evidence of the quantitative relationship between the amount consumed and the risk of cancer, partly because of the unreliability of the histories given by heavy drinkers and possibly also by light drinkers in communities where the consumption of alcohol is discouraged, as both groups may underestimate their consumption; and partly because of the rarity of the cancers most closely related to alcohol consumption in non-drinkers, who commonly tend also to be non-smokers. The latter has

---

[1] Throughout this chapter, "drink" refers specifically to alcohol use, and alcohol implies alcoholic beverages. When reference to the chemical C_2H_5OH is intended, it will be called "ethanol".

meant that very large numbers of people have had to be recruited to the studies if adequate numbers of cases (or deaths) were to be observed.

Many aspects of the relationship between the consumption of alcohol and the risk of developing cancer have, therefore, had to be examined in case-control studies in which histories of alcohol consumption are obtained from cancer patients after the cancer has developed or, in some cases, from their relatives after the patients have died. This introduces a further element of uncertainty into the quantitative estimates of risk, as histories may not be given with equal reliability by the cancer patients and their controls (regardless of whether the controls are patients with other diseases or healthy members of the general population), and allowance has to be made for the possibility that "recall bias" may have influenced the results.

No useful quantitative evidence can be obtained from the few ecological studies: that is, from correlations between the incidence of or mortality from specific cancers in different populations and the average amounts of alcohol estimated to be consumed per person in these populations. Such studies have, however, occasionally suggest hypotheses for investigation by other methods (as was the case with the correlation observed between cancer of the rectum and beer consumption; Enstrom 1977), and the results obtained in these studies contribute to the totality of the evidence that justifies the conclusion that an association observed in case-control and cohort studies implies cause and effect.

Cancers of the Mouth, Pharynx, Oesophagus and Larynx

A massive body of epidemiological evidence has accumulated to show (1) that in smokers, consumption of alcoholic beverages increases the risk of cancers of the mouth, pharynx, oesophagus and larynx (other than cancers of the salivary glands and nasopharynx); (2) that the risk increases roughly proportionally with the quantity drunk; (3) that, in each case, alcoholic beverages act synergistically with smoking, each agent approximately multiplying the effects of the other; and (4) that the main component of alcoholic beverages that determines the risk of cancer is ethanol. Cancers of the salivary glands and nasopharynx are excluded from these statements, even though they have constituted a small proportion of the cancers of the mouth and pharynx in some series, because enough is known about their aetiology to be sure that other factors are more important and because no direct evidence has been obtained to indicate that they are related to alcohol use.

The evidence on which these statements are based has been obtained mainly from Europe and North America, where these diseases are rare in non-smokers and non-drinkers; but very similar findings have also been recorded in South America (Franco et al. 1989, De Stefani et al. 1990b) and Asia (Sankaranarayanan et al. 1990, 1991, Choi and Kahyo 1991a, b). In some parts of Africa and Asia other factors cause some of these diseases to be exceptionally common, and the role of alcohol and tobacco may be quite small. There is, however, no reason to suppose that alcoholic beverages do not have a similar qualitative effect in all societies.

Most of the many studies that have led to these conclusions have been summarized by the International Agency for Research on Cancer (1988), in one of the Agency's series of monographs on the evaluation of carcinogenic risks to man, and are not listed here. Studies reported subsequently led to similar conclusions (Adami et al. 1992, Barra et al. 1990, Blot et al. 1988, Boffeta et al. 1990, Brown et al. 1988, Choi et al. 1991a, b, De Stefani et al. 1990b, Falk et al. 1990, Franco et al. 1989, Kabat et al. 1989, La Vecchia e al. 1989, McLaughlin et al. 1988, Merletti et al. 1990, Sankaranarayanan et al. 1990, 1991, Talamini et al. 1990, Tuyns et al. 1988, Zatonski et al. 1991, Zheng et al. 1990), and none has contradicted them. The results described below provide examples of the type of evidence obtained.

DOSE-RESPONSE RELATIONSHIP

An indication of the dose-response relationship for two types of upper digestive tract cancer, free from recall bias, is provided by the results of the American Cancer Society's cohort study of 1 million men and women over 30 years of age (Boffeta et al. 1990). Results relating to alcohol have been published so far for only 12 years of observations on 276,802 men aged 40–59 years who had provided detailed drinking histories. Mortality data have been given separately for oral cancer and for oesophageal cancer, standardized for age, smoking, and education. These are shown in Table 1. For both types of cancer, the mortality increases regularly (with one exception in the case of oral cancer) from that in non-smokers through three cat-egories of occasional or light drinkers to "heavy drinkers" (in the American sense) in whom the mortality is increased about six-fold.

Table 1
Relative risk of developing oral[a] or oesophageal cancer by drinking habit (after Boffeta et al. 1990)

Drinks per day	Type of cancer	
	oral	oesophageal
0	1.0 (55)[b]	1.0 (59)
≤1	0.7 (16)	1.3 (29)
2–3	1.4 (25)	2.2 (37)
4–5	3.1 (18)	4.8 (25)
6+	6.2 (26)	5.8 (22)

[a] Including cancer of the salivary glands.
[b] Numbers of deaths in parenthesis.

Table 2
Relative risk of oral or pharyngeal cancer by level of smoking and drinking (after Rothman et al. 1972)

Drinking, ml/day[a]	Smoking, cigarette equivalents per day			
	0	<20	20–39	≥40
0	1.0	1.5	1.4	2.4
<12	1.4	1.7	3.2	3.3
12–44	1.6	4.4	4.5	8.2
≥45	2.3	4.1	9.6	15.5

[a] The authors' "ounces per day" have been converted to ml for comparison with other tables.

Table 3
Relative risk of oesophageal cancer by level of smoking and drinking (after Tuyns et al. 1977)

Drinking, g/day	Smoking, g/day		
	0–10	10–30	≥30
0–40	1.0	3.9	7.8
40–80	7.3	8.6	33.6
80–120	11.7	13.1	87.0
≥121	49.7	78.7	149.1

Table 4
**Relative risk of cancers of larynx and hypopharynx by drinking
level and the site within the larynx
and standardized for smoking**

Drinking, g/day	Relative risk for cancer of			
	glottis	supraglottis	epilarynx	hypopharynx
Series 1a				
0–40	1.0	1.0	1.0	1.0
40–100	0.8	2.6	1.9	3.3
100–160	1.5	11.0	18.7	28.6
≥160	6.1	42.1	101.4	143.1
Cancer patients (n)	240	224	217	366
Series 2b				
0–20	1.0	1.0	1.0	1.0
20–40	0.8	0.9	0.9	1.6
40–80	1.1	1.1	1.5	3.2
80–120	1.7	1.7	5.1	5.6
>120	3.4	2.0	10.6	12.5
Cancer patients (n)	270	426	118	281

[a] Brugère et al. (1986): alcohol use measured as average daily current consumption.
[b] Tuyns et al. (1988): alcohol use measured as average daily consumption in adult life.

SYNERGISM WITH SMOKING

In the above example, the effect of smoking was effectively eliminated by standardization. To see how the two factors interact large numbers are needed, and these have been obtained only in case-control studies. Typical results were obtained by Rothman et al. (1972) in a study of 598 men with squamous carcinomas of the mouth and pharynx, matched one-for-one with men of the same ages in the same hospital. The results given in Table 2 suggest that each factor contributes about equally, having perhaps a greater relative effect when the other is present than when it is absent.

For oesophageal cancer in Normandy, where much larger quantities of alcohol are consumed, the relative risk (RR) for heavy drinkers and heavy smokers rises to a much stronger extent, as is shown in Table 3.

Observations on laryngeal cancer are confused by the fact that, despite the small size of the larynx as defined for anatomical and clinical purposes, its different parts react differently to different aetiological factors. Aetiologically it is best divided into the glottis and subglottis, which lie wholly within the respiratory system, and the supraglottis and epilarynx, which border on the hypopharynx. Two large case-control studies in France (Brugère et al. 1986) and in France, Italy, Spain, and Switzerland (Tuyns et al. 1988) have obtained similar results. These are summarized in Table 4. They show that cancers in all parts of the larynx and the hypopharynx are closely related to the amount smoked, but that the glottis is sharply distinguished from the epilarynx in its relationship with alcohol, the latter being closely related to alcohol consumption, like the hypopharynx, while the former is related to alcohol only when the consumption is what would be regarded as exceptionally heavy in many other countries (that is, 100 g or more per day). The results for the supraglottic area differed, however, being more like those for the epilarynx in one series and more like those for the glottis in the other. This is not easily explained by the use of different definitions in the two series. The very different relative risks for heavy consumption can be explained, however, as Brugère et al. (1986) compared levels of current consumption, while Tuyns et al. (1988) compared average levels over all adult life.

EFFECT IN THE ABSENCE OF SMOKING

In Europe and North America, all cancers of the upper respiratory and digestive tracts are rare in the absence of smoking, and only very few studies have included enough cases to provide any useful information about the effect of alcohol by itself. Groups of non-smokers who are defined as not being current smokers (Elwood et al. 1984) or even as not having smoked for the past 20 years (Wynder et al. 1957a) are inadequate in view of the strong effect of tobacco, which is liable to persist for many years after smoking has been stopped.

Table 5A
Relative risk (number of cases) for oropharyngeal cancer in non-smokers by drinking level

Reference	Drinking level	Relative risk (number of cases)	
		men	women
Blot et al. 1988	<1 drink/week	1.0 (12)	1.0 (36)
	1–4 drinks/week	1.3 (12)	0.7 (11)
	5–14 drinks/week	1.6 (15)	1.3 (7)
	15–29 drinks/week	1.4 (4)	0.0 (0)
	≥30 drinks/week	1.4 (4)	0.0 (0)
Talamini et al. 1990[a]	<14 drinks/week	1.0 (1)	1.0 (1)
	≥14 drinks/week	1.2 (5)	1.6 (11)
Merletti et al. 1989[b]	0–20 g/day		1.0 (6)
	20–40 g/day		1.1 (5)
	>40 g/day		0.8 (2)

[a] Relative risks were given for men and women combined (RR 1.0 for <14 drinks/week, RR 1.5 for 14-55 drinks/week, RR 2.2 for >55 drinks/week). The calculated χ^2 for trend was 4.08 ($P = 0.04$) on four levels (0, <14, 14-55 and >55 drinks/week).
[b] Oral cancer only.

Table 5B
Relative risk (number of cases) for oesophageal cancer in non-smokers by drinking level

Reference	Drinking level	Relative risk (number of cases)	
		men	women
Tuyns 1983a	0-40 g/day	1.0 (7)	1.0 (25)
	40-80 g/day	3.8 (15)	5.6 (8)
	80-120 g/day	10.2 (9)	11.0 (3)
	>120 g/day	101.0 (8)	–
La Vecchia et al. 1989[a]	<4 drinks/day	1.0 (5)	1.0 (22)
	>4 drinks/day		4.3 (5)
	4-8 drinks/day	1.1 (3)	
	>8 drinks/day	3.3 (3)	

[a] Relative risks were directly calculated from published data. La Vecchia et al. gave relative risks for men and women combined, adjusted for age and sex, of 1.0 for >4 drinks/day, 2.1 for 4-8 drinks per day, and 3.6 for >8 drinks/day. χ^2 for trend 0.09.

Table 5C
Relative risk (number of cases) for laryngopharyngeal cancer in male non-smokers by drinking level (after Tuyns et al. 1988)

Drinking level (g/day)	Epilarynx and hypopharynx	Endolarynx
0–40	1.0 (1)	1.0 (7)
>40	6.7 (8)	
40-80		1.5 (3)
>80		1.7 (6)

The few data available for oropharyngeal, oesophageal and laryngo-pharyngeal cancer are summarized in Tables 5A, 5B and 5C. Little or no increase in risk with amount consumed is seen for oropharyngeal cancer in three out of five sets of data or in the one set for cancer of the endolarynx (glottis), but the increases seen for oesophageal cancer are substantial. The differences are hard to explain by bias or confounding, but they can be explained by paucity of numbers and, if one drink is taken to equal ca. 10 g alcohol, by differences in the amount consumed. Acceptance of a causal relationship does not necessarily imply that ethanol is a complete carcinogen, however. There is no reason to suppose that tobacco smoke is the only carcinogenic agent to which the human upper respiratory and digestive tracts are exposed (indeed there is clear evidence that in parts of Asia and Africa it is not the only agent), and ethanol may facilitat the effect of other unrecognized carcinogenic agents in non-smokers, just as it commonly facilitates the effect of tobacco smoke.

DIFFERENTIAL EFFECTS OF DIFFERENT ALCOHOLIC BEVERAGES

Many attempts have been made to separate the effects of different types of alcoholic beverages. Some authors have concluded that no separation is possible (e.g. Williams et al. 1977, Breslow et al. 1980, Burch et al. 1981, Kabat et al. 1989, Merletti et al. 1990). Others have recorded greater risks with spirits, regardless of type, than with wine or beer (Wynder et al. 1956, 1957a, 1961, Hirayama 1979, Pottern et al. 1981). In Normandy, Tuyns et al. (1979) recorded a greater risk with apple-based drinks (digestives and cider) than with wine, beer or aperitifs. In Italy, however, Barra et al. (1990) found greater risks of oropharyngeal and oesophageal cancer in wine drinkers than in wine drinkers who also drank spirits or beer after adjustment for amount consumed. It is doubtful, however, whether histories regarding the quantity consumed can be equally accurate (or inaccurate) when described in tots of spirits, glasses of wine and bottles of beer, and Barra et al. (1990) point out that the most frequently consumed beverage in each area tends to be the one with the highest estimated relative risk. It may be that "strong" drinks are more deleterious, in grams of pure alcohol, than other alcoholic beverages, but the evidence is weak and inconclusive.

That ethanol itself, independent of any congeners present in different alcoholic beverages, may act to increase the risk of cancer in mucosal tissues with which it comes into contact is also demonstrated by the observation that the risk of oropharyngeal cancer increases in both men and women who regularly use mouthwashes with a high alcohol content (Winn et al. 1991).

NUTRITION

The evidence that nutrition affects the incidence of a wide variety of cancers, if not of all, is mounting steadily. There is now reason to believe that the risks from exposure to many carcinogenic agents can be reduced by the regular consumption of fruit and green vegetables. Early evidence has suggested that this might be particularly true for cancers of the hypopharynx, which have been associated with the Plummer-Vinson syndrome (Wynder et al. 1957b), and a deficiency of such foods seems to be a major cause of the exceptionally high risk of oesophageal cancer in parts of Asia (Day 1975). Heavy drinking is commonly associated with poor nutrition, and poor nutrition may be held to increase the risk of particularly pharyngeal and oesophageal cancers in heavy drinkers. Direct evidence of the role of nutritional deficiencies in the risk of alcohol-associated cancers has been obtained for cancers of the mouth and pharynx by Winn et al. (1984), McLaughlin et al. (1988), La Vecchia et al. (1991), and Franco et al. (1989); for cancers of the larynx by Zatonski et al. (1991); and for cancers of the oesophagus by Ziegler et al. (1981), Tuyns (1983b), Decarli et al. (1987), Tuyns et al. (1987), and Brown et al. (1988).

Conclusion

There is consensus that the use of alcoholic beverages increases the risk of developing cancers of the mouth (other than the salivary glands), pharynx (other than the nasopharynx), oesophagus and larynx; that the risks are principally due to the presence of ethanol and increase with the amount consumed; that the risks are increased by increased smoking, each agent approximately multiplying the effects of the other; and that, in the absence of smoking, the risks in developed countries are all small unless alcohol use is exceptionally heavy. There is also evidence that the risks are diminished by a diet rich in fruit and green vegetables.

Whether the cocarcinogenic effects of different alcoholic beverages depend solely on the presence of ethanol and are unaffected either by the concentration of ethanol or the presence of congeners is uncertain.

Cancer of the Stomach

As early as 1833 it was recognized that excessive drinking can cause an acute inflammation of the stomach lining (gastritis), and it is now believed that repeated insults of excess alcohol (in alcoholics, for example) leads to a persistent inflammatory response (chronic gastritis) (Taylor 1987). Because chronic gastritis is thought to pre-dispose to later cancerous changes in the stomach (Correa 1988), it has been suggested that alcohol consumption might increase the risk of stomach cancer. Apart from the association with gastritis, alcohol might also affect stomach cancer risk by altering gastric juice physiology (e.g. by changing acidity) or by occasional contamination with carcinogenic substances (e.g. N-nitroso compounds in certain beers and whiskies) (MAFF 1987).

Stomach cancer is invariably more common in men than in women, by a factor of around two, and this has been attributed to comparable differences in alcohol consumption (Flamant et al. 1964). There has, however, been a dramatic worldwide decline in the incidence of stomach cancer (Muñoz 1988), a finding in contrast to the general increases in alcohol consumption and alcohol-related diseases such as cirrhosis of the liver. The male excess is much the same in different countries regardless of drinking levels, and the attribution of the male excess to alcohol cannot be sustained.

Table 6
Cohort studies of alcohol consumption in relation to cancers of the stomach, colon, rectum and pancreas

Study, country	Relative risk (number of cancer cases or deaths)				Comments
	stomach	colon	rectum	pancreas	
Studies of alcoholics					
Sundby 1967, Norway	1.3 (45)	1.0 (9)	1.9 (12)	0.9 (5)	1722 men compared with local rates
Hakulinen et al. 1974, Finland	0.8 (6)	1.8 (3)	—	1.8 (4)	>16,000 men vs. national incidence rates
Hakulinen et al. 1974, Finland	—	1.0 (82)	—	—	205,000 men vs. national incidence rates
Monson et al. 1975, USA	1.0 (15)	0.6 (7)	0.7 (4)	0.6 (3)	1139 men and 143 women vs. National mortality rates
Adelstein et al. 1976, UK	0.8 (8)	1.3 (9)	0.9 (4)	1.5 (7)	1595 men and 475 women vs. National mortality rates
Robinette et al. 1979, USA	1.0 (9)	0.8 (7)	3.3 (6)	0.9 (4)	4401 men compared with national mortality rates
Schmidt et al. 1981, Canada	1.0 (19)	1.0 (19)	1.0 (10)	1.2 (11)	9889 men (mean intake 200 g/day) relative to local mortality rates
Adami et al. 1992, Sweden	M 0.9 (23), F 0.7 (1)	M 1.2 (26), F 1.7 (4)	M 0.8 (12), F 0.8 (1)	M 1.4 (19), F 2.6 (3)	8340 men and 1013 women, vs. Local incidence rates
Studies of brewery workers					
Dean et al. 1979, Ireland	0.8 (40)	1.3 (32)	1.6* (32)	1.2 (17)	3600 men (mean intake 58 g/day) vs. local mortality rates
Jensen 1980, Denmark	0.9 (92)	1.1 (87)	1.0 (85)	1.1 (44)	14,313 men (allowance 78 g/day) vs. national incidence rates
Carstensen et al. 1990, Sweden	1.1 (53)	1.2 (48)	1.7* (49)	1.7* (38)	6230 men (allowance 1 litre/day) vs. national incidence rates
Study of waiters					
Andersen et al. 1989, Norway	0.6* (14)	1.1 (24)	2.0 (28)	1.0 (11)	2413 men compared with national incidence rates

Table 6 (continued)

Follow-up studies of populations with known consumption

Study					Description
Gordon et al. 1984, USA	* (18)	n.s. (36)	—	—	2106 men an 2641 women, RR not estimated, mortality
Kono et al. 1986, 1987, Japan	1.2 (116)	a	1.4 (39)	1.5 (14)	5130 male physicians, ≥2 drinks/day vs. Non-drinkers, mortality
Blackwelder et al. 1980, Stemmermann et al. 1980, Hawaii	1.2 (174)	1.4* (211)	1.9* (101)	n.a. (13)	8006 Japanase men, RR for 112 g/month vs. non-drinkers, incidence
Hirayama 1989, 1992, Japan	0.9 (5247)	1.7* (574)	1.4 (n.a.)	1.0 (n.a.)	122,261 men and 142,857 women, RR for daily drink-ing vs. Non-drink-ing, significant for sigmoid colon only
Kneller et al. 1991, USA	1.1 (75)	—	—	—	17,818 men, mainly European descent, RR for ≥14 drinks per month vs. non-drinkers, mortality
Kato et al. 1992, Japan	2.8* (57)	—	—	—	9753 subjects, RR for ≥50 g/day vs. non-drinkers, mortality; trend n.s.
Wu et al. 1987, USA	—	1.3 (76)	1.6 (51)	—	11,888 subjects, RR for >27 g/day vs. non-drinkers, incidence
Klatsky et al. 1981, 1988, Hiatt et al. 1988, USA	n.s. (13)	1.6 (203)	2.5 (66)	09 (48)	>100,000 subjects, RR for daily dirnking vs. non-drinking, incidence; signfilcant trend for rectal cancer
Heuch et al. 1983, Norway	—	—	—	10.8* (18)	4995 men, RR for "frequent" drinking vs. non-drinking, incidence; significant trend

* $P<0.05$; n.s., not significant.
a Combined with rectal cancer.
n.a., data not available

COHORT STUDIES

The relationship between alcohol intake and cancer at a variety of sites has been assessed in several cohort studies, the results of which are summarized in Table 6. In most studies, detailed information on type of beverage, amount consumed and smoking habits was not available. Most of the cohort studies were of the retrospective (historical) type, comparing cancer incidence in groups with high alcohol intake with that of the general population.

In 11 studies, stomach cancer rates in groups with an established high intake of alcohol were compared with appropriate rates from the general population. Seven of these were groups of clinically diagnosed alcoholics (Adami et al. 1992, Adelstein et al. 1976, Hakulinen et al. 1974, Monson et al. 1975, Robinette et al. 1979, Schmidt et al. 1981, Sundby 1967), three were groups of brewery workers (Carstensen et al. 1990, Dean et al. 1979, Jensen 1980), and one a group of waiters (Andersen et al. 1989). The results are summarized in Table 6. Not one of these studies showed a significant increase in stomach cancer rate, and the small study of waiters showed a significant decrease. Combining the findings of all the studies, 325 cases of stomach cancer were observed, while 352 were expected from the comparison populations; that is, there were less cases of stomach cancer than expected, overall, though not significantly less.

There have also been seven published cohort studies in which alcohol use was recorded, by interview or questionnaire, in cross-sections of various populations (Gordon et al. 1984, Hirayama 1989, 1992, Kato et al. 1992, Klatsky et al. 1981, Kneller et al. 1991, Kono et al. 1987, Stemmermann et al. 1990). The subsequent rate of stomach cancer in drinkers was then compared with that in non-drinkers. These results are also summarized in Table 6. Two studies (Gordon et al. 1984, Kato et al. 1992) reported a significant increase with heavy drinking, of which one was based on a total of only 18 deaths from stomach cancer (Gordon et al. 1984). In contrast, the largest study, in Japan, was based on 5247 male deaths from stomach cancer and showed that the RR in daily drinkers was 0.92 compared with non-drinkers (Hirayama 1989, 1992).

CASE-CONTROL STUDIES

There have been at least 37 published case-control studies in which the relationship between alcohol consumption and stomach cancer has been reported. Of these, seven showed a significant positive relationship (Agudo et al. 1992, Correa et al. 1985, De Stefani et al. 1990a, Hoey et al. 1981, Hu et al. 1988, Lee et al. 1990, Wu-Williams et al. 1990), while 30 did not (Acheson et al. 1964, Armijo et al. 1981, Bjelke 1974, Boeing et al. 1991, Buiatti et al. 1989, 1990, Palli et al. 1992, Burr et al. 1989, Demirir et al. 1990, Ferraroni et al. 1989, Graham et al. 1967, 1972, Haenszel et al. 1972, 1976, Higginson 1966, Hoshiyama et al. 1992, Jedrychowski et al. 1986, Kato et al. 1990a, Kono et al. 1988, Modan et al. 1974, Risch et al. 1985, Stocks 1957, Tajima et al. 1985, Tominaga et al. 1991, Trichopoulos et al. 1985, Tuyns et al. 1992, Unakami et al. 1989, Williams et al. 1977, Wynder et al. 1963, You et al. 1988, Yu et al. 1991).

Among the negative studies, there were some that showed an effect in a particular subgroup. Thus, positive effects were reported for sake drinkers in a study of Japanese in Hawaii (Haenszel et al. 1972), beer drinkers in Germany (Boeing et al. 1991), and vodka drinkers (but only before breakfast) in Poland (Jedrychowski et al. 1986). None of these three studies showed a positive effect for overall alcohol consumption.

The seven positive studies were from a variety of countries: China (Hu et al. 1988), France (Hoey et al. 1981), Spain (Agudo et al. 1992), Taiwan (Lee et al. 1990), Uruguay (De Stefani et al. 1990a) and the USA (Correa et al. 1985, Wu-Williams et al. 1990). The RR for drinkers as compared to non-drinkers was reported in four studies (Agudo et al. 1992, Correa et al. 1985, Lee et al. 1990, Wu-Williams et al. 1990) and varied between 1.5 and 1.7. The results were all of borderline statistical significance. Five studies (Agudo et al. 1992, Correa et al. 1985, De Stefani et al. 1990a, Lee et al. 1990, Wu-Williams et al. 1990) reported on the trend in relative risk with increasing drinking level, which was significant in all except one (Agudo et al. 1992), albeit in one US study the significance was restricted to blacks (Correa et al. 1985).

Two of the seven positive studies were made difficult to interpret by combining non-drinkers and "low" drinkers into a single baseline group. In one study (Hu et al. 1988) the "low" drinkers were individuals who drank up to 4000 g alcohol per year (equivalent to about 1 drink per day), while in the other study (Hoey et al. 1981) this cut-off point was 568 g/week (equivalent to 7 litres of wine per week).

The type of alcoholic beverage consumed and its relationship to risk was reported in four of the seven positive studies. In these studies, wine had the strongest effect in two studies (Agudo et al. 1992, De Stefani et al. 1990a), spirits in one (Correa et al. 1985), and beer in the fourth (Wu-Williams et al. 1990).

Two studies (Agudo et al. 1992, De Stefani et al. 1990a) reported positive results for men but not for women.

Most of the positive results have been adjusted for tobacco smoking, but the extent to which other potential confounding factors (notably related to diet and socioeconomic status) were controlled for was variable. Many such confounding factors are related to both alcohol use and gastric cancer risk and could hence have given rise to false-positive findings.

CANCER OF THE GASTRIC CARDIA

The cardia region of the stomach is the uppermost area where the stomach adjoins the oesophagus. There has recently been interest in cancer at this site because, unlike the more distal regions of the stomach, cardia cancer rates have been increasing. It has been suggested that this cancer resembles a specific type of cancer (adenocarcinoma) of the lower oesophagus and may share common risk factors, notably tobacco and alcohol exposure. Three of the case-control studies have analysed alcohol use in relation to cardia cancer. One US study (Wu-Williams et al. 1990) found an extremely strong effect of alcohol in the cardia, whereas Italian (Palli et al. 1992) and Japanese (Unakami et al. 1989) studies found no effect in comparison with cancer elsewhere in the stomach. The US study also found an increased effect of alcohol in the upper part of the non-cardia stomach (the corpus) compared with the lower part (the antrum). A further study from Uruguay (De Stefani et al. 1990a), in which cardia and corpus cases were combined, found that the alcohol association with these was no stronger than that in the antrum. Finally, a Canadian study (Gray et al. 1992), which did not have a control group, found no difference between alcohol use in patients with cardia cancer and those with cancer in other sites of the stomach, while both groups consumed less than oesophageal cancer patients.

Conclusion

The evidence reviewed pertaining to the relationship between alcohol use and stomach cancer derives from 18 cohort and 37 case-control studies. The existing balance of the evidence indicates that alcohol use is unlikely to be involved in the aetiology of the disease. The absence of recall bias means that particular emphasis should be placed on the cohort studies, only two of which were positive. In addition, less than a quarter of the case-control studies reported positive findings and, in most of these, the size of the effect was relatively small and of borderline statistical significance.

Our conclusion is slightly less cautious than that reached by the IARC (1988) that "there is little in the aggregate data to suggest a causal role for drinking of alcoholic beverages in stomach cancer". There is likely to be general consensus in favour of the IARC conclusion, but a minority of investigators might dissent from that conclusion and suggest that alcohol could have an aetiological role in stomach cancer, albeit minor and unproven.

As yet there is insufficient evidence to draw conclusions about subsidiary hypotheses, such as whether alcohol use is a risk factor for cancer of the gastric cardia.

Cancer of the Pancreas

Pancreas cancer is reported to occur more frequently in men than in women, more in blacks than in whites, and more in urban than in rural populations. At present, epidemiological and toxicological studies have not consistently identified any specific factor responsible for the development of pancreatic cancer except cigarette smoking (Levison 1979, Morgan et al. 1977, Wynder 1975). Consequently, it is believed that combinations of dietary and life-style factors such as fat, protein and alcohol, which are thought to promote the effects of environmental carcinogens, may play a role in the pathogenesis of this highly fatal form of cancer. Alcohol as a possible cause of pancreas cancer was proposed for the first time by Dörken (1964) and has been extensively studied since then. This review summarizes the epidemiological data available to 1993 about the role of alcohol in the development of pancreas cancer.

COHORT STUDIES

Heuch et al. (1983) have reported a significant dose-response effect of alcohol (based on the frequency of consumption of beer and spirits) in a cohort of 16,713 Norwegians, which persisted after controlling for smoking of cigarettes in 18 cases with pancreas cancer. Based on these findings, the authors concluded that there exists a strong causal relationship between alcohol use and pancreatic cancer. However, the apparent high non-participation rate of heavy drinkers during the formative phase of the cohort, and the conflicting evidence derived from histologically confirmed and unconfirmed pancreatic cancer cases (among the latter, the association with alcohol intake appears to be negative), makes a causal interpretation of the findings difficult (IARC 1988). One of three studies of brewery workers (Carstensen et al. 1990) showed a significant 70% excess of pancreatic cancers, but none of the other cohort studies reviewed reported a significant association between consumption of alcoholic beverages and pancreatic cancer risk (Sundby 1967, Hakulinen et al. 1974, Monson et al. 1975, Adelstein et al. 1976, Dean et al. 1979, Jensen 1979, 1980, Robinette et al. 1979, Hirayama 1992, Kono et al. 1983, 1986, Blackwelder et al. 1980, Schmidt et al. 1981, Hiatt et al. 1988, Adami et al. 1992, Andersen et al. 1989).

CASE-CONTROL STUDIES

At least 23 case-control studies have been reported in which pancreas cancer patients or their relatives ("proxy respondents") were queried as to their life-style, and in which their responses were compared with those of people without the disease. The number of cases in the various studies ranged from 18 to 901. Controls were usually hospital-based, but occasionally population-based or community-based controls were used. Patients were usually classified into several drinking categories, but the definition of these categories was not always explicitly stated. A significant positive association of alcohol use with pancreatic cancer was found in five studies. Burch et al. (1968) reported that 54 (65%) of 83 patients with pancreatic cancer diagnosed in the New Orleans Veterans Hospital between 1960 and 1966 had an average daily alcohol use of 57–85 g. Cuzick et al. (1989) reported evidence of a positive trend in the association between risk of pancreatic cancer and total alcohol use. They found a threefold risk of pancreatic cancer among heavy beer drinkers and demonstrated a dose-response relation. Moreover, they found that the effect of alcohol appeared to be largely confined to smokers. No significant trend with amount of alcohol was found in non-smokers. Furthermore, Durbec et al. (1983) found a positive association between total alcohol intake (especially in the case of wine with a high alcohol content) and pancreatic cancer risk (RR 2.4 for drinkers versus non-drinkers). The risk was reduced after controlling for fat and carbohydrate intake; there was no increased risk with regular drinking of aperitifs or spirits. Raymond et al. (1987) reported a significantly increased pancreatic cancer risk among beer drinkers. After pooling the data from the population-based case-control study performed by Raymond et al. (1987) and two negative hospital-based case-control studies conducted in Paris (Clavel et al. 1989) and Greater Milan (Ferraroni et al. 1989), no association with alcohol use was found (Bouchardy et al. 1990). Recently, Olsen et al. (1989) conducted a case-control study in the Minneapolis-St. Paul area and observed that heavy drinking (4 or more drinks per day), adjusted for several potential confounding variables, was positively associated with pancreatic cancer. All exposure data of this study, however, were obtained from proxy respondents, which may lead to misclassification of risk factors, as has recently been pointed out by Lyon et al. (1992).

Other groups did not find a consistent significant association between alcohol intake and cancer of the pancreas (Bueno de Mesquita et al. 1992, Clavel et al. 1989, Bouchardy et al. 1990, Wynder et al. 1973, 1983, Williams et al. 1977, MacMahon et al. 1981, Manousos et al. 1981, Haines et al. 1982, Kodama et al. Mori 1983a, b, Gold et al. 1985a, Falk et al. 1988, Farrow et al. 1990, Jain et al. 1991). Some reported an inverse association between alcohol intake and the relative risk for pancreas cancer (Baghurst et al. 1991, Ghadirian et al. 1991, Gold et al. 1985b, Mack et al. 1986, Norell et al. 1986, Falk et al. 1988, Hiatt et al. 1988). The earliest report of an inverse relationship between pancreatic cancer and wine was that of Gold et al. (1985b). In a population-based case-control study in Los Angeles, Mack et al. (1986) found a non-significant inverse association between cancer of the pancreas and alcohol intake from any source; the inverse relationship being most pronounced for table wine. Norell et al. (1986) performed a population-based case-control study in Sweden and found an inverse association with RRs for frequent versus infrequent alcohol use of 0.5 (hospital controls) and 0.7 (population controls). Falk et al. (1988) found decreased risks for all types of alcoholic beverages among women and among the heaviest male beer drinkers. The pooled analysis of three case-control studies (Bouchardy et al. 1990) did not reveal a relationship with wine, but the data from the Paris study (Clavel et al. 1989) showed a significant inverse dose-response effect. No biologically plausible explanation for a protective effect of alcohol is apparent.

THE ROLE OF (CALCIFYING) PANCREATITIS

It is generally accepted that chronic alcohol abuse, whether or not in combination with a high-fat diet, is the most common cause of chronic (calcifying) pancreatitis (Ishii et al. 1973, Johnson et al 1979, Sarles et al. 1974, 1980, Singh 1986, Ammann et al. 1988, Singh et al. 1990).

Several mechanisms have been proposed for the pathogenesis of alcoholic pancreatitis. There is mounting evidence from both animal and human studies that alcohol has a direct effect on pancreatic cells. Light and electron microscopy of pancreatic tissue from alcoholic patients with chronic pancreatitis revealed dedifferentiation of acinar cells to tubular complexes (Singh 1986). In addition to the loss of acinar cells, there is loss of ductal cells.

The association between chronic pancreatitis and pancreatic cancer has been described by Mikal et al. (1950) in autopsies and by Paulino-Netto et al. (1960) and Becker (1978) in surgical patients. The data are inadequate to draw conclusions, however, especially since pancreatitis may be the consequence, rather than the cause, of pancreatic cancer. Although chronic pancreatitis microscopically surrounding pancreatic carcinoma is common, cancer developing in chronic pancreatitis has rarely been shown. Recently, Haas et al. (1990) presented four male patients with pancreatic cancer who had had surgery for complications of chronic pancreatitis. Chronic pancreatitis, including calcifications, had been caused by alcohol in three cases.

Conclusions

Cohort studies of people with high alcohol intake provide no strong evidence for an association between alcohol consumption and the risk of pancreatic cancer. Population-based cohort studies as well as case-control studies produce inconsistent results. The level of alcohol intake reported in the various studies does not account for the inconsistency. The average alcohol intake in the studies that reported a positive association was lower than in studies where no association between alcohol consumption and pancreatic cancer risk was reported.

It is generally accepted, however, that chronic alcohol abuse is associated with chronic (calcifying) pancreatitis. Recurrent tissue damage and repair is an important phenomenon in this disease. There is, moreover, substantial evidence that cancer may be associated with chronically injured tissue (Feron et al. 1989). Colon cancer is frequently seen in patients with chronic colitis (Laroye 1974), skin cancer may occur in burn scars (Berenblum 1944), and many lung tumours grow in areas of scarring (Bennett et al. 1969). A large body of animal data also suggests that chronic tissue injury induced by chemical or physical agents could be a major factor in tumour development in connective tissue and epithelial tissues (Grasso 1987). For example, malignant tumours induced in the nasal epithelium by irritating substances such as acetaldehyde and formaldehyde have been found to arise only from epithelium that is severely damaged (Woutersen et al. 1986a, Kerns et al. 1983).

Taking into account all the epidemiological data now available, it can be concluded that it is unlikely that a causal relationship between consumption of alcohol and the risk of pancreas cancer exists. An indirect association via the induction of chronic (calcifying) pancreatitis, however, cannot be completely excluded.

Cancer of the Large Bowel

A relationship between alcohol use and colorectal cancer was originally suggested, in the 1970s, by correlational studies in populations. At least five studies showed positive correlations between measures of alcohol disappearance or consumption and colorectal cancer incidence or mortality rates, both between populations (McMichael et al. 1979) and within them (Breslow et al. 1974, Enstrom 1977, Kono et al. 1979, Decarli et al. 1986). Such correlational studies, however, are of value only in formulating hypotheses worth further consideration in analytical studies.

COHORT STUDIES

At least 15 cohort studies gave some data on colorectal and large bowel cancer (IARC 1988), the results of which are summarized in Table 6. Of these, however, seven included fewer than 50 cases of (or deaths from) colorectal cancer combined and are not very informative. The main findings from the other eight cohort studies are described below (Hakulinen et al. 1974, Dean et al. 1979, Jensen 1979, Pollack et al. 1984, Stemmermann et al. 1990, Wu et al. 1987, Klatsky et al. 1988, Hirayama 1989, Carstensen et al. 1990).

The geographic area, the identification of the study cohorts, the main type of alcoholic beverage, and the pattern of drinking (i.e. regular versus binge) varied from study to study. It is remarkable, therefore, that all the RR estimates for colon cancer varied within the relatively narrow range of 1.0 to 1.7, with most between 1.1 and 1.3. This overall consistency of results is only in apparent contrast with several heterogeneities observed within studies. For instance, in the large Japanese cohort (Hirayama 1989), the RR for daily alcohol drinking was 5.4 for the sigmoid colon without any significant association for the proximal colon or rectum. These apparent discrepancies are not surprising, however, since several combinations of alcoholic beverages and cancer sub-sites were examined.

For rectal cancer, the RRs for alcohol use in eight cohort studies (Hakulinen et al. 1974, Dean et al. 1979, Jensen 1979, Pollack et al. 1984, Stemmermann et al. 1990, Wu et al. 1987, Klatsky et al. 1988, Carstensen et al. 1990) ranged from 1.0 to 2.5, and in most studies were between 1.0 and 1.7. Beer drinking was a specific concern for rectal cancer because of the findings in some correlation studies, and three cohorts of brewery workers are, therefore, of particular interest: they gave RRs of 1.0, 1.6 (significant) and 1.7 (significant).

Thus, the overall evidence from these eight cohort studies providing data on alcohol and colorectal cancer risk excludes an excess risk among alcohol drinkers of a factor of 2 or more. Inclusion of seven smaller studies (IARC 1988, Adami et al. 1992) did not modify this conclusion: a total of 133 cases were observed in seven studies versus 115 expected, giving a summary RR of 1.2. The total evidence, therefore, indicates a weak positive association. The information from cohort studies is not easy to interpret, however, since several studies were based on highly selected populations, and most of them permitted only limited (or no) allowance for major covariates. In this respect, data from case-control studies may be more informative.

CASE-CONTROL STUDIES

At least 18 case-control studies (Wynder et al. 1967, Williams et al., 1977, Tuyns et al. 1982, Manousos et al. 1983, Miller et al. 1983, Potter et al. 1986, Kabat et al. 1986, Kune et al. 1987, Tuyns 1988, Freudenheim et al. 1990, Longnecker 1990, Slattery et al. 1990, Kato et al. 1990b, Hu et al. 1991, Choi et al. 1991a, Riboli et al. 1991, Barra et al. 1992, Peters et al. 1992), each based on 100 or more cases of colorectal cancer, provided information on the potential relationship of alcohol use with large bowel cancer. Eight were hospital-based studies, and 10 used community or neighbourhood controls. The number of cases ranged from 100 to over 1400. Eight studies were from North America, five from Europe, two from Australia, and one each from Japan, China, and Korea.

Among these, four studies were totally negative and showed no evidence of association between cancer at any of the large bowel sub-sites or sex strata with alcohol or any type of alcoholic beverage (Wynder et al. 1967, Tuyns et al. 1982, Manousos et al. 1983, Slattery et al. 1990). Three other studies showed overall statistically significant direct associations. Of two studies from North America, one showed an association for beer (Kabat et al. 1986) with rectal cancer (RR 2.7 for the highest drinking level), and one (Freudenheim et al. 1990) found an association for total alcohol use, again only for rectal cancer, but with RR estimates below 2 in both sexes. A third study, from China, showed significant trends in risk both for colon and rectum cancer (Hu et al. 1991), but numbers of regular drinkers were small, leaving open the possibility of selection mechanisms. The remaining 11 studies showed no consistent and significant overall association, but the RRs were elevated in some specific strata. Also, these apparent associations were of moderate strength, the RRs being generally below 2 for the highest drinking levels.

In most case-control studies, and in particular in the most recent ones, the results were adjusted for major covariates, specifically for indicators of socio-economic status and, in several studies, for selected foods or nutrients as well. Even after these adjustments, however, the inherent problem remains that diet in drinkers is probably different in several aspects (including higher fat and total energy intake) from that of non-drinkers (La Vecchia et al. 1992). Persisting confounding is therefore possible and may partly or largely explain a pattern of risk characterized by several moderate and inconsistent associations.

Beer drinking, particularly in relation to rectal cancer, was a specific issue in several studies. While some North American studies (Kabat et al. 1986, Freudenheim et al. 1990, Longnecker 1990) and one Australian investigation (Kune et al. 1987) found elevated risks, these were not confirmed by studies from Europe, including one from Belgium (Tuyns 1988), where beer is the main alcoholic beverage. It may be, therefore, that different correlates of beer drinking in different populations may account for some of the elevated risks, rather than there being a carcinogenic effect of beer itself on the rectal epithelium.

Conclusions

The majority of cohort and case-control studies suggest a positive relationship between alcohol use and colorectal cancer. A formal meta-analysis of published data (Longnecker et al. 1990) led to an estimate of overall RR of 1.1 (95% CI 1.05–1.14) for total alcohol use, which was consistent for both men and women and for both colon and rectum. The relationship is quantitatively moderate, and there is consensus that a twofold risk for both colon and rectum cancer can be excluded, even with high drinking levels. There is also consensus that there is no appreciable and consistent difference in risk between the sexes, between cancer sites (colon and rectum) and among types of alcoholic beverage. Apparent discrepancies in the results of the various studies can be easily accounted for by random variation.

Despite the large body of epidemiological research, including the provision of data for several thousand cases, no consensus has emerged on the interpretation of the observations. The issue remains open and continues to attract research interest.

It is possible that alcohol causes some small risk of colorectal cancer. While some obvious biases and sources of confounding can be excluded, it is conceivable that some differences in diet between drinkers and non-drinkers may account for the observed association. Moreover, a moderate association may be produced, at least in part, by the selective publication of positive results. Thus, the epidemiological evidence regarding a causal role for alcohol use in the production of colorectal cancer remains inconclusive.

Recommendation for Research

The principal uncertainty in the relationship between alcoholic beverages and cancers of the digestive tract and larynx is whether the observed weak association between their consumption and the development of cancers of the large bowel is causal or a secondary effect of the type of diet commonly associated with heavy drinking. It is recommended to encourage research aimed at discovering whether the association can be explained by confounding with dietary patterns.

References

Acheson ED, Doll R (1964) Dietary factors in carcinoma of the stomach: study of 100 cases and 200 controls. Gut 5: 126–31

Adami HO, McLaughlin JK, Hsing AW, et al. (1992) Alcoholism and cancer risk: a population-based cohort study. Cancer Causes Control 3: 419–25

Adelstein A, White G (1976) Alcoholism and mortality. Popul Trends 6: 7–13

Agudo A, Gonzalez CA, Marcos G, et al. (1992) Consumption of alcohol, coffee, and tobacco, and gastric cancer in Spain. Cancer Causes Control 3: 137–43

Ammann RW, Muench R, Otto R, et al. (1988) Evolution and regression of pancreatic calcification in chronic pancreatitis. A prospective long-term study of 107 patients. Gastroenterology 95:1018–28

Andersen AA, Bjelke E, Langmark F (1989) Cancer in waiters. Br J Cancer 60: 112–15

Armijo R, Orellana M, Medina E, et al. (1981) Epidemiology of gastric cancer in Chile I: case-control study. Int J Epidemiol 10: 53–56

Baghurst PA, McMichael AJ, Slavotinek AH, et al. (1991) A case-control study of diet and cancer of the pancreas. Am J Epidemiol 134: 167–79

Barra S, Franceschi S, Negri E, et al. (1990) Type of alcoholic beverage and cancer of the oral cavity, pharynx and oesophagus in an Italian area with high wine consumption. Int J Cancer 46: 1017–20

Barra S, Negri E, Franceschi S, et al. (1992) Alcohol and colorectal cancer: a case-control study from northern Italy. Cancer Causes Control 3: 153–59

Becker V (1978) Cancer of the pancreas and chronic pancreatitis, a possible relationship. Acta Hepatogastroenterol 25: 257–59

Bennett DE, Sasser WF, Ferguson TB (1969) Adenocarcinoma of the lung in men. Cancer 23: 431–39

Berenblum I (1944) Irritation and carcinogenesis. Arch Pathol 38: 233–44

Bjelke E (1974) Epidemiological studies of cancer of the stomach, colon, and rectum; with special emphasis on the role of diet. Scand J Gastroenterol 9: 1–235

Blackwelder WC, Yano K, Rhoads GG, et al. (1980) Alcohol and mortality: the Honolulu Heart Study. Am J Cancer 68: 164–69

Blot WH, McLaughlin JK, Winn DM, et al. (1988) Smoking and drinking in relation to oral and pharyngeal cancer. Cancer Res 48: 3282–87

Boeing H, Frentzel-Beyme R, Berger M, et al. (1991) Case-control study on stomach cancer in Germany. Int J Cancer 47: 858–64

Boffeta P, Garfinkel L (1990) Alcohol drinking and mortality among men enrolled in an American Cancer Society prospective study. Epidemiology 1: 342–48

Bouchardy C, Clavel F, La Vecchia C, et al. (1990) Alcohol, beer and cancer of the pancreas. Int J Cancer 45: 842–46

Breslow NE, Enstrom JE (1974) Geographical correlations between cancer mortality rates and alcohol-tobacco consumption in the United States. J Natl Cancer Inst 53: 631–39

Breslow NE, Day N (1980) Statistical methods in cancer research, vol. 1. The analysis of case-control studies. IARC Scientific Publications 32. International Agency for Research on Cancer, Lyon, France pp. 227–33.

Brown LM, Blot WJ, Schuman SH, et al. (1988) Environmental factors and high risk of esophageal cancer among men in coastal South Carolina. J Natl Cancer Inst 90: 1620–25

Brugère J, Guenel P, Leclerc A, et al. (1986) Differential effects of tobacco and alcohol in cancer of the larynx, pharynx, and mouth. Cancer 57: 391–95

Bueno de Mesquita HB, Maisonneuve P, Moerman CJ, et al. (1992) Lifetime consumption of alcoholic beverages, tea and coffee and exocrine carcinoma of the pancreas: a population-based case-control study in The Netherlands. Int J Cancer 50: 514–22

Buiatti E, Palli D, Decarli A, et al. (1989) A case-control study of gastric cancer and diet in Italy. Int J Cancer 44: 611–16

Buiatti E, Palli D, Decarli A, et al. (1990) A case-control study of gastric cancer and diet in Italy. II. Association with nutrients. Int J Cancer 45: 896–901

Burch GE, Ansari A (1968) Chronic alcoholism and carcinoma of the pancreas: a correlative hypothesis. Arch Intern Med 122: 273–75

Burch JD, Howe GR, Miller AB, et al. (1981) Tobacco, alcohol, asbestos, and nickel in the etiology of cancer of the larynx: a case-control study. J Natl Cancer Inst 67: 1219–24

Burr ML, Holliday RM (1989) Fruit and stomach cancer. J Hum Nutr Diet 2: 273–77

Carstensen JM, Bygren LO, Hatschek T (1990) Cancer incidence among Swedish brewery workers. Int J Cancer 45: 393–96

Castonguay A, Rivenson A, Trushin N, et al. (1984) Effects of chronic ethanol consumption on the metabolism and carcinogenicity of N'-nitrosonornicotine in F344 rats. Cancer Res 44: 2285–90

Choi SY, Kahyo H (1991a) Effect of cigarette smoking and alcohol consumption in the aetiology of cancers of the digestive tract. Int J Cancer 49: 381–86

Choi SY, Kahyo H (1991b) Effect of cigarette smoking and alcohol consumption in the aetiology of cancer of the oral cavity, pharynx, and larynx. Int J Epidemiol 20: 845–51

Clavel F, Benhamou E, Auquier A, et al. (1989) Coffee, alcohol, smoking and cancer of the pancreas: a case-control study. Int J Cancer 43: 17–21

Correa P (1988) A human model of gastric carcinogenesis. Cancer Res 48: 3554–60

Correa P, Fontham E, Pickle LW, et al. (1985) Dietary determinants of gastric cancer in south Louisiana inhabitants. J Natl Cancer Inst 75: 645–54

Cuzick J, Babiker AG (1989) Pancreatic cancer, alcohol, diabetes mellitus and gall-bladder disease. Int J Cancer 43: 415–21

Day NE (1975) Some aspects of the epidemiology of esophageal cancer. Cancer Res 35: 3304–07

Dean G, MacLennan R, McLoughlin H, et al. (1979) Causes of death of blue-collar workers at a Dublin brewery. Br J Cancer 40: 581–89

Decarli A, La Vecchia C (1986) Environmental factors and cancer mortality in Italy: correlational exercise. Oncology 43: 116–26

Decarli A, Liati P, Negri E, et al. (1987) Vitamin A and other dietary factors in the etiology of esophageal cancer. Nutr Cancer 10: 39–47

Demirer T, Icli F, Üzunalimoglu O, et al. (1990) Diet and stomach cancer incidence: a case-control study in Turkey. Cancer 65: 2344–48

De Stefani E, Correa P, Fierro L, et al. (1990a) Alcohol drinking and tobacco smoking in gastric cancer: A case-control study. Rev Epidemiol Santé Publique 38: 297–307

De Stefani E, Muñoz N, Esteve J, et al. (1990b) Male drinking, alcohol, tobacco, diet, and esophageal cancer in Uruguay. Cancer Res 50: 426–31

Dörken H (1964) Einige Daten bei 280 Patienten mit Pancreaskrebs. Gastroenterologia 102: 47–77

Durbec JP, Chevillotte G, Bidart JM, et al. (1983) Diet, alcohol, tobacco, and risk of cancer of the pancreas: a case-control study. Br J Cancer 47: 463–70

Elwood JM, Pearson JCG, Skippen DH, et al. (1984) Alcohol, smoking, social and occupational factors in the aetiology of cancer of the oral cavity, pharynx, and larynx. Int J Cancer 34: 603–12

Enstrom JE (1977) Colorectal cancer and beer drinking. Br J Cancer 35: 674–83

Falk RT, Williams PL, Fontham ET, et al. (1988) Life-style risk factors for pancreatic cancer in Louisiana: a case-control study. Am J Epidemiol 128: 324–36

Falk RT, Pickle LW, Brown LM, et al. (1990) Effect of smoking and alcohol consumption on laryngeal cancer risk in coastal Texas. Cancer Res 49: 4024–29

Farrow DC, Davis S (1990) Risk of pancreatic cancer in relation to medical history and the use of tobacco, alcohol and coffee. Int J Cancer 45: 816–20

Feron VJ, Woutersen RA (1989) Role of tissue damage in nasal carcinogenesis. In: Feron VJ, Bosland MC (eds), Nasal carcinogenesis in rodents: relevance to human health risk., Proceedings of the TNO-CIVO/NYU Nose Symposium, Veldhoven, Netherlands, 24–28 October 1988. Pudoc, Wageningen, pp. 76–84

Ferraroni M, Negri E, La Vecchia C, et al. (1989) Socioeconomic indicators, tobacco and alcohol in the aetiology of digestive tract neoplasms. Int J Epidemiol 18: 556–62

Flaks BJ, Moore MA, Flaks A (1980) Ultrastructural analysis of pancreatic carcinogenesis. I. Morphological characterization of N-nitroso-bis(2-hydroxo-propyl)amine-induced neoplasms in Syrian hamster. Carcinogenesis 1: 423–38

Flaks BJ, Moore MA, Flaks A (1981) Ultrastructural analysis of pancreatic carcinogenesis. IV. Pseudoductular transformation of acini in the hamster pancreas during N-nitroso-bis(2-hydroxopropyl)amine carcinogenesis. Carcinogenesis 2: 1241–53

Flamant R, Lasserre O, Lazar P, et al. (1964) Differences in sex ratio according with use of tobacco and alcohol. Review of 65,000 cases. J Natl Cancer Inst 32: 1309–16

Franco EL, Kowalski LP, Oliveira BV, et al. (1989) Risk factors for oral cancer in Brazil: a case-control study. Int J Cancer 43: 992–1000

Freudenheim JL, Graham S, Marshall JR, et al. (1990) Lifetime alcohol intake and risk of rectal cancer in Western New York. Nutr Cancer 13: 101–9

Ghadirian P, Simard A, Baillargeon J (1991) Tobacco, alcohol, and coffee and cancer of the pancreas. Cancer 67: 2664–70

Gibel W (1967) Experimental studies on syncarcinogenesis in oesophageal carcinoma (Ger.). Arch Geschwulstforsch 30: 181–89

Gold EB, Gordis L, Diener MD, et al. (1985a) Diet and other risk factors for cancer of the pancreas. Cancer 44: 460–67

Gold EB, Gordis L, Diener MD, et al. (1985b) Diet and other risk factors for cancer of the pancreas: a case-control study. Cancer 55: 460–67

Gordon T, Kannel WB (1984) Drinking and mortality: the Framingham study. Am J Epidemiol 120: 97–107

Graham S, Lilienfeld AM, Tidings JE (1967) Dietary and purgation factors in the epidemiology of gastric cancer. Cancer 20: 2224–34

Graham S, Schotz W, Martino P (1972) Alimentary factors in the epidemiology of gastric cancer. Cancer 30: 927–38

Grasso P (1987) Persistent organ damage and cancer production in rats and mice. Arch Toxicol 11: 75–83

Gray JR, Coldman AJ, MacDonald WC (1992) Cigarette and alcohol use in patients with adenocarcinoma of the gastric cardia or lower esophagus. Cancer 69: 2227–31

Griciuté L, Castegnaro M, Béréziat J-C (1982) Influence of ethyl alcohol on the carcinogenic activity of N-nitrosodi-n-propylamine. In: Bartsch H, Castegnaro M, O'Neill IK, Okada M (eds), N-nitroso compounds: occurrence and biological effects, IARC Scientific Publication 41. International Agency for Research on Cancer, Lyon, France, pp. 643–48

Griciuté L, Castegnaro M, Béréziat J-C (1984) Influence of ethyl alcohol on carcinogenesis induced with N-Nitrosodiethylamine. In: Börzsönyi M, Day NE, Lapis K, et al. (eds), Models, mechanisms and aetiology of tumour promotion, IARC Scientific Publication 56. International Agency for Research on Cancer, Lyon, France, pp. 413–17

Haas O, Guillard G, Rat P, et al. (1990) Pancreatic carcinoma developing in chronic pancreatitis: a report of four cases. Hepatogastroenterology 37: 350–51

Haenszel W, Kurihara M, Segi M, et al. (1972) Stomach cancer among Japanese in Hawaii. J Natl Cancer Inst 49: 969–88

Haenszel W, Kurihara M, Locke FB, et al. (1976) Stomach cancer in Japan. J Natl Cancer Inst 56: 265–78

Haines AP, Moss AR, Whittemore A, et al. (1982) A case-control study of pancreatic carcinoma. J Cancer Res Clin Oncol 103: 93–97

Hakulinen T, Lehtimäki L, Lehtonen M, Tet al. (1974) Cancer morbidity among two male cohorts with increased alcohol consumption in Finland. J Natl Cancer Inst 52: 1711–14

Hamilton SR, Sohn OS, Fiala ES (1987) Effects of timing and quantity of chronic dietary ethanol consumption on azoxymethane-induced colonic carcinogenesis and azoxymethane metabolism in Fischer 344 rats. Cancer Res 47: 4305–11

Hamilton SR, Sohn OS, Fiala ES (1988) Inhibition by dietary ethanol of experimental colonic carcinogenesis induced by high-dose azoxymethane in F344 rats. Cancer Res 48: 3313–18

Heuch I, Kvale G, Jacobsen BK, et al. (1983) Use of alcohol, tobacco and coffee, and risk of pancreatic cancer. Br J Cancer 48: 637–43

Hiatt RA, Klatsky AL, Armstrong MA (1988) Pancreatic cancer, blood glucose, and beverage consumption. Int J Cancer 41: 794–97

Higginson J (1966) Etiological factors in gastrointestinal cancer in man. J Natl Cancer Inst 37: 527–45

Hirayama T (1979) Diet and cancer. Nutr Cancer 1: 67–81

Hirayama T (1981) A large-scale cohort study on the relationship between diet and selected cancers of digestive organs. In: Bruce WR, Correa P, Lipkin M, et al. (eds), Gastrointestinal cancer: endogenous factors; Banbury Report 7. Cold Spring Harbor Laboratory, Cold Spring Harbor, NY, pp. 409–26

Hirayama T (1989) Association between alcohol consumption and cancer of the sigmoid colon: observations from a Japanese cohort study. Lancet ii: 725–27

Hirayama T (1992) Life-style and cancer: from epidemiological evidence to public behaviour change to mortality reduction of target cancers. J Natl Cancer Inst 12: 65–74

Hoey J, Montvernay C, Lambert R (1981) Wine and tobacco: risk factors for gastric cancer in France. Am J Epidemiol 113: 668–74

Horie A, Kohchi S, Kuratsune M (1965) Carcinogenesis in the esophagus. II. Experimental production of esophageal cancer by administration of ethanolic solution of carcinogens. Gann (Jpn J Cancer Res) 56: 429–41

Hoshiyama Y, Sasaba T (1992) A case-control study of stomach cancer and its relation to diet, cigarettes, and alcohol consumption in Saitama Prefecture, Japan. Cancer Causes Control 3: 441–48

Howarth AE, Pihl E (1985) High-fat diet promotes and causes distal shift of experimental rat colonic cancer, beer and alcohol do not. Nutr Cancer 6: 229–35

Hu J, Liu Y, Yu Y, et al. (1991) Diet and cancer of the colon and rectum: a case-control study in China. Int J Epidemiol 20: 362–67

Hu J, Zhang S, Jia E, et al. (1988) Diet and cancer of the stomach: a case-control study in China. Int J Cancer 41: 331–35

IARC (1988) Alcohol drinking. IARC Monographs on the Evaluation of Carcinogenic Risks for Humans Vol. 44. International Agency for Research on Cancer, Lyon, France

Ishii K, Takeuchi T, Hirayama T (1973) Chronic calcifying pancreatitis and pancreatic carcinoma in Japan. Digestion 9: 429–37

Jain M, Howe GR, St Louis P, et al. (1991) Coffee and alcohol as determinants of risk of pancreas cancer: a case-control study from Toronto. Int J Cancer 47: 384–89

Jedrychowski W, Wahrendorf J, Popiela T, et al. (1986) A case-control study of dietary factors and stomach cancer risks in Poland. Int J Cancer 37: 837–42

Jensen OM (1979) Cancer morbidity and causes of death among Danish brewery workers. Int J Cancer 23: 454–63

Jensen OM (1988) Cancer morbidity and causes of death among Danish brewery workers. In: Alcohol drinking, IARC Monograph on the Evaluation of Carcinogenic Risks for Humans, Vol. 44. International Agency for Research on Cancer, Lyon, France, p. 216

Johnson JR, Zintel HA (1979) Pancreatic calcification and cancer of the pancreas. Surg Gyn Obst 117: 585–88

Kabat GC, Howson CP, Wynder EL (1986) Beer consumption and rectal cancer. Int J Epidemiol 15: 494–501

Kabat GC, Wynder EL (1989) Type of alcoholic beverage and oral cancer. Int J Cancer 43: 190–94

Kato I, Tominaga S, Ito Y, et al. (1990a) A comparative case-control analysis of stomach cancer and atrophic gastritis. Cancer Res 50: 6559–64

Kato I, Tominaga S, Matsuura A, et al. (1990b) A comparative case-control study of colorectal cancer and adenoma. Jpn J Cancer Res 81: 1101–08

Kato I, Tominaga S, Matsumoto K (1992) A prospective study of stomach cancer among a rural Japanese population: a 6-year survey. Jpn J Cancer Res 83: 568–75

Kerns WD, Pavkov KL, Donofrio DJ, et al. (1983) Carcinogenicity of formaldehyde in rats and mice after long-term inhalation exposure. Cancer Res 43: 4382–92

Klatsky AL, Friedman GD, Siegelaub AB (1981) Alcohol and mortality: a ten-year Kaiser-Permanente experience. Ann Intern Med 95: 139–45

Klatsky AL, Armstrong MA, Friedman GD, et al. (1988) The relations of alcoholic beverage use to colon and rectal cancer. Am J Epidemiol 128: 1007–15

Kneller RW, McLaughlin JK, Bjelke E, et al. (1991) A cohort study of stomach cancer in a high-risk American population. Cancer 68: 672–78

Kodama T, Mori W (1983a) Morphological behaviour of carcinoma of the pancreas. I. Histological classification and electron microscopical observation. Acta Pathol Jpn 33: 467–81

Kodama T, Mori W (1983b) Morphological lesions of the pancreatic ducts. Significance of pyloric gland metaplasia in carcinogenesis of exocrine and endocrine pancreas. Acta Pathol Jpn 33: 645–60

Konishi N, Kitahori Y, Shimoyama T, et al. (1986) Effects of sodium chloride and alcohol on experimental esophageal carcinogenesis induced by n-nitrosopiperidine in rats. Jpn J Cancer Res (Gann) 77: 446–51

Kono S, Ikeda M (1979) Correlation between cancer mortality and alcoholic beverage in Japan. Br J Cancer 40: 449–55

Kono S, Ikeda M, Ogata M, et al. (1983) The relationship between alcohol and mortality among Japanese physicians. Int J Epidemiol 12: 437–41

Kono S, Ikeda M, Tokudome S, et al. (1988) A case-control study of gastric cancer and diet in northern Kyushu, Japan. Jpn J Cancer Res 79: 1067–74

Kono S, Ikeda M, Tokudome S, et al. (1986) Alcohol and mortality: a cohort study of male Japanese physicians. Int J Epidemiol 15: 527–32

Kono S, Ikeda M, Tokudome S, et al. (1987) Cigarette smoking, alcohol and cancer mortality: a cohort study of male Japanese physicians. Jpn J Cancer Res 78: 4656–58

Kune S, Kune GA, Watson LF (1987) Case-control study of alcoholic beverages as etiological factors: the Melbourne colorectal cancer study. Nutr Cancer 9: 43–56

Lamy L (1910) Statistical clinical study of 134 cases of cancer of the oesophagus and cardia (French). Arch Mal Appar Dig Mal Nutr 4: 451–75

Laroye GJ (1974) How efficient is immunological surveillance against cancer and why does it fail? Lancet 1: 1097–1100

La Vecchia C, Negri E (1989) The role of tobacco in oesophageal cancer in non-smokers and of tobacco in non-drinkers. Int J Cancer 43: 784–85

La Vecchia C, Negri E, d'Avonzo B, et al. (1991) Dietary indicators of oral and pharyngeal cancer. Int J Epidemiol 20: 39–44

La Vecchia C, Negri E, Franceschi S, et al. (1992) Differences in dietary intake with smoking, alcohol and education. Nutr Cancer 17: 297–304

Lee HH, Wu HY, Chuang YC, et al. (1990) Epidemiologic characteristics and multiple risk factors of stomach cancer in Taiwan. Anticancer Res 10: 875–82

Levison DA (1979) Carcinoma of the pancreas. J Pathol 129: 203–23

Levitt MH, Harris CC, Squire R, et al. (1977) Experimental pancreatic carcinogenesis. I. Morphogenesis of pancreatic adenocarcinoma in the Syrian golden hamster induced by N-nitroso-bis(2-hydroxypropyl)amine. Am J Pathol 88: 5–28

Longnecker MP (1990) A case-control study of alcoholic beverage consumption in relation to risk of cancer of the right colon and rectum in men. Cancer Causes Control 1: 5–14

Longnecker MP, Orza MJ, Adams ME, et al. (1990) A meta-analysis of alcoholic beverage consumption in relation to risk of colorectal cancer. Cancer Causes Control 1: 59–68

Lyon JL, Egger MJ, Robison LM, et al. (1992) Misclassification of exposure in a case-control study: the effects of different types of exposure and different proxy respondents in a study of pancreatic cancer. Epidemiology 3: 223–31

Mack TM, Yu MC, Hanisch R, et al. (1986) Pancreas cancer and smoking, beverage consumption, and past medical history. J Natl Cancer Inst 76: 49–60

MacMahon B, Yen S, Trichopoulos D, et al. (1981) Coffee and cancer of the pancreas. New Engl J Med 304: 630–33

MAFF (1987) Nitrate, nitrite and N-nitroso compounds in food. Food surveillance paper 20, Ministry of Agriculture, Fisheries and Food. HMSO, London

Manousos O, Trichopoulos D, Koutseliinis A, et al. (1981) Epidemiologic characteristics and trace elements in pancreatic cancer in Greece. Cancer Det Prev 4: 439–42

Manousos O, Day NE, Trichopoulos D, et al. (1983) Diet and colorectal cancer: a case-control study in Greece. Int J Cancer 32: 1–5

McLaughlin JK, Gridley G, Block G, et al. (1988) Dietary factors in oral and pharyngeal cancer. J Natl Cancer Inst 80: 1237–43

McMichael AJ, Potter JD, Hetzel BS (1979) Time trends in colo-rectal cancer mortality in relation to food and alcohol consumption: United States, United Kingdom, Australia and New Zealand. Int J Epidemiol 8: 295–303

Meijers M, Bruijntjes JP, Hendriksen EGJ, et al. (1989) Histogenesis of early preneoplastic lesions induced by N-nitrosobis(2-oxopropyl)amine in exocrine pancreas of hamsters. Int J Pancreatol 4: 127–37

Merletti F, Boffeta P, Ciccone G, et al. (1989) Role of tobacco and alcoholic beverages in the etiology of cancer of the oral cavity/oropharynx in Torino, Italy. Cancer Res 49: 4919–24

Mikal S, Campbell A (1950) Carcinoma of pancreas: diagnostic and operative criteria based on 100 consecutive autopsies. Surgery 28: 961–69

Miller AB, Howe GR, Jain M, et al. (1983) Food items and food groups as risk factors in a case-control study of diet and colo-rectal cancer. Int J Cancer 32: 155–61

Modan B, Lubin F, Barell B, et al. (1974) The role of starches in the etiology of gastric cancer. Cancer 34: 2087–92

Monson RR, Lyon JL (1975) Proportional mortality among alcoholics. Cancer 36: 1077–79

Morgan GGH, Wormsley KG (1977) Cancer of the pancreas. Gut 18: 580–96

Mufti SI, Becker G, Sipes IG (1989) Effect of chronic dietary ethanol consumption on the initiation and promotion of chemically-induced esophageal carcinogenesis in experimental rats. Carcinogenesis 10: 303–09

Muñoz N (1988) Descriptive epidemiology of gastric cancer. In: Reed PI, Hill MJ (eds), Gastric carcinogenesis. Excerpta Medica, Amsterdam, pp. 51–69

Nelson RL, Samelson SL (1985) Neither dietary ethanol nor beer augments experimental colon carcinogenesis in rats. Dis Colon Rectum 28: 460–62

Norell SE, Ahlbom A, Erwald R, et al. (1986) Diet and pancreatic cancer: a case-control study. Am J Epidemiol 124: 894–902

Olsen GW, Mandel JS, Gibson RW, et al. (1989) A case-control study of pancreatic cancer and cigarettes, alcohol, coffee and diet. Am J Public Health 79: 1016–19

Palli D, Bianchi S, Decarli A, et al. (1992) A case-control study of cancers of the gastric cardia in Italy. Br J Cancer 65: 263–66

Paulino-Netto A, Dreiling DA, Boronofsky ID (1960) The relationship between pancreatic calcification and cancer of the pancreas. Ann Surg 151: 530–37

Peters RK, Pike MC, Garabrant D, et al. (1992) Diet and colon cancer in Los Angeles County, California. Cancer Causes Control 3: 457–73

Pollack ES, Nomoura AMY, Lance K, et al. (1984) Prospective study of alcohol consumption and cancer. N Engl J Med 310: 617–21

Potter JD, McMichael AJ (1986) Diet and cancer of the colon and rectum: a case-control study. J Natl Cancer Inst 76: 557–69

Pottern LM, Morris LE, Blot WJ, et al. (1981) Esophageal cancer among black men in Washington DC: Alcohol, tobacco, and other risk factors. J Natl Cancer Inst 71: 1085–87

Pour PM (1984) Histogenesis of exocrine pancreatic cancer in the hamster model. Environ Health Perspect 56: 229–43

Pour PM (1988) Mechanism of pseudoductular (tubular) formation during pancreatic carcinogenesis in the hamster model. An electron-microscopic and immuno-histochemical study. Am J Pathol 130: 335–44

Pour PM, Reber HA, Stepan K (1983) Modification of pancreatic carcinogenesis in the hamster model. XII. Dose-related effect of ethanol. J Natl Cancer Inst 71: 1085–87

Raymond L, Infante F, Tuyns AJ, et al. (1987) Diet and pancreatic cancer (French). Gastroenterol Clin Biol 11: 488–92

Riboli E, Cornée J, Macquart-Moulin G, et al. (1991) Cancer and polyps of the colorectum and lifetime consumption of beer and other alcoholic beverages. Am J Epidemiol 133: 157–66

Risch HA, Jain M, Choi NW, et al. (1985) Dietary factors and the incidence of cancer of the stomach. Am J Epidemiol 122: 947–59

Robinette CD, Hrubec Z, Fraumeni Jr, JF (1979) Chronic alcoholism and subsequent mortality in World War II veterans. Am J Epidemiol 109: 687–700

Rothman K, Keller R (1972) The effect of joint exposure of alcohol and tobacco on risk of cancer of the mouth and pharynx. J Chron Dis 25: 711–16

Sankaranarayanan R, Duffy SW, Nair MK, et al. (1990) Tobacco and alcohol as risk factors in cancer of the larynx in Kerala, India. Int J Cancer 45: 879–82

Sankaranarayanan R, Duffy SW, Padmakumary G, et al. (1991) Risk factors for cancer of the oesophagus in Kerala, India. Int J Cancer 49: 485–89

Sarles H, Lebreuil G, Tasso F, et al. (1971) A comparison of alcoholic pancreatitis in rat and man. Gut 12: 377–88

Sarles H, Tiscornia O (1974) Ethanol and chronic calcifying pancreatitis. Med Clin North Am 58:1333–46

Sarles H, Figarella C, Tiscornia O, et al. (1980) Chronic calcifying pancreatitis (CCP). Mechanism of formation of the lesions. New data and critical study. In: Fitzgerald PJ, Morrison AB (eds), The pancreas. Williams and Wilkins, Baltimore, pp. 48–66

Schmidt W, Popham RE (1981) The role of drinking and smoking in mortality from cancer and other causes in male alcoholics. Cancer 47: 1031–41

Seitz HK, Czygan P, Waldherr R, et al. (1984) Enhancement of 1,2-dimethylhydrazine-induced rectal carcinogenesis following chronic ethanol consumption in the rat. Gastroenterology 86: 886–91

Singh M (1986) Ethanol and the pancreas. In: Go VLW, et al.(eds), The exocrine pancreas: biology, pathobiology, and disease. Raven Press, New York, pp. 423–37

Singh M, Simsek H (1990) Ethanol and the pancreas: current status. Gastroenterology 98: 1051–62

Slattery ML, West DW, Robison LM, et al. (1990) Tobacco, alcohol, coffee, and caffeine as risk factors for colon cancer in a low-risk population. Epidemiology 1: 141–45

Stemmermann GN, Nomura AMY, Chyou PH, et al. (1990) Prospective study of alcohol intake and large bowel cancer. Dig Dis Sci 35: 1414–20

Stocks P (1957) Cancer in North Wales and Liverpool regions. In: Thirty-fifth annual report: supplement to part II. British Empire Cancer Campaign, London, pp. 51–113

Sundby P (1967) Alcoholism and mortality. Universitetsforlaget, Oslo

Tajima K, Tominaga S (1985) Dietary habits and gastro-intestinal cancers: a comparative case-control study of stomach and large intestinal cancers in Nagoya, Japan. Jpn J Cancer Res (Gann) 76: 705–16

Takahashi M, Arai H, Kokubo T, et al. (1980) An ultrastructural study of precancerous and cancerous lesions of the pancreas in Syrian golden hamsters induced by N-nitroso-bis(2-oxopropyl)amine. Gann (Jpn J Cancer Res) 71: 825–31

Takahashi M, Hasegawa R, Furukawa F, et al. (1986) Effects of ethanol, potassium metabisulfite, formaldehyde and hydrogen peroxide on gastric carcinogenesis in rats after initiation with n-methyl-N'-nitro-N-nitrosoguanidine. Jpn J Cancer Res (Gann) 77: 118–24

Talamini R, Franceschi S, Barra S, et al. (1990) The role of alcohol in oral and pharyngeal cancer in non-smokers and non-drinkers. Int J Cancer 46: 391–93

Taylor KB (1987) Gastritis. In: Weatherall DG, Ledingham JGG, Worrall, DA (eds), Oxford Textbook of Medicine, 2nd ed., vol. 12. Oxford University Press, London, pp. 77–86.

Tominaga K, Koyama Y, Sasagawa M, et al. (1991) A case-control study of stomach cancer and its genesis in relation to alcohol consumption, smoking, and familial cancer history. Jpn J Cancer Res (Gann) 82: 974–79

Trichopoulos D, Ouranos G, Day NE, et al. (1985) Diet and cancer of the stomach: a case-control study in Greece. Int J Cancer 36: 291–97

Tuyns AJ (1983a) Oesophageal cancer in non-smoking drinkers and in non-drinking smokers. Int J Cancer 32: 443–44

Tuyns AJ (1983b) Protective effects of citrus fruit on esophageal cancer. Nutr Cancer 5: 195–200

Tuyns AJ (1988) Beer consumption and rectal cancer. Rev Epidemiol Santé Publique 36: 144–45

Tuyns AJ, Pequignot G, Jensen OM (1977) Les cancers de l'oesophage en Ille-et-Villaine en fonction des niveaux de consommation d'alcool et de tabac, Des risques qui se multiplient. Bull Cancer 64:45–60

Tuyns AJ, Pequignot G, Abbatucci JS (1979) Oesophageal cancer and alcohol consumption: importance of type of beverage. Int J Cancer 23: 443–47

Tuyns AJ, Pequignot G, Gignoux M, et al. (1982) Cancers of the digestive tract, alcohol and tobacco. Int J Cancer 30: 9–11

Tuyns AJ, Riboli E, Doornbus G, et al. (1987) Diet and esophageal cancer in Calvados (France). Nutr Cancer 9: 81–92

Tuyns AJ, Estève J, Raymond L, et al. (1988) Cancer of the larynx/ hypolarynx, tobacco and alcohol. IARC international case-control study in Turin and Varese (Italy), Zaragoza and Navarra (Spain), Geneva (Switzerland) and Calvados (France). Int J Cancer 41: 483–91

Tuyns AJ, Kaaks R, Haelterman M, et al. (1992) Diet and gastric cancer. A case-control study in Belgium. Int J Cancer 51: 1–6

Tweedie JH, Reber H, Pour PM, et al. (1981) Protective effect of ethanol on the development of pancreatic cancer. Surg Forum 32: 222–24

Unakami M, Hara M, Fukuchi S, et al. (1989) Cancer of the gastric cardia and the habit of smoking. J Jpn Soc Pathol 39: 420–24

Williams RR, Horm JW (1977) Association of cancer sites with tobacco and alcohol consumption and socioeconomic status of patients: interview study from the Third National Cancer Survey. J Natl Cancer Inst 58: 525–47

Winn DM, Blot WJ, McLaughlin JK, et al. (1991) Mouthwash use and oral conditions in the risk of oral and pharyngeal cancer. Cancer Res 51: 3041–47

Winn DM, Ziegler RG, Pickle LW, et al. (1984) Diet in the etiology of oral and pharyngeal cancer among women from the Southern United States. Cancer Res 44: 1216–22

Woutersen RA, Appelman LM, Wilmer JWGM, et al. (1986a) Inhalation toxicity of acetaldehyde in rats. III. Carcinogenicity study. Toxicology 41: 213–31

Woutersen RA, van Garderen-Hoetmer A, Bax J, et al. (1986b) Modulation of putative preneoplastic foci in exocrine pancreas of rats and hamsters. I. Interaction of dietary fat and ethanol. Carcinogenesis 7: 1587–93

Woutersen RA, van Garderen-Hoetmer A, Bax J et al. (1989) Modulation of dietary fat-promoted pancreatic carcinogenesis in rats and hamsters by chronic ethanol ingestion. Carcinogenesis 10: 453–59

Wu AH, Paganini-Hill A, Ross RK, et al. (1987) Alcohol, physical activity and other risk factors for colorectal cancer: a prospective study. Br J Cancer 55: 687–94

Wu-Williams AH, Yu MC, Mack TM (1990) Life-style, workplace, and stomach cancer by subsite in young men of Los Angeles County. Cancer Res 50: 2569–76

Wynder EL (1975) An epidemiologic evaluation of the causes of cancer of the pancreas. Cancer Res 35: 2228–33

Wynder EL, Bross IJ, Day E (1956) A study of environmental factors in cancer of the larynx. Cancer 9: 86–110

Wynder EL, Bross IJ, Feldman RM (1957a) A study of etiological factors in cancer of the mouth. Cancer 10: 1300–23

Wynder EL, Hultberg S, Jacobsen E, et al. (1957b) Environmental factors in cancer of upper alimentary tract: Swedish study with special reference to Plummer-Vinson (Paterson-Kelly) syndrome. Cancer 10: 470–87

Wynder EL, Bross IJ (1961) A study of etiological factors in cancer of the esophagus. Cancer 14: 389–413

Wynder EL, Kmet J, Dungal N, et al. (1963) Epidemiological investigation of gastric cancer. Cancer 15: 1461–96

Wynder EL, Shigematsu T (1967) Environmental factors of cancer of the colon and rectum. Cancer 20: 1520–63

Wynder EL, Mabuchi K, Maruchi N, et al. (1973) A case-control study of cancer of the pancreas. Cancer 31: 641–48

Wynder EL, Hall NEL, Polansky M (1983) Epidemiology of coffee and pancreatic cancer. Cancer Res 43: 3900–06

You WC, Blot WJ, Chang YS, et al. (1988) Diet and high risk of stomach cancer in Shandong, China. Cancer Res 48: 3518–23

Young M, Russell WT (1926) An investigation into the statistics of cancer in different trades and professions. Medical Research Council, special report series. HMSO, London, p. 99

Yu GP, Hsieh CC (1991) Risk factors for stomach cancer: population-based case-control study in Shanghai. Cancer Causes Control 2: 169–74

Zatonski W, Becher H, Lissowska J, et al. (1991) Tobacco, alcohol, and diet in the etiology of laryngeal cancer: a population-based case-control study. Cancer Causes Control 2: 3–10

Zheng T, Boyle P, Hu H, et al. (1990) Tobacco smoking, alcohol consumption and risk of oral cancer: a case-control study in Beijing, People's Republic of China. Cancer Causes Control 1: 173–79

Ziegler RG, Morris LE, Blot WJ, et al. (1981) Esophageal cancer among black men in Washington DC. II. Role of nutrition. J Natl Cancer Inst 67: 1199–1206

Appendix 2

Alcohol and Liver Disease

J. Rodés
University of Barcelona, Spain

M. Salaspuro
University of Helsinki, Finland

T.I.A. Sorensen
Copenhagen Health Services, Denmark

Abstract

It is well established that excess alcohol consumption in man is associated with increased risk of developing liver disease. However, the pathogenesis of alcoholic liver injury is not well understood. At present, many questions still remain unanswered. This report presents an analysis of knowledge on the effects of excess alcohol ingestion on the liver. For this purpose, the mechanisms involved in alcoholic liver damage, the clinical manifestations and pathology of alcoholic liver disease (ALD), the epidemiology of chronic alcoholism and liver disease, and a list of the associations between liver disease and chronic consumption of alcohol are critically reviewed.

At present there is strong evidence for the relation of the pathogenesis of alcohol-related liver damage to the direct toxicity of ethanol, its metabolism and metabolites, obtained from experiments done with animal models. However, it is important to take into account that in these models the energy derived from alcohol varies from 30–50% of total energy. Therefore, nutritional deficiencies as major patho-genic factors cannot be excluded in the development of liver injury.

The liver plays a dominant role in alcohol metabolism, with its main pathway for oxidation being alcohol dehydrogenase (ADH) activity. By the action of ADH, ethanol is transformed to acetaldehyde, which in turn is rapidly oxidized in the liver to acetate by the action of aldehyde dehydrogenase (ALDH). Acetaldehyde is a very potent and reactive compound, and it has been suggested that it is one of the major factors in the pathogenesis of ALD.

Excessive alcohol ingestion produces the development of hepatic steatosis. A key mechanism in the genesis of fatty liver is due to the alcohol-induced change in the redox state of the liver. It has also been suggested that excessive alcohol intake may produce liver damage by other mechanisms such as promotion of lipid peroxidation and toxicity associated with an activation of the microsomal ethanol-oxidizing system. Although there is some evidence that both mechanisms may play a role in the development of alcoholic liver injury, further studies are required to reach definitive consensus. Finally, nutritional factors have also been implicated in association with excessive alcohol ingestion; however, the data obtained until now are not sufficient to establish a critical role for nutritional factors.

It is considered that chronic alcoholics may exhibit a wide spectrum of hepatic lesions, the most frequent being fatty liver, alcoholic hepatitis, and hepatic cirrhosis. The deposition of fat in the hepatocytes is very frequent (90% of the cases) among chronic alcoholics. The deposition of a single large lipid droplet in hepatocytes is the histological lesion defining alcoholic fatty liver. A micro-vesicular form may also be observed, although less frequently. Chronic alcoholics may also develop an increase of collagen content, particularly in the perivenular area (perivenular fibrosis), and the association with steatosis (steatofibrosis) is relatively frequent. Alcoholic hepatitis is the most characteristic hepatic lesion found in heavy drinkers. This lesion is characterized by hepatocellular necrosis associated with an inflammatory cell infiltrate constituted by neutro-phils and in many cases with Mallory bodies. The clinical picture starts with fatigue, anorexia, nausea and vomiting. A few days later, abdominal pain, jaundice and fever appear. Tender hepatomegaly may be detected. Biochemical tests reveal a moderate increase in trans-aminases; the γ-glutamyltransferase (GGT) level is very high and may be associated with hyperbilirubinaemia and high alkaline phosphatase levels. It has recently been reported that chronic alcoholism may produce chronic hepatitis; however, it is possible that this lesion among alcoholics is due to viral infection (hepatitis C virus). The prevalence of hepatic cirrhosis in chronic alcoholics varies from study to study and is usually of the micronodular type. The clinical manifestations are identical to those observed in hepatic cirrhosis of other aetiologies. It is important to note that abstinence will reverse, improve or delay progression of ALD, depending on the stage of the lesion indicating that, in fact, alcohol in these cases is responsible for liver damage.

It is considered that chronic alcoholism presently constitutes a significant public health problem. The incidence of alcoholic cirrhosis has recently been estimated at 190 per million person-years in Danish men and 85 in Danish women, with the age-specific incidence rates peaking at 50–60 years. Similar results have been found in the UK and in the USA. The sex difference in incidence of ALD may be due to the greater frequency of heavy drinkers among men, but it has also been suggested that women are more sensitive to develop liver injury due to chronic alcohol ingestion. Further prospective control studies are required to obtain a full consensus. The average duration of excessive alcohol ingestion until diagnosis of alcoholic cirrhosis may be between 10 and 20 years. Among excessive drinkers, the rate of development of cirrhosis may be at about 2–3% per year, and, accordingly, the prevalence of cirrhosis is greater the longer the duration of excessive alcohol use. A large number of aggregate population studies have assessed the changes over time within populations and the differences among populations in mortality from cirrhosis in relation to total per capita alcohol use. These studies have shown very high correlations between mortality from cirrhosis and alcohol use. However, despite the strikingly high correlation, the risk function for development of cirrhosis cannot be clearly derived from these relationships. Several retrospective case-control studies have been conducted showing that the probability of becoming a hospitalized cirrhotic patient increases exponentially with increased daily alcohol consumption ranging from 20 to160 g. However, the interpretation of these studies in terms of risk function for the development of cirrhosis is very difficult. On the other hand, other retrospective, cross-sectional studies have been performed in which the study population was defined as alcoholics. One of these studies defined a threshold for cumulated alcohol use below which there seemed to be no risk of cirrhosis (the theoretical threshold of 1 g alcohol per day per kg body weight over 15 years). The interpretation of these results, in terms of the risk function for cirrhosis, is also very difficult.

Five prospective studies of general populations have assessed the relationship between daily consumption reported at the start of the study and subsequent cirrhosis mortality during long-term follow-up. It was found that the risk increased steadily by increasing daily dirnking level. In one study it was found that the development of cirrhosis after 10–15 years with a minimum alcohol use of 50 g/day was about 2% per year. This study also showed that individuals drinking intermittently had a lower risk of liver damage. The studies performed so far do not allow a consensus about a precise threshold of safe alcohol use below which there is no risk of development of cirrhosis. On the other hand, there may be a levelling off of the risk at about 2–3% per year by increasing drinking level above ca. 70 g/day.

There is firm consensus about the association between chronic drinking and the development of fatty liver, perivenular fibrosis, acute alcoholic hepatitis and hepatic cirrhosis. This consensus implies that the probability of developing these conditions is higher in individuals who, for a period of time, have drunk excessively. This is based on vast clinical experience and numerous systematic studies. In addition, the frequency of death attributed to liver disease in the general population is correlated across time and place with measures of the total alcohol use by these populations. Whereas the consensus about the qualitative association between excessive alcohol consumption and the development of the above-mentioned hepatic lesions is well established, there is much uncertainty about the dose-effect relationship.

The fact that only a minor proportion of individuals drinking excessive amounts of alcohol develop the most severe forms of liver damage, cirrhosis in particular, indicates that other causal factors are involved. Despite years of research, no consensus has been achieved on any one such factor. Current research focuses on genetic factors, viral infections and specific nutritional disturbances.

Mechanism of Liver Disease Induced by Chronic Alcoholism: General Overview

In the late 1940s, the pathogenesis of alcoholic liver injury was assumed to be associated almost exclusively with a secondary protein and choline deficiency (Best et al. 1949). Since then, strong evidence has accumulated for the relation of the pathogenesis of alcohol-related liver damage to the direct toxicity of ethanol, its metabolism and its metabolites (Lieber 1988b, 1991b, Lieberet al. 1991, 1992, French 1989, Salaspuro 1989, 1991). However, many questions still remain unanswered. Why do only a proportion of heavy drinkers or alcoholics develop liver injury? What is the basic mechanism behind the "cell death" caused by alcohol? What is the most important toxic factor: ethanol, its metabolism or its metabolites? Can we indeed entirely exclude nutritional deficiency in the pathogenesis of alcoholic liver injury? During the past few decades, the pathways and principles of ethanol oxidation in the liver and other tissues have been extensively characterized. Numerous reviews and books cover epidemio-logical (Grant et al. 1988, Hall 1985a, Lelbach 1976, Paton 1988, Schmidt 1977, Sörensen 1989), metabolic, aetiopathological (Agarwal et al. 1989, Bird et al. 1988, French 1989, Goedde et al. 1989, Hall 1985a, Israel et al. 1981, Lieber 1977a, b, 1984, 1988a, b, 1991a, b, c, 1992, Lieber et al. 1992, Mezey 1989, 1991, Salaspuro 1989, 1991, Seitz et al. 1985), as well as clinical aspects of ALD (Burnett et al. 1981, Diehl 1989, Fisher et al. 1977, Hall 1985a, Morgan 1981, 1991, Saunders 1989, Wallgren et al. 1970). On the basis of expanding information, many hypotheses regarding the pathogenesis of ALD have been presented, but so far none of these many theories has gained general acceptance or solid scientific basis.

Animal Models of Alcohol-Related Organ Damage

A lot of evidence supporting the direct hepatotoxicity of ethanol has been obtained from experiments done with animal models of alcohol-induced organ damage (Salaspuro et al. 1980, Israel et al. 1984, Lieber et al. 1986, 1991). One of the major advances has been the introduction of a technique of feeding alcohol to rats as a part of nutritionally adequate totally liquid diet (Lieber et al. 1965). However, even with the "liquid diet model", the rat will not consume more than 36% of total energy as alcohol. Consequently, liver lesions more advanced than fatty liver cannot be produced by the "Lieber-DeCarli diet" in rats.

More advanced ALD has been produced in baboons by applying a liquid-diet feeding technique to this animal (Lieber et al. 1974). The alcohol intake of baboons can be increased to 50% of total energy. Furthermore, the primates are phylogenetically close to man, and their lifespan is long enough for the development of cirrhosis to occur. In this animal model, the biochemical and morphological alterations in the liver (even liver cirrhosis) are comparable to those seen in man, despite the fact that a complete histological spectrum of alcoholic hepatitis as seen in man has not been produced in baboons (Popper et al. 1980). However, the opinions vary greatly with regard to the respective roles of alcohol and/or nutritional deficiencies as major pathogenetic factors behind the liver injury in this animal model. Nevertheless, the establishment of the animal models of ALD has had its greatest contribution in the improved understanding of the multifactorial biochemical alterations produced in the liver during chronic feeding of alcohol.

Role of the Liver in the Metabolism of Ethanol

The importance of the liver in the elimination of ethanol was established in several studies in the 1930s (Chapheau 1934, Fiessinger et al. 1936, Mirsky et al. 1939), and subsequently the incomplete hepatic oxidation of ethanol to acetate was also demonstrated (Lundsgaard 1938, Leloir et al. 1938). Though the liver plays a dominant role in the metabolism of ethanol, other tissues such as the kidney (Leloir et al. 1938), the stomach (Carter et al. 1971), the intestine (Lamboeuf et al. 1981), and bone marrow cells (Bond et al. 1983) have also been shown to oxidize ethanol to a small extent. More recently, diminished gastric alcohol dehydrogenase (ADH) activity in females has been related to higher susceptibility to ethanol (DiPadova et al. 1988), but the magnitude and importance of the gastric metabolism of ethanol is still largely unknown.

Pathways of Ethanol Oxidation

ADH-mediated oxidation of ethanol to acetaldehyde represents the main pathway for ethanol oxidation. During the past two decades, the multiple molecular forms and characteristics of ADH have been established (Agarwal et al. 1989, Yoshida et al. 1991). Various ADH isoforms appear in different frequencies in different racial populations, which explains, at least in part, individual variations in the rate of ethanol elimination (Martin et al. 1985, Bosron et al. 1988). These have been related to the production of acetaldehyde and to the extent of the first-pass elimination of ethanol (von Wartburg et al. 1984). A possible relationship between ADH genotype and the susceptibility to alcoholism or alcohol-related organ injury, however, remains to be established.

Pathways of Acetaldehyde Oxidation

Over 90% of the acetaldehyde formed from ethanol is rapidly oxidized in the liver to acetate by aldehyde dehydrogenase (ALDH). Two major ALDH isozymes exist in human beings (Goedde et al. 1989). Interestingly, the mitochondrial isozyme (ALDH1) has been found to be missing in about 50% of Oriental populations (Goedde et al. 1979, Agarwal et al. 1981). This loss of enzyme activity is due to a change of one amino acid in the enzyme molecule (Hsu et al. 1985, Yoshida et al. 1991). The deficiency of ALDH1 in Orientals results in marked elevations of blood acetaldehyde levels after alcohol ingestion (Mizoi et al. 1979). These individuals then develop facial flushing and tachycardia as a direct consequence of acetaldehyde-induced catecholamine release (Ijiri 1974, Inoue et al. 1980). Accordingly, homozygotic Japanese with the atypical ALDH1 allele are at a much lower risk of developing ALD than those with homozygotic

Caucasian ALDH1 (Shibuya et al. 1988).

Microsomal Ethanol-Oxidizing System

The existence of a distinct and adaptive microsomal ethanol-oxidizing system (MEOS) is, after two decades of lively debate, generally accepted (Lieber et al. 1968, 1970a, 1992, Lieber 1988b). Chronic alcohol exposure results in the induction of a unique cytochrome P450 that has been designated cytochrome P4502E1 or CYP2E1 (Ohnishi et al. 1977, Lieber et al. 1988, Nebert et al. 1987). In addition to its role in ethanol metabolism, MEOS may have signif-icant consequences for the pathogenesis of liver injury, either directly (through the production of active and potentially toxic acetaldehyde) or indirectly (through the microsomal activation of other xenobiotics).

Alterations in Metabolism of Ethanol and Acetaldehyde During Chronic Alcohol Consumption

Most studies show that chronic alcohol consumption enhances ethanol clearance, except in the presence of significant liver damage or severe food restriction. The biochemical background for the enhanced clearance is still the subject of debate and has variably been attributed to increased ADH activity (Hawkins et al. 1966), to increased mitochondrial reoxidation of NADH (Videla et al. 1970), to a hypermetabolic state in the liver (Israel et al. 1975), to increased MEOS (Lieber et al. 1970a, Alderman et al. 1989), and to catalase (Handler et al. 1987, 1988a, b). The theory on the hypermetabolic state of the liver produced by chronic alcohol consumption has been assumed to produce ALD via hypoxia-induced liver damage in the centrilobular area, and treatment by propylthiouracil has been suggested (Orrego et al. 1987).

Acetaldehyde is both pharmacologically and chemically a very potent and reactive compound, and accordingly it has been suggested as one of the major initiating factors in the pathogenesis of ALD (Salaspuro et al. 1985, Lieber 1988a, b, 1991b, Lauterburg et al. 1988). Enhanced hepatic oxidation of ethanol associated with chronic alcohol use may lead to both increased blood and tissue acetaldehyde concentrations (Lindros et al. 1980). This may be further potentiated by a reduction in the capacity of mitochondria to oxidize acetaldehyde, at least in rats (Hasumura et al. 1975). In addition, hepatic ALDH activity has been shown to be decreased in chronic alcoholics as compared to non-alcoholic controls (Nuutinen et al. 1983).

Pathogenesis of Alcoholic Liver Injury: Specific Associations

Animal Models of Alcohol-Related Organ Damage

As previously stated, one of the major advances in the research on the pathogenesis of ALD has been the introduction of a technique of feeding alcohol to rats as a part of a nutritionally adequate totally liquid diet (Lieber et al. 1965, 1967, Salaspuro and Lieber 1980, Israel et al. 1984, Lieber and DeCarli 1986, 1991). With the Lieber-DeCarli diet, which in addition to ethanol (36% of total energy) contains rather large amounts of fat (35–43% of total energy), it is possible to produce fatty liver in rats (Lieber et al. 1965). However, if the fat content of the alcohol-containing liquid diet is reduced from 32% to 25%, hepatic triglyceride accumulation significantly decreases (Lieber et al. 1970b). Accordingly, others have questioned the direct hepatotoxicity of alcohol in this animal model and have attributed the pathological liver changes to nutritional factors (such as dietary proportions of protein, fat, and carbohydrate or lipotropic deficiency) rather than to alcohol itself (Porta et al. 1965, 1967, Patek et al. 1976, Barak et al. 1988, Derr et al. 1990).

Severe and progressive steatosis with focal necrosis has been produced in rats by continuous intragastric infusion of alcohol and nutritionally defined low-fat liquid diet (Tsukamoto et al. 1986, French et al. 1986). Furthermore, this damage is potentiated with the development of early hepatic fibrosis by increasing the fat content of the diet to 25% of energy (Tsukamoto et al. 1986). In this animal model, the severity of alcohol-induced liver injury appeared to be related to a high blood alcohol concentration (BAC). Feeding an alcohol-containing liquid diet together with a small dose of 4-methylpyrazole (ADH inhibitor) to rats potentiates alcoholic liver injury in this animal model (Lindros et al. 1983). By following BACs, this effect could be related to the uninterrupted and prolonged presence of alcohol in the animal. Alcohol feeding to rats subjected to a jejunoileal bypass leads to marked liver injury, which mimics that of ALD in man but without zonal distribution (Bode et al.

1987).

With regard to rats as an animal model of alcoholic liver injury, two major conclusions can be drawn: (1) the Lieber-DeCarli diet has been accepted as a standard in the studies on alcoholic fatty liver in rats, but the degree of hepatic fatty infiltration in this animal model may be modified by dietary factors such as the fat and lipotropic content of the diet; and (2) continuous intragastric infusion of alcohol and a nutritionally defined low-fat liquid diet to rats is a promising new experimental model of ALD. After confirmation in other labora-tories, the use of this animal model should be encouraged.

By feeding a totally liquid diet containing 50% of energy as alcohol, Lieber and co-workers have been able to produce significant hepatic fibrosis or cirrhosis in about one-third of baboons (Lieber et al. 1974, 1991). In this animal model, hepatitis is unusual and is not necessary for the development of fibrosis and cirrhosis (Popper et al. 1980). However, some other groups have not been able to produce significant hepatic fibrosis or cirrhosis in primates, giving large amounts of alcohol and adequate diet up to 5 years (Rogers et al. 1981, Mezey et al. 1980, 1983, Ainley et al. 1988). The discrepancies in these results have been attributed to the higher nutrient value of the diet in the latter studies (Ainley et al. 1988) or to the much smaller number of animals used by others as compared to Lieber's group (Lieber et al. 1991).

It can be concluded that a consensus does not exist with respect to the major pathogenetic factor (direct effect of alcohol or nutritional deficiency) behind the fibrosis and cirrhosis produced in baboons by the Lieber-DeCarli diet. Further studies on the topic are warranted.

Hepatotoxic Factors Associated With Ethanol and its Oxidation

TOXICITY OF ETHANOL TO LIVER MEMBRANES

Hepatocytes isolated from alcohol-fed animals exhibit pronounced morphological alterations of their plasma membranes on scanning electron microscopy (Yamada et al. 1985). Ethanol directly "fluidizes" membrane lipid bilayers, and it has been proposed that during chronic alcohol exposure, cell surface membranes may resist this effect of ethanol (i.e. "adapt") by changing their membrane lipid composition. Chronic alcohol feeding, however, has been shown to increase – even when ethanol is not present – the fluidity of liver plasma membranes of rats (Yamada et al.

1985) and mice (Zysset et al. 1985) and in cell cultures (Polokoff et al. 1985). The membrane alterations are associ-ated with a decrease in membrane vitamin A and an increase in the cholesteryl ester content (Kim et al. 1988).

Changes in the enzyme activities of liver plasma membrane include a decrease in cytochrome a and b, succinic dehydrogenase, cytochrome oxidase, as well as in the total respiratory capacity of the mitochondria (Taraschi et al. 1985). Furthermore, chronic alcohol use potentiates the release of alkaline phosphatase from the liver plasma membranes (Yamada et al. 1985) and produces changes in the oligosaccharide chains of plasma membrane glycoproteins (Metcalf et al. 1987).

In conclusion, ethanol may have direct effects on liver plasma membranes. However, the exact biochemical mechanisms behind the phenomenon are unknown, and the possible associations with the pathogenesis of ALD are still hypothetical.

ALCOHOLIC FATTY LIVER

Interactions of ethanol with lipids are multiple and complex (Lieber et al. 1984, Lieber and Pignon 1989). Fatty liver can be produced by either acute or chronic administration of alcohol both in laboratory animals and man and is potentiated by increased fat content of the diet (Lieber et al. 1970b, French et al. 1986).

Lipids accumulating in the liver may originate from dietary lipids or adipose tissue. Alcohol may increase peripheral fat mobilization, enhance hepatic triglyceride synthesis, decrease lipid oxidation in the liver and increase hepatic lipoprotein release (Lieber et al. 1992). In each case the prevailing major mechanism is dependent on the experimental conditions.

The ethanol-induced increase in the NADH/NAD ratio (redox state) is a sign of a major change in hepatic metabolism during ethanol oxidation. Many of the acute changes in the intermediary metabolism of the liver can be explained by the action of ethanol on the hepatic redox state. These include the inhibition of tricarboxylic acid cycle (Forsander et al. 1985) and gluconeogenesis. The redox-related inhibition of fatty acid oxidation (Lieber et al. 1961, 1967) and the enhancement of triglyceride synthesis (Nikkilä et al. 1963) are important mechanisms in the development of alcoholic fatty liver. A major site of inhibition by this mechanism is 2-oxoglutarate dehydrogenase (Ontko 1973). After chronic ethanol use, the acute inhibition of fatty-acid oxidation is attenuated (Salaspuro et al. 1981), resulting in a levelling off in the accumulation of hepatic fat.

It can be concluded that consensus exists with respect to most of the pathogenetic mechanisms leading to alcoholic fatty liver. However, some conflicting results still exist, which are most probably due to different experimental conditions.

THE ROLE OF GASTRIC ADH IN THE HEPATOTOXICITY OF ETHANOL

ADH is present in the mucosa of the stomach, and it has been suggested to be responsible for the gastric oxidation of ethanol (Hempel et al. 1979, 1984, Lambouef et al. 1981, 1983, Pestalozzi et al. 1983). However, the magnitude of gastrointestinal ethanol metabolism was long assumed to be small or almost negligible (Lin et al. 1980, Wagner 1986). It has recently been suggested, however, that a significant fraction (up to 20%) of alcohol ingested by rats (in doses in keeping with usual "social drinking") does not enter the systemic circulation in the rat and is oxidized mainly in the stomach (Julkunen et al. 1985a, b, Caballeria et al. 1987, 1989b). This process was also shown to occur in man (DiPadova et al. 1987, 1988) and has been suggested to partly determine the bioavailability of alcohol and thus to modulate its potential hepatotoxicity.

This gastric barrier may be low in women (DiPadova et al. 1988, Frezza et al. 1990) and may thus contribute to their increased susceptibility to alcohol. Commonly used H2 antagonists such as cimetidine decrease the activity of gastric ADH (Caballeria et al. 1989a, Hernandez-Munoz et al. 1990) and may thereby enhance peripheral blood alcohol levels. The existence of first-pass gastric metabolism of alcohol in the rat, however, has again been recently questioned (Smith et al. 1992). Moreover, the studies in man should be repeated, since it has been demonstrated that *Helicobacter pylori* also contains significant amounts of ADH (Roine et al. 1992a, b), which may obviously interfere with gastric alcohol metabolism in individuals carrying the bacteria (Salmela et al. 1993). The finding of "gastric" first-pass metabolism of ethanol is most interesting, but conflicting results and some new findings warrant further studies on the topic.

HEPATOTOXICITY OF ACETALDEHYDE

Acetaldehyde is both pharmacologically and chemically a very potent and reactive compound and has accordingly been suggested to be a major initiating factor in the pathogenesis of ALD (Salaspuro et al. 1985, Lieber

1988a, 1991a, Sorrell et al. 1985, Lauterberg et al. 1988).

COVALENT BINDING OF ACETALDEHYDE AND ACETALDEHYDE ADDUCTS

In vitro, acetaldehyde has been shown to form adducts with phospholipids (Kenney 1982). However, the most probable target macromolecules are proteins (Gaines et al. 1977), including liver proteins such as hepatic microsomal proteins (Nomura et al. 1981), other hepatic proteins (Medina et al. 1985), and liver tubulin (Jennett et al. 1989, Tuma et al. 1991). Evidence for the formation of acetaldehyde adducts with liver proteins, also *in vivo*, has been recently presented (Barry et al. 1985, Lin et al. 1988). The target molecule for acetaldehyde binding can, for instance, be the microsomal ethanol-inducible CYP2E1 (Behrens et al. 1988).

Acetaldehyde adducts may serve as antigens and generate an immune response in the centrilobular region of the liver of individuals consuming excessive amounts of alcohol (Niemelä et al. 1990). In addition, acetaldehyde adducts may (1) inhibit hepatic protein secretion produced by both acute and chronic ethanol administration (Matsuda et al. 1979, 1985, Valentine et al. 1987), (2) displace pyridoxal phosphate from its binding sites on proteins (Lumeng 1978), (3) impair biological functions of proteins (Mauch et al. 1984), or (4) combine with tissue macromolecules and thereby cause severe tissue injury, as in the case of acetaminophen.

Acetaldehyde has been related to hepatotoxicity of ethanol in many ways. After the establishment of reliable analytical methods for the determination of blood and tissue acetaldehyde levels, consensus exists in most of the biochemical changes and associations observed to date. However, the true pathogenetic role of acetaldehyde in the development of ALD still remains hypothetical.

HEPATOTOXICITY ASSOCIATED WITH MEOS

Theoretically, MEOS may cause enhanced hepatotoxicity by several means. MEOS contributes to the production of the potentially hepatotoxic agent acetaldehyde. MEOS may enhance oxygen consumption and provide so-called "empty calories" (Lieber 1991b) which may, at least in part, potentiate hypoxia. Both of these factors may be more crucial in the centrilobular (perivenous) areas of the hepatic acinus, since the ethanol-inducible microsomal CYP2E1 is predominantly localized to the perivenous region of the liver (Tsutsumi et al. 1989). MEOS may activate hepatotoxic agents such as carbon tetrachloride (Hasumura et al. 1974) or acetaminophen (Teschke et al. 1979). In accordance with this hypothesis, the history of alcohol consumption in human individuals has been shown to increase the hepatotoxicity of acetaminophen (Seeff et al. 1986).

Both in experimental animals and in man, chronic alcohol use has been shown to be associated with vitamin A depletion (Sato et al. 1981, Leo et al. 1982). This is caused by the induction of a new pathway of microsomal retinol oxidation that is inducible by ethanol and that may degrade an amount of retinol comparable to the daily intake (Leo et al. 1985). Decreased hepatic vitamin A levels may lead to some functional and structural abnormalities in the liver (Leo et al. 1983, Ray et al. 1988). However, the possible therapeutic use of vitamin A in ALD may be complicated by its own potential hepatotoxicity (Leo et al. 1982, 1983).

Although the existence of MEOS is generally accepted, its role in the pathogenesis of ALD is still open for further studies.

PROMOTION OF LIPID PEROXIDATION

Enhanced lipid peroxidation as a mechanism of ALD was proposed in 1966 by Kalish et al.. Free radicals (superoxide and hydroxyl radicals) may damage a wide range of cellular components via lipid peroxidation, including proteins, nucleic acids, free amino acids and lipoproteins (Cross et al. 1987, Cederbaum 1987).

In addition to the cytochrome P450 pathway, microsomes may oxidize ethanol by a separate pathway involving formation of hydroxyl radicals (Cederbaum 1987). Reactive oxygen intermediates are also produced when acetaldehyde is oxidized to acetate via xanthine oxidase (Lewis et al. 1982). Free radicals are scavenged by superoxide dismutase and glutathione peroxidase. On the other hand, binding of acetaldehyde with cysteine or glutathione (GSH) may contribute to the depression of liver GSH (Shaw et al. 1981, 1983). Chronic alcohol feeding increases GSH turnover and the cellular requirements for GSH (Morton et al. 1985). Furthermore, there is an increased loss of GSH from cells (Callans et al. 1987), especially from mitochondria (Fernandez-Checa et al. 1987). Evidence of GSH depletion and lipid peroxidation has also been found in human liver biopsies (Shaw et al. 1983).

In naive rats large amounts of ethanol (5–6 g/kg) are required to produce lipid peroxidation (Di Luzio et al. 1967). After chronic alcohol consumption, however, even smaller doses of alcohol administered acutely produce lipid peroxidation, which can be partly prevented by the GSH precursor methionine (Shaw et al. 1981). Ethanol-induced microsomal induction and iron mobilization have been suggested as potentiating factors in lipid peroxidation reactions in rats (Shaw et al. 1988).

In chronic alcoholics there is an increase in both serum and liver lipoperoxide levels (Suematsu et al. 1981). The content of hepatic reduced GSH is decreased, especially in patients with histological liver necrosis (Videla et al. 1984). As an integral part of the enzyme GSH peroxidase, selenium has a central role in the protection against the tissue damage caused by lipid peroxides. In this respect the decrease of selenium (not only in blood but also in liver) in patients with ALD may also play a significant role (Välimäki et al. 1987). Low vitamin E intake may also potentiate hepatic lipid peroxidation (Kawase et al. 1989).

There is consensus that lipid peroxidation is associated with the experimental models of ALD. Furthermore, there is some evidence supporting the existence of this damaging mechanism in man.

PERIVENULAR HYPOXIC INJURY

A characteristic feature of liver injury in alcoholics is the predominance of steatosis and other lesions in the perivenular (also called centrilobular) zone, i.e. zone 3 of the hepatic acinus. It has been postulated that the increased uptake of oxygen increases the gradient of oxygen tensions along the sinusoids to the extent of producing anoxic injury of perivenular hepatocytes (Israel et al. 1975, French et al. 1984). These findings have led to the theory of alcohol-induced liver necrosis secondary to a "hypermetabolic" state of the liver and consequently to therapeutic trials with propylthiouracil (Orrego et al. 1987, Orrego et al. 1989).

Slight decreases in hepatic venous oxygen saturation and PO_2 have been reported both in experimental animals and in human alcoholics (Kessler et al. 1954, Jauhonen et al. 1982, Sato et al. 1983). However, results in baboons suggest that increased hepatic oxygen consumption is offset by increased blood flow, resulting in unchanged hepatic venous oxygen tension (Jauhonen et al. 1982). In baboons, defective O_2 utilization rather than lack of O_2 blood supply characterizes liver injury produced by high alcohol concentrations (Lieber et al. 1989).

An alternative hypothesis to explain the selective perivenular hepatotoxicity of ethanol postulates that the low oxygen tensions normally prevailing in perivenular zones could exaggerate the redox shift produced by ethanol (Jauhonen et al. 1982, 1985).

Perivenular fibrosis has been suggested to be an early warning sign and a predictor of the development of more advanced liver fibrosis and cirrhosis, both in baboons and in man (Van Waes et al. 1977, Nasralah et al. 1980, Worner et al. 1985). No consensus exists regarding the mechanism and pathogenetic relevance of decreased oxygen tension in the perivenular area of the hepatic acinus. Consequently, confirming clinical studies with propylthiouracil in the treatment of ALD are still needed before it can be recommended for general use. Further studies are also needed to establish the true clinical significance of perivenular fibrosis.

NUTRITIONAL FACTORS

Excess weight has been shown to be a risk factor or a predictive sign of histological liver damage in alcoholics (Iturriaga et al. 1988). In epidemiological studies of populations at the aggregate level, the amount of pork consumed appears to correlate with mortality from cirrhosis (Nanji et al. 1985). Further evaluation has suggested that both saturated fat and cholesterol may protect against alcoholic cirrhosis, while polyunsaturated fat may promote it (Nanji et al. 1986b). In accordance with these findings, a high-fat diet has been shown to potentiate, and beef fat to prevent, alcohol-induced hepatic fibrosis and ALD in rats (French et al. 1986, Nanji et al. 1989, Takahashi et al. 1991).

Deficiencies in lipotropic factors (choline and methionine) may produce fatty liver and cirrhosis in growing rats (Daft et al. 1941, Best et al. 1949). In later studies, hepatic injury induced by choline deficiency was suggested to be primarily an experimental disease of rats with little if any relevance to ALD, particularly in mans (Lieber 1982). More recently, rats have been shown to be more resistant to choline deficiency than man, since human beings have a reduced ability to produce betaine (the main donator of methyl groups) from choline (Barak et al. 1985). Furthermore, choline has been suggested to be an essential nutrient for man when excess methionine and folate are not available in the diet (Zeisel et al. 1991). Therefore betaine, the first metabolite of choline, has been suggested for the treatment of ALD in man (Barak et al. 1988).

With respect to the protection of ALD in subhuman primates by choline, the results are controversial as stated previously (Lieber et al. 1974, 1991, Popper et al. 1980, Rogers et al. 1981, Mezey et al. 1983, Ainley et al. 1988). The discrepancy in the results has also been related to the differences in the choline content of the diets. Accordingly, it has been suggested that chronic alcohol feeding may exaggerate choline requirements of monkeys (Mezey et al. 1983, Ainley et al. 1988). However, additional choline failed to prevent the development of fibrosis in baboons (Lieber et al. 1985). On the other hand, S-adenosyl-L-methionine (Lieber et al. 1990) and polyunsaturated lecithin (Lieber et al. 1990) have recently been shown to attenuate alcohol-induced hepatic injury in baboons. Because of the high phosphatidylcholine content of polyunsaturated lecithin, the prepara-tion contained additional choline (400 mg/l), which is about four times more than the original "Lieber-DeCarli" diet.

From these studies it can be concluded that there is no consensus with regard to the role of choline in the prevention of ALD, either in experimental animals or in man. Accordingly, further controlled studies both in baboons, and perhaps also in man, are needed in order to establish the possible therapeutic value of choline, S-adenosyl-L-methionine, betaine and polyunsaturated lecithin in the prevention of ALD.

It has been claimed that ALD is frequently recognized among well-nourished alcoholics manifesting no nutritional deficiency. On the other hand, cirrhotic alcoholics have been reported to have a significantly lower total food energy intake, and a significantly lower daily protein intake, than non-cirrhotic chronic alcoholics (Patek et al. 1975). Using established criteria to diagnose and classify protein-energy malnutrition, all 248 patients with ALD were shown to have some evidence of malnutrition (Mendenhall et al. 1984, Mendenhall 1985). The prevalence of the malnutrition correlated closely with the severity of the liver disease, with a prevalence of 72% of both kwashiorkor and marasmus in severe disease. It should be noted, however, that in neither study was the cause-effect relationship between malnutrition and liver disease established; malnutrition, at least in part, might have been secondary to the liver injury and not its cause.

Data on the nutritional status of heavy drinkers is also controversial. Only subtle nutritional alterations have been document-ed in several studies (Neville et al. 1986, Hurt et al. 1981, Goldschmith et al. 1983, Rissanen et al. 1987). Nevertheless, these drinkers also frequently develop laboratory signs of ALD (Rissanen et al. 1987). In some other studies, significantly reduced protein, fat and cholesterol intake has been documented in heavy drinkers (Jones et al. 1982, Hillers et al. 1985), and there is some epidemiological evidence pointing to the possible protective effect of a high-protein diet on alcohol-induced cirrhosis (Raymond et al. 1985).

It can be concluded that no firm consensus exists with regard to the occurrence of protein-energy malnutrition among chronic alcoholics. In order to resolve this question, properly controlled prospective studies using modern nutritional techniques are needed.

Clinical Manifestations and Pathology of Alcoholic Liver Disease

Chronic alcoholics may present a wide spectrum of hepatic lesions, the most frequent being fatty liver, alcoholic hepatitis and hepatic cirrhosis (Baptista et al. 1981, Hall 1985b, McSween et al. 1986, Ishak et al. 1991). Other lesions more recently described, such as chronic hepatitis and fibrosis (Van Waes et al. 1977, Nasralah et al. 1980), are less frequent. These hepatic lesions may be found isolated or in combination, and the clinical manifestations are very variable, ranging from asymptomatic forms to severe hepatic failure. Therefore, to establish the exact diagnosis of hepatic diseases induced by chronic alcohol consumption, liver biopsy is required (Bruguera et al. 1977a).

Alcoholic Fatty Liver

The deposition of fat in the cytoplasm of hepatocytes is common among chronic alcoholics (Edmondson et al. 1967, Christoffersen et al. 1971). This lesion may be seen isolated or in combination with more severe hepatic lesions (alcoholic hepatitis) (Morgan et al. 1978), particularly in patients with recent and high alcohol intake. The prevalence of fatty liver in alcoholic patients is about 90% of the cases (Edmondson et al. 1967).

The deposition of a single large lipid droplet in hepatocytes is the histological lesion defining alcoholic fatty liver. This lipid droplet may occupy all the hepatic cytoplasm, and the nucleous is displaced (macrovesicular steatosis) (Christoffersen et al. 1971). Occasionally, as a consequence of cellular damage secondary to cell distension induced by intracellular lipid deposition or to cell membrane alteration, an inflammatory response may occur with the presence of lymphocytes and macrophages, resulting in the development of lipogranulomas (Christoffersen et al. 1971). The degree of hepatic steatosis varies from patient to patient. In the moderate forms it is frequently localized to the perivenular areas, while in the massive forms lipid deposition occupies the entire hepatic acinus.

A microvesicular form of fatty liver has been described (Uchida et al. 1983). This lesion is characterized by the presence of multiple small droplets of fat in the hepatocellular cytoplasm. In these cases the nuclei of hepatic cells are not displaced. Microvesicular steatosis is usually present in the perivenular areas. The frequency of this lesion is very low and may be associated with other alcoholic liver lesions, such as alcoholic hepatitis, cholestasis or fibrosis (Montull et al. 1989).

Fatty liver is usually asymptomatic, and in most cases the only sign is the presence of smooth, regular and minimally tender hepato-megaly (Leevy et al. 1968). The biochemical tests are usually normal, and an overt increase of γ-glutamyltransferase (GGT), a slight increase in serum aspartate (ASAT) and alanine (ALAT) transaminase (amino-transferase) activity is observed (Morgan 1991). In those patients in whom steatosis is associated with other hepatic lesions, the sympto-matology observed is due to these latter lesions and not to fatty liver.

Massive hepatic steatosis is less common, and clinical manifestations are more evident. The development of severe hepatic failure with encephalopathy and marked decrease of prothrombin time has been described (Morgan et al. 1978). In these patients cholestasis may develop.

Microvesicular steatosis usually presents with fatigue, anorexia, nausea, vomiting, and occasionally abdominal pain. Hepatomegaly is very frequent. There is a marked increase in plasma cholesterol and triglycerides, and in about half of the patients a decrease in prothrombin time and conjugated hyperbilirubinaemia is observed (Montull et al. 1989).

Hepatic Fibrosis

Chronic alcoholics may exhibit an increase in collagen content in the space of Disse (perisinusoidal space) around the hepatocytes (pericellular fibrosis), particularly in the perivenular area (perivenular fibrosis) (Edmondson et al. 1963, Nakano et al. 1982). This lesion may be observed isolated or in combination with fatty liver (fibrosteatosis) and alcoholic hepatitis (Van Waes et al. 1977). However, it has been found that chronic alcoholics may develop hepatic fibrosis without other associated hepatic lesions. This finding is a consequence of an increase in hepatic fibrogenetic activity. The prevalence of hepatic fibrosis is not known and probably varies from country to country; in Japan it is the most frequent lesion induced by chronic alcohol use (Takada et al. 1982).

Most patients are asymptomatic. Some may present hepatomegaly, with moderate abdominal pain and jaundice. These patients usually show a slight increase of ALAT, ASAT and GGT.

There is no consensus in considering alcoholic fibrosis as a new form of ALD independent of steatosis, alcoholic hepatitis and cirrhosis. Further, the prognostic value of the different forms of alcoholic fibrosis must be further clarified (Nasralah et al. 1980, Worner et al. 1985, Parés et al. 1987).

Alcoholic Hepatitis

Alcoholic hepatitis is the most characteristic hepatic lesion found in chronic alcoholism, particularly in heavy drinkers. It is estimated that the prevalence of alcoholic hepatitis is about 40% of chronic alcoholics, although this figure may also vary from country to country (Hislop et al. 1983).

Histologically, the lesion is characterized by the presence of areas of hepatocellular necrosis associated with an inflammatory cell infiltrate constituted by neutrophil polymorphs (Baptista et al. 1981, McSween et al. 1986). The lesion is generally located in the peri-venular areas. In the necrotic areas hepatocytes are large and ballooned with a clear cytoplasm. Within the hepatocytes homogeneous eosinophilic, perinuclear inclusion bodies with irregular appearance may be seen. This lesion constitutes the Mallory bodies or alcoholic hyaline. Ultrastructurally, the Mallory bodies are made up of clusters of proteinic fibrils with a special chemotactism for neutrophils (French 1981). This explains why neutrophils usually surround the Mallory bodies. Alcoholic hepatitis is usually associated with fatty liver and portal and pericellular fibrosis. Other lesions observed are giant mito-chondria, acidophil bodies and perivenular fibrosis (Bruguera et al. 1977a). This latter lesion may produce portal hypertension without the presence of cirrhosis. Perivenular fibrosis may be an important precursor of development of cirrhosis, although more studies are needed (Worner et al. 1985).

The clinical picture of alcoholic hepatitis is variable (Parés et al. 1978, Maddrey 1988). Alcoholic hepatitis usually develops when chronic alcoholics increase their alcohol intake. The most common clinical picture of this lesion initiates with fatigue, anorexia, nausea and vomiting. A few days later, abdominal pain localized to the upper right abdominal quadrant, jaundice and fever appear. Tender hepato-megaly and other signs of ALD (spider nevi, cutaneous telangiectasia, palmar erythema, parotid enlargement, gynaecomastia, testicular atrophy, peripheral neuropathy, Dupuytren's contracture) may be detected. Biochemical tests reveal a moderate increase in trans-aminases, usually less than 300 U/l. Among patients with alcoholic hepatitis ASAT is usually greater than ALAT, and the ASAT/ ALAT ratio is higher than 2 (Nanji et al. 1989). GGT is very high and may be associated with conjugated hyperbilirubinaemia and high alkaline phosphatase. Macrocytosis is frequent and is probably due to the toxic effect of alcohol on developing erythrocytes (Morgan et al. 1981). Thrombocytopenia, leukocytosis and neutrophilia are also frequent. Fever and leukocytosis could be secondary to hepatic necrosis and inflammation or bacterial infections (Parés et al. 1978). In a few cases the hepatic surface may be irregular, and a murmur may be detected. This is a consequence of intrahepatic arteriovenous anastomosis and an increase in hepatic arterial flow. These cases should be differentiated from hepatocellular carcinoma. A few patients may develop acute hepatic failure (Parés et al. 1978). Other patients may present clinical features similar to hepatic cirrhosis (ascites, gastrointestinal bleeding). To establish differential diagnosis in these patients, liver biopsy is required. Alcoholic hepatitis may also be asymptomatic, being detected by routine examination in chronic alcoholics (Bruguera et al. 1977b). Very few patients may develop acute hepatic failure with deep jaundice, encephalopathy, very low prothrombin time and progressive renal failure. The prognosis of these patients is very poor, and death occurs within a short period of time. Acute alcoholic hepatitis may be associated with massive fatty liver, haemolysis and hyperlipidaemia (hypertriglyceridaemia).

Chronic Alcoholic Hepatitis

It has been suggested that alcohol may produce chronic hepatitis (Goldberg et al. 1977, Crapper et al. 1983, Adelasco et al. 1987, Laskus et al. 1990, Corrao et al. 1991b). This suggestion was inspired by the fact that chronic hepatitis among alcoholics improves after the suppression of alcohol ingestion (Takase et al. 1991). Clinical manifestations in these patients are very slight, with a moderate increase in transaminase levels being observed. At present there is no clear evidence indicating that chronic hepatitis may be due to chronic alcoholism. It is possible that chronic hepatitis described in chronic alcoholic patients may be due to viral infection, particularly hepatitis C virus infection (Brillanti et al. 1989, Parés et al. 1990).

There is no consensus about the role of alcohol as an aetiological agent in chronic hepatitis. The normalization of transaminases and liver lesions after abstinence suggests that this role may be important in some cases of chronic hepatitis; in other cases the hepatitis C virus could be predominant. This point should be clarified in the future.

Hepatic Cirrhosis

The prevalence of hepatic cirrhosis in the chronic alcoholic population varies from study to study. Histologically, there are no differences between this and other types of cirrhosis. Alcoholics usually exhibit a micronodular type (McSween et al. 1986). Other alcoholic hepatic lesions, particularly fatty liver and alcoholic hepatitis, are frequently observed in alcoholic cirrhosis. Clinical manifestations of these patients are identical to those observed in other cirrhotic patients. Portal hypertension, ascites, gastro-intestinal bleed-ing by oesophageal varices and encephalopathy appear at the end stage of the disease. Symptoms and signs directly related to chronic alcoholism are also frequently observed.

Hepatocellular Carcinoma

It has been suggested that chronic alcohol consumption may lead to development of primary hepatocellular carcinoma (IARC 1988). It is also considered that hepatocellular carcinoma develops in about 15% of patients with alcoholic cirrhosis (Ishak et al. 1991). The role played by alcohol consumption in development of liver cancer seems complex: liver cirrhosis is definitely associated with increased risk of liver cancer; but when cirrhosis has developed, the role of alcohol in carcinogenesis is unclear (Colombo et al. 1992). It is also unknown whether cirrhosis caused by excessive alcohol use carries a greater risk of cancer development than cirrhosis caused by other factors (except for chronic hepatitis B infection, which results in a very high cancer risk). The high prevalence of antibodies against hepatitis C virus in alcoholic patients with liver cirrhosis and hepatocellular carcinoma (Bruix et al. 1989, Colombo et al. 1989, Chiaramonte et al. 1990, Kaklamani et al. 1991) suggests that this virus is responsible for the tumour. A large Italian case-control study showed no influence on development of hepatocellular carcinoma of alcohol abuse per se, either among cirrhotics or noncirrhotics (Pagliaro et al. 1983). Another prospective Italian study also did not support the hypothesis that the alcoholic aetiology is of particular importance for the development of carcinoma (Colombo et al. 1991). Some studies suggest that the macronodular cirrhosis that develops in abstaining alcoholics is particularly prone to carcinogenesis (Lee 1966). However, the role of alcohol, hepatitis virus or their association in the development of hepatocellular carcinoma in alcoholics needs further investigation.

Abstinence in the Treatment of Alcoholic Liver Disease

The main treatment for ALD is abstinence from alcohol. Abstinence will reverse, improve or delay the progression of ALD, depending on the stage of the lesion. Even when cirrhosis is established, prognosis is improved with alcohol abstinence (D'Amico et al. 1986, Saunders et al. 1981b, Morgan 1977, Ginés et al. 1987, Orrego et al. 1987, Tygstrup et al. 1971).

Epidemiological Aspects of Chronic Alcoholism and Liver Disease

There is no doubt that alcohol consumption in man is associated with a risk of liver disease with the characteristic features of the diagnostic categories of "alcoholic liver disease" (International Group 1981), which constitutes a significant public health problem (Grant et al. 1988). The incidence of the end-stage of alcoholic cirrhosis has recently been estimated at 190 per million person-years in Danish men and 85 in Danish women, with the age-specific incidence peaking at 50–60 years in both sexes (Almdal et al. 1991, Prytz et al. 1980). Comparable results have previously been obtained in the UK, the USA and Canada (Garagliano et al. 1979, Saunders et al. 1981b, Hunter et al. 1988). The overall 5-year survival upon diagnosis of cirrhosis is 50–35% but depends heavily on the degree of decompensation and continued drinking (Borowsky et al. 1981, Bouchier et al. 1992, Christensen et al. 1986, Orholm et al. 1985, Saunders et al. 1981b, Tygstrup et al. 1971).

Even among the heaviest drinkers, however, some remain free of liver disease throughout their life (Klatskin 1961, Lelbach 1975, 1976). This means that alcohol consumption is not a sufficient cause of ALD. Alcohol use is also not a necessary cause: the morphological features of "alcoholic liver disease" are found, albeit very rarely, without preceding excessive dirnking.

The Risk Function

The epidemiological analysis of the relationship between alcohol use and liver disease has three requirements: (1) measurement of alcohol use, (2) diagnosis of liver disease, and (3) estimation of their association implying estimation of the risk of liver disease upon alcohol consumption. Since the amount of alcohol consumed differs among individuals and within individuals over time, the measure of the association is the risk for different given amounts of alcohol consumed for different given periods of time. The risk of liver disease should be specified as the risk or probability of occurrence of the liver disease at issue per unit of time from a given point in time (Sorensen 1989). The combination of this measure of alcohol use with the risk estimate is the risk function.

There are two important reservations to be made when applying the concept of risk function to the relationship between alcohol use and liver disease. First, no data are, and will probably never become, available that allow a direct estimation of the values of the risk function as defined here. Second, even though data allowing proxy estimates of the risk function may be available from observations of populations of individuals with different drinking patterns, the question of whether a given individual, by deliberately changing drinking behaviour, changes the affiliated risk of liver disease concordantly will remain unanswered. The scientific evidence for this link would require unfeasible and unethical large-scale human experiments with increases and decreases in alcohol consumption and no changes in other conditions for prolonged periods of time. The closest approximation to such evidence would be the conduct of large-scale, population-based longitudinal studies with repeated assessment of alcohol intake and recording of ALD development. In this design, the actual changes in alcohol use that do occur may be related to the subsequent risk of liver disease.

The Time Relationship

Using various epidemiological methods, a number of studies have approached an indirect estimation of the risk function. These studies have revealed two sets of specific problems: (1) the time relationship between alcohol use and the development of liver disease, and (2) the effect of alcohol use at the various stages of development and manifestation of liver disease (Sorensen 1989). The questions about time relationship deal with the minimum period of time of alcohol use required for development of liver injury, the duration of its damaging effect, and the possible time lag and cumulative effect of consumed alcohol.

The shortest period of time of excessive alcohol consumption reported to have caused fatty liver is a few days (Rubin et al. 1968), and three months for development of alcoholic hepatitis and cirrhosis (Lischner et al. 1971). Cirrhosis has been seen developing during a 12-month period of abstinence following excessive alcohol consumption (Galambos 1987), and the tendency to progress despite abstinence seems to be particularly strong in women (Parés et al. 1986).

The average duration of excessive drinking until diagnosis of alcoholic cirrhosis is 10 to 20 years, and the prevalence of cirrhosis is greater the longer the duration of excessive drinking. This has been interpreted as a combination of a time lag and a cumulative effect. However, this interpretation is probably wrong (Sorensen 1989). First, the distribution among patients of the duration of excessive drinking before diagnosis of cirrhosis is flat rather than bell-shaped (Lischner et al. 1971), indicating that the average has no meaning in terms of a shared characteristic among the patients. Second, even if there were no cumulative effect at all, but only a constant, short-lasting effect, the prevalence of the irreversible cirrhosis steadily increases just by the passage of time. Third, a prospective study of alcoholics has shown that the future risk of development of cirrhosis is independent of the duration of excessive drinking before entry to the study (Sorensen et al. 1984). Finally, it seems unlikely that alcohol in some individuals has no short-term damaging effect, but only damaging effects that suddenly emerge many years later.

Stage of Alcoholic Liver Disease

At the time of first diagnosis, ALD manifests itself in a variety of morphological changes in the liver, ranging from slight steatosis through end-stage macronodular cirrhosis with liver cancer; and a broad spectrum of clinical manifestations, from asymptomatic conditions through severe liver failure and death (Alves et al. 1982, Bruguera et al. 1977b, Lelbach 1967, Lischner et al. 1971). It is assumed that the more severe stages of the disease are reached by progression through less severe forms (Galambos 1987, Junge et al. 1988, Lieber 1975, 1983, Maier et al. 1979, Parés et al. 1986, Sorensen et al. 1984). Most studies addressing the risk function have evaluated the development of cirrhosis, not necessarily applying to cirrhosis as such or clinical manifestations of cirrhosis. However, it is possible that the risk function is different for different stages and that the risk function for clinical manifestations at given stages of liver damage, including death, may be different from the risk function for developing these stages (Sorensen 1989). This means that a risk function estimated for the current and preceding stages, for example, the risk function for death from cirrhosis is a mixture of the risk function for cirrhosis and for death given that cirrhosis necessarily applies to cirrhosis as such. These problems have obvious consequences for recommendations about alcohol use, both at the public health level and in the clinical setting.

Studies of the Risk Function

The studies addressing the risk function may be subdivided into those conducted at population aggregates and those based on examina-tion of individual subjects.

AGGREGATE POPULATION STUDIES

A large number of studies have assessed the changes over time within populations and differences between populations in mortality or morbidity from cirrhosis, as assessed by national statistics, in relation to total per capita consumption of alcohol, usually determined from sales statistics or population surveys (Capocaccia et al. 1988, Colón 1981, Colón et al. 1982, Coppéré et al. 1986, Gallagher et al. 1980, Hunter et al. 1988, 1989, Israel et al. 1991, Joliffe et al. 1941, Klatskin 1961, McGlashan 1980, Norstrom 1987, Parrish et al. 1991, Prytz et al. 1988, Qiao et al. 1988, Romelsjo et al. 1985, Sales et al. 1989, Schmidt 1977, Smart 1988, Smart et al. 1987,

1991, Skinhoj et al. 1981, Skog 1985, Smith et al. 1985, Svendsen et al. 1977, La Vecchia et al. 1986, Williams et al. 1988, Wilson 1984). With few exceptions, these studies have shown very high correlations between mortality or morbidity from cirrhosis and alcohol consumption.

Departures from this close direct relation may be due to changes or differences (1) in sex and age composition of the populations (sex and age standardization may not always eliminate the problem); (2) in the procedures for recording death from cirrhosis, including distinction between alcoholic and non-alcoholic cirrhosis; (3) in unregistered alcohol use; (4) in the distribution of consumption among the members of the populations including treatment of alcoholism; (5) in exposure of the populations to co-factors for development of cirrhosis or progression of a fatal course; and (6) to a time lag from changes in consumption until changes in mortality (Duffy et al. 1986, Furst et al. 1981, Graudal et al. 1991, Haberman et al. 1990, Halliday et al. 1991, Hyman 1981, Kreitman et al. 1989, Lint 1981a, b, Mann et al. 1988, 1991, Maxwell 1985, Nanji et al. 1985, 1986a, Natta et al. 1985, Norstrom 1987, Parrish et al. 1991, Prytz et al. 1988, Qiao et al. 1988, Romelsjo et al. 1985, Skinhoj et al. 1981, Skog 1980, 1984, 1985, Smart et al. 1987, 1991, Williams et al. 1988, Wilson 1984).

Despite the strikingly high correlations, it is of note that the risk function for death from cirrhosis cannot be derived from such relationships. Thus, the mere existence of a risk function implying that there is no reduction in risk by increasing consumption by the individual will, regardless of the shape of the risk function, produce this kind of statistics at the aggregate level (Sorensen 1989).

SUBJECT POPULATION STUDIES

Proper interpretation of these studies requires a distinction between prospective studies and retrospective studies and, among the latter group, distinction between cross-sectional and case-control studies. In prospective studies, the assessment of alcohol use is carried out before development of liver disease in a study population, which then is followed with regard to development of liver disease. In retrospective studies, alcohol use is assessed at the same time the diagnosis of liver disease is made or later. The cross-sectional study assesses alcohol use in a study population that is selected regardless of the presence of liver disease and in which the assessment of the presence of liver disease takes place at the same time. In case-control studies, patients with liver disease are identified and their preceding alcohol consumption is compared with selected controls, usually matched to the cases by other characteristics possibly influencing alcohol use (e.g. sex and age).

Retrospective Case-Control Studies

A large number of case-control studies have been conducted (Batey et al. 1992, Bourliere et al. 1991, Coates et al. 1986, Corrao et al. 1991a, b, Durbec et al. 1979, Norton et al. 1987, Pagliaro et al. 1982, Pequignot 1961, 1978, Rotily et al. 1990, Tuyns et al. 1984). The controls have been either other hospitalized patients or various samples from the general population. The studies showed that the probability of becoming a hospitalized cirrhotic patient increased exponentially by increasing daily alcohol use throughout a range from about 20 g to 160 g. Some studies showed that women developing cirrhosis have drunk smaller daily alcohol doses and/or a shorter duration of excessive drinking than men developing cirrhosis. Interpretation of these studies in terms of risk function for development of cirrhosis is hampered for several reasons (Sorensen 1989). First, the risk function involves the risk of becoming hospitalized for symptomatic and even complicated cirrhosis and having this disease diagnosed (Corrao et al. 1991a). Second, the recorded intake may be a poor reflection of alcohol intake before cirrhosis developed (Corrao et al. 1991b). The daily intake may not be constant, and there may very well be a recall bias in the reporting of previous consumption. The potential bias is accentuated by the fact that the liver disease probably developed at some unknown time before diagnosis, or the relevant time period of consumption cannot be identified. Third, daily consumption usually increases by duration of excessive drinking, so that the greater probability of cirrhosis at high drinking levels is, at least to some extent, due to the trivial explanation that the subjects have been at risk for a longer time.

These difficulties may also blur the comparison of men and women (Batey et al. 1992, Bourliere et al. 1991, Norton et al. 1987, Pagliaro et al. 1982, Tuyns and Pequignot 1984). It should be noted that the frequently made comparison between male and female patients with ALD (Morgan et al. 1977, Saunders et al. 1981a, 1984) without including relevant male and female controls is not informative with regard to differences in the risk function (expressing different susceptibility) because of the great difference in distribution of alcohol consumption among men and women in the general population. If we assume that the risk function is the same for men and women, this difference in distribution would result in smaller and shorter excessive drinking by women than by men developing cirrhosis.

Retrospective Cross-Sectional Studies

Four such studies have been conducted in which the study population was defined as alcoholic, either identified in special clinics for alcoholics or in general hospitals (Eghöje et al. 1973, Lelbach 1967, 1975, 1976, Saunders et al. 1984, Wilkinson et al. 1969). In these populations, there was increasing prevalence of cirrhosis the longer the duration of excessive drinking, the greater the drinking level, and hence the greater the cumulated quantity of alcohol drunk. One of the studies defined a threshold for cumulated consumption below which there seemed to be no risk of cirrhosis (the theoretical amount of 15 g/day per kg body weight for 1 year, or 1 g for 15 years, in a man of 70 kg).

The reservation that must be made before interpreting these results in terms of the risk function for cirrhosis is the same as for the case-control study, except that the possible effect of alcohol on the manifestation of cirrhosis is less likely to confound the result (Sorensen 1989).

An important difference between case-control studies and cross-sectional studies conducted among alcoholics is that the former group can address the relationship between alcohol use and cirrhosis at lower daily drinking levels than seen among subjects identified as alcoholics.

Prospective Studies

Several studies of general populations or special subpopulations defined according to criteria not related to their alcohol use have assessed the relationship between daily drinking reported at the start of the study to subsequent cirrhosis mortality during long-term follow-up (Blackwelder et al. 1980, Farchi et al. 1992, Klatsky 1981, Kono et al. 1983, 1989). They found that the risk increased steadily by increasing drinking level up to 30 and 60 g more alcohol, respectively. A recent study of 129,000 subjects followed for up to 10 years with regard to mortality from cirrhosis showed that, compared to non-daily drinking, those drinking 1–2, 3–5 and 6 or more drinks per day had a RR of 3.5, 6.1, and 23.6, with no consistent differences between men and women (Klatsky et al. 1992).

In none of the studies was the absence of liver disease histo-logically verified at the start of the study, and the development of cirrhosis during follow-up was not recorded. The estimated risk function is thus a mixture of the risk function for development of cirrhosis and death from cirrhosis.

In one study (Sorensen et al. 1984), alcoholics reporting a minimum alcohol use of 50 g/day for at least 1 year had liver biopsy performed in addition to an inquiry about the duration and level of their previous alcohol use at the start of the observation. Development of cirrhosis which was followed over the subsequent 10–13 years occurred at a rate of about 2% per year, regardless of the level and duration of alcohol use before the start of the study. This finding indicates that there are no long-term cumulative effects of previous alcohol use.

This study also showed that those who were drinking intermittently at the start of the study later had a lower risk of liver damage than those drinking continuously. This is in accordance with an interpretation implying that the risk of damage exists when drinking, vanishes while drinking is interrupted, and emerges again when drinking is resumed. The evidence is rather weak, however, because intermittent and continuous drinkers may not be comparable in terms of other aspects of their drinking behaviour.

Another study (Marbet et al. 1987) among hospitalized alcoholics, which was prospective with regard to recent development of cirrhosis among patients shown to be non-cirrhotic at the start of the study but retrospective with regard to quantitative assessment of alcohol use (at follow-up), found no relationship between the amount of daily intake and the development of cirrhosis.

These two studies did not allow assessment of the relationship between alcohol use and the risk of cirrhosis on a short-term basis or at daily consumption below 50 g/day. None of the prospective studies addressed the risk of other types of ALD or the possible difference between men and women in risk of liver disease at a given drinking level.

List of Specific Associations Between Liver Disease and Consumption of Alcohol

Progress in Achievement of Scientific Consensus

EXISTING CURRENT CONSENSUS

There is a firm consensus about the association between excessive drinking and the development of the following conditions: fatty liver, hepatic centrilobular fibrosis, alcoholic hepatitis and liver cirrhosis.

SPECIFIC CONTENT OF THE CONSENSUS

Consensus about the qualitative association between excessive drinking and the development of fatty liver, hepatic centrilobular fibrosis, alcoholic hepatitis and liver cirrhosis implies that the likeli-hood that these conditions develop is much higher in individuals who, for a period of time, have drunk excessively than in individuals who have drunk little or no alcohol or have drunk excessively only for a short period of time. It is also implied that, for a given consumption over a given period of time, the likelihood is greatest for development of fatty liver and lower for the other conditions listed above. There is consensus about these associations being only one of likelihood, since some individuals may consume huge amounts of alcohol for decades without developing any of the conditions.

RESEARCH ALLOWING CONSENSUS

The consensus about the qualitative association between excessive drinking and the development of fatty liver, hepatic centrilobular fibrosis, alcoholic hepatitis or liver cirrhosis is based on vast clinical experience and numerous systematic studies showing either a higher frequency of these conditions among individuals who have drunk excessively than among other individuals, or a much higher frequency of excessive alcohol use among patients with these diseases than among individuals without the diseases.

In addition, the frequency of death attributed to liver disease in the general population is correlated over time and place with measurement of the total alcohol use by these populations.

These four types of liver damage may have distinct causes other than alcohol use. However, they exhibit a variety of histopathological features, of which sets can be defined that are very rarely seen in patients who have not drunk excessively.

Although the studies may have methodological problems of various sorts in the selection of the study populations, in the diagnosis of liver disease and in the assessment of alcohol use, none of these problems provides grounds for raising doubt about the qualitative association between the diseases and alcohol use.

Most of these studies are retrospective in design, in that the diagnosis of liver disease at one point in time has been related to reports on alcohol use during preceding periods of time. Since development of the conditions precedes the diagnosis by some unknown time interval, this kind of evidence leaves open the question about the time sequence of excessive drinking and development of the condition. The main argument supporting that the liver disease develops after excessive drinking is the observation that the specific histopathological changes, as mentioned, are very rarely seen without excessive alcohol use, and that symptoms and signs associated with the conditions appear some time after the patients have been engaged in excessive drinking.

Accepting that excessive drinking leads to an increased risk of liver damage, the association may be either a direct cause-effect relationship or an indirect apparent relationship resulting from confounding by another factor causing the liver damage and co-occurring with excessive drinking. Such a confounding effect, itself being of merely methodological and not genuine scientific interest, must be clearly distinguished from a possible mediation of the damaging effect of alcohol through some other consequences of the excessive drinking, or the possible requirement of other causal factors, acting together with alcohol in damaging the liver. Mediating or co-acting factors are of great scientific interest and could be, for example, specific nutritional disturbances.

No convincing confounding factors have yet been identified. As reflected in the synonym of alcoholic cirrhosis, nutritional cirrhosis, poor nutrition has been suspected of being involved. Severe malabsorption, probably mainly of protein, induced by intestinal bypass surgery for massive obesity may rarely result in liver damage of a similar type (Peters 1977). This is an extreme situation, and exposure to alcohol, perhaps of intestinal origin, has not been definitely excluded. There is no evidence indicating that poor nutrition by itself without alcohol use is associated with development of the type of liver damage seen after excessive drinking. Moreover, the association of alcohol and liver damage has been observed in many different populations varying in genetic background and life-style under such diverse conditions that it is extremely unlikely that confounding is responsible.

For fatty liver, observational studies have been supplemented by a few controlled human experimental studies that confirm the direct causal relationship with alcohol use (Rubin et al. 1968).

CONSENSUS ON DOSE-EFFECT RELATIONSHIPS

Whereas consensus about the qualitative association between excessive alcohol use and the development of fatty liver, hepatic centrilobular fibrosis, acute alcoholic hepatitis and liver cirrhosis is well established, there is much uncertainty about the more complex issue of a dose-effect relationship, including a possible threshold effect or safe limit (Anderson et al. 1984), and no clear operational conclusion can be drawn from the available evidence.

Missing Scientific Consensus and Need of Research

The lack of consensus on the quantitative association (i.e. dose-effect relationships) between excessive drinking and the development of fatty liver, hepatic centrilobular fibrosis, alcoholic hepatitis and liver cirrhosis is due to several substantial, both theoretical and practical, difficulties in the study of this matter.

To identify the problems, it is important to specify the question further in order to interpret the results of the available studies as answers to the question. Existence of a dose-effect relationship will imply that the current risk per unit of time of development of any of the conditions is dependent on current or preceding doses of alcohol consumed by the individual. Denoting this as the "risk function" we may proceed by asking about its position or shape in relation to particular measures of alcohol consumption.

Most studies have dealt with liver cirrhosis. The information on dose-effect relationship for the other three conditions is scarce. This is particularly regrettable in view of their role as possibly reversible precursor states of cirrhosis. A dose-effect relationship has been found in one study of fatty liver (Coates et al. 1986). Another case-control study of asymptomatic "chronic hepatitis" (Corrao et al. 1991b) showed a clear dose-effect relationship, the strength of which declined, however, with increasing duration of alcohol use and disappeared at durations exceeding 30 years, possibly suggesting a selection effect.

The measure of alcohol use involves the fundamental question about the possible effect on the current risk of liver damage caused by previous alcohol use. The studies relating reported previous alcohol use to the current diagnosis of liver damage indicate that the damage does not occur unless the individual has been consuming alcohol daily for at least a number of days, the minimum period reported for fatty liver being 10 days, and for alcohol hepatitis and cirrhosis about 3 months. This demonstrates that a "memory" spanning at least 3 months is implicit in the risk function, in that the risk may be related to the consumption up to 3 months back in time. In agreement with this interpretation, intermittent or binge drinking seems to be associated with a lower risk of liver damage than steady drinking (Brunt et al. 1974, Grant et al. 1988, Sorensen et al. 1984).

Whether alcohol consumption before this minimum period of time also influences the current risk of liver damage is still disputed. It is a common finding in retrospective studies that the longer the duration of excessive drinking, the greater is the proportion of individuals who suffer from liver damage. This has been taken as evidence of a cumulative effect of alcohol use. It does not necessarily imply, however, that current risk is greater in those who have drunk excess alcohol for a long time as compared to those who have drunk only during the minimum time required for the risk to be established (Sorensen 1989). The finding may be a simple consequence of studying individuals subject to a constant risk incurred by current or immediately preceding drinking for variable periods of time. Even if the risk is constant per unit of time, it is obvious that the longer the individuals are at this risk, the greater is the number that will suffer from liver damage. The resolution of the problem requires prospective studies, of which only one addressing this problem has so far been conducted (Sorensen et al. 1984). The results suggested that how long alcohol-abusing men had been drinking in the past had no influence on their future risk of developing alcoholic cirrhosis.

The next question is about the relationship between the shape of the risk function and the amount of alcohol drunk per day over the minimum period of time required for the risk to be manifest. Implicit in this question is the special question about whether a drinking threshold exists below which there is no risk of liver damage.

Several studies based on retrospective assessment of alcohol use at the time of diagnosis of liver damage, particularly liver cirrhosis, have addressed this question. Most of them found that the risk of liver damage increased by amount of alcohol consumed throughout the range reported. The daily amount below which no cirrhosis was found varied considerably between the studies and ranged from 20 to 160 g.

There are, as previously mentioned, several difficulties in interpreting these studies as answers to the question about the risk function, and about safe limits in particular. In principle, the prospective study design, including longitudinal monitoring, will take away these difficulties.

The fact that only a minor proportion of individuals consuming excessive amounts of alcohol do develop the most severe form of liver damage, cirrhosis in particular, indicates that differences exist in exposure to other causal factors, among which at least one must be time-dependent and thereby determines the occasion at which the damage begins. Despite years of research, no consensus has been reached on any one such factor (Bird et al. 1988, Brunt 1988, Galambos 1987, Grant et al. 1988, Johnson et al. 1985, Lieber 1991, Saunders 1984). Current research focuses on genetic factors (Devor et al. 1988, Hrubec et al. 1981), viral infections (Fong et al. 1988, Pagliaro et al. 1982, Parés et al. 1990, Saunders et al. 1983), and specific nutritional disturbances (Ainley et al. 1988, Derr et al. 1990, Nanji et al. 1985, 1986b, Qiao et al. 1988, Rao et al. 1986, 1989, Rotily et al. 1990).

The type of alcoholic beverage (beer, wine, spirits) consumed has, in several studies, been excluded as vehicle of such a co-factor (Tuyns and Pequignot 1984). One exception is that the proportion of females among cirrhotics is higher in beer-drinking countries than in spirit-and wine-drinking countries (Nanji et al. 1984).

To achieve progress in most of the areas lacking scientific consensus, we need substantial investment in prospective studies with proper assessment of alcohol use and liver pathology and, where appropriate, subsequent experimental intervention studies (Grant et al. 1988).

References

Adelasco L, Monarca A, Dantes M, et al. (1987) Features of chronic hepatitis in alcoholics. A survey in Milan. Liver 7: 283–89

Agarwal DP, Goedde HW (1989) Enzymology of alcohol degradation. In: Goedde HW, Agarwal DP (eds), Alcoholism: biomedical and genetic aspects. Pergamon Press, New York, pp. 3–20

Agarwal DP, Harada S, Goedde HW (1981) Racial differences in biological sensitivity to ethanol: the role of alcohol dehydrogenase and aldehyde dehydrogenase isoenzymes. Alcohol Clin Exp Res 5: 12–16

Ainley CC, Senapati A, Brown IMH, et al. (1988) Is alcohol hepatotoxic in the baboon? J Hepatol 7: 85–92

Alderman J, Kato S, Lieber CS (1989) The microsomal ethanol oxidizing system mediates metabolic tolerance to ethanol in deermice lacking alcohol dehydrogenase. Arch Biochem Biophys 271: 33–39

Almdal TP, Sorensen TIA (1991) Incidence of parenchymal liver disease in Denmark, 1981 to 1985: analysis of hospitalization registry data. Hepatology 13: 650–55

Alves PS, Correia JP, Borda d'Agua C, et al. (1982) Alcoholic liver diseases in Portugal. Clinical and laboratory picture, mortality and survival. Alcohol Clin Exp Res 6: 216–24

Anderson P, Cremona A, Wallace P (1984) What are safe levels of alcohol consumption? Br Med J 289: 1657–58

Baptista A, Bianchi L, De Groote J (1981) Alcoholic liver disease: Morphological manifestations. Review by an international group. Lancet i: 707–11

Barak AJ, Beckenhauer HC (1988) The influence of ethanol on hepatic transmethylation. Alcohol Alcoholism 23: 73–77

Barak AJ, Tuma DJ, Beckenhauer HC (1985) Ethanol, the choline requirement, methylation and liver injury. Life Sci 37: 789–91

Barry RE, McGivan JD (1985) Acetaldehyde alone may initiate hepatocellular damage in acute alcoholic liver disease. Gut 26: 1065–69

Batey RG, Burns T, Benson RJ, et al. (1992) Alcohol consumption and the risk of cirrhosis. Med J Aust 153: 413–16

Behrens UJ, Hoerner M, Lasker JM, et al. (1988) Formation of acetaldehyde adducts with ethanol-inducible P450IIE1 in vivo. Biochem Biophys Res Commun 154: 584–90

Best CH, Hartroft WS, Lucas SS, et al. (1949) Liver damage produced by feeding alcohol or sugar and its prevention by choline. Br Med J 2: 1001–06

Bird GLA, Williams R (1988) Factors determining cirrhosis in alcoholic liver disease. Mol Aspects Med 10: 97–105

Blackwelder WC, Yano K, Rhoads GG, et al. (1980) Alcohol and mortality: the Honolulu Heart Study. Am J Med 68: 164–69

Bode C, Gast J, Zelder O, et al. (1987) Alcohol-induced liver injury after jejunoileal bypass operation in rats. J Hepatol 5: 75–84

Bond AN, Wickramasinghe SN (1983) Investigations into the production of acetate from ethanol by human blood and bone marrow cells in vitro. Acta Haematol 69: 303–13

Borowsky SA, Strome S, Lott E (1981) Continued heavy drinking and survival in alcohol cirrhotics. Gastroenterology 80: 1405–09

Bosron WF, Lumeng L, Li T-K (1988) Genetic polymorphism and susceptibility to alcoholic liver disease. Mol Aspects Med 10: 147–58

Bouchier IAD, Hislop WS, Prescott RJ (1992) A prospective study of alcoholic liver disease and mortality. J Hepatol 16: 290–97

Bourliere M, Barthet H, Berthenzene P, et al. (1991) Is tobacco a risk factor for chronic pancreatitis and alcoholic cirrhosis? Gut 32: 1392–95

Brillanti S, Barbara L, Miglioli M, et al. (1989) Hepatitis C virus: a possible cause of chronic hepatitis in alcoholics. Lancet ii: 1390–91

Bruguera M, Bertrán A, Bombí JA, et al. (1977a) Giant mitochondria in hepatocytes. A diagnostic hint for alcoholic liver diseases. Gastro-enterology 73: 1383–87

Bruguera M, Bordas JM, Rodés J (1977b) Asymptomatic liver disease in alcoholics. Arch Pathol Lab Med 101: 644–47

Bruix J, Barrera JM, Calvet X, et al. (1989) Prevalence of antibodies to hepatitis C virus in Spanish patients with hepatocellular carcinoma and cirrhosis. Lancet ii: 1004–06

Brunt P (1988) The liver and alcohol. J Hepatol 7: 377–83

Brunt PW, Kew MC, Scheuer PJ, et al. (1974) Studies in alcoholic liver disease in Britain. Gut 15: 52–58

Burnett, DA, Sorrell, MF (1981) Alcoholic cirrhosis. Clin Gastroenterol 10: 443–55

Caballeria J, Baraona E, Lieber CS (1987) The contribution of the stomach to ethanol oxidation in the rat. Life Sci 41: 1021–27

Caballeria J, Baraona E, Rodmilans M, et al. (1989a) Effects of cimetidine on gastric alcohol dehydrogenase activity and blood ethanol levels. Gastroenterology 96: 388–92

Caballeria J, Frezza M, Hernandez-Munoz R, et al. (1989b) The gastric origin of the first pass metabolism of ethanol in man: effect of gastrectomy. Gastroenterology 97: 1205–09

Callans DJ, Wacker LS, Mitchell MC (1987) Effects of ethanol feeding and withdrawal on plasma glutathione elimination in the rat. Hepatology 7: 496–501

Capocaccia R, Farchi G (1988) Mortality from liver cirrhosis in Italy: proportion associated with consumption of alcohol. J Clin Epidemiol 41: 347–57

Carter EA, Isselbacher KJ (1971) The metabolism of ethanol to carbon dioxide by stomach and small intestinal slices. Proc Soc Exp Biol Med 138: 817–19

Cederbaum AI (1987) Microsomal generation of hydroxyl radicals: its role in microsomal ethanol oxidising system (MEOS) activity and requirement for iron. Ann NY Acad Sci 492: 35–49

Chapheau M (1934) Action de la phlorizine et de l'acide iodoacetique sur la combustion de l'alcool ethylique chez le lapin. C R Soc Biol 116: 887–89

Chiaramonte M, Farinati F, Fagiouli S, et al. (1990) Antibody to hepatitis C virus in hepatocellular carcinoma. Lancet i: 301–02

Christensen E, Schlichting P, Andersen PK, et al. (1986) Updating prognosis and therapeutic effect evaluation in cirrhosis with Cox's multiple regression model for time-dependent variables. Scand J Gastroenterol 21: 163–74

Christoffersen P, Braendstrup O, Juhl E (1971) Lipogranulomas in human liver biopsies with fatty liver. A morphological, biochemical and clinical investigation. Acta Pathol Microbiol Scand 79: 150–58

Coates RA, Halliday ML, Rankin JG, et al. (1986) Risk of fatty infiltration or cirrhosis of the liver in relation to ethanol consumption: a case-control study. Clin Invest Med 9: 26–32

Colombo M, Kwo G, Choo QL, et al. (1989) High prevalence of antibody to hepatitis C virus in patients with hepatocellular carcinoma. Lancet ii: 1006–08

Colombo M, Franchis Rd, Ninno ED, et al. (1991) Hepatocellular carcinoma in Italian patients with cirrhosis. New Engl J Med 325: 675–80

Colombo M (1992) Hepatocellular carcinoma. J Hepatol 15: 225–36

Colón I (1981) Alcohol availability and cirrhosis mortality rates by gender and race. Am J Public Health 71: 1325–28

Colón I, Citter HSG, Jones WC (1982) Prediction in alcoholism from available alcohol consumption and demographic data. J Stud Alcohol 43: 1199–1213

Coppéré H, Audigier JC (1986) Evolution de la mortalité par cirrhose en France entre 1925 et 1982. Gastroenterol Clin Biol 10: 468–74

Corrao G, Arico S, Carle F (1991a) A case-control study on alcohol consumption and the risk of chronic liver disease. Rev Epidemiol Santé Publique 39: 333–43

Corrao G, Arico S, Russo R (1991b) Alcohol consumption and non-cirrhotic chronic hepatitis: a case-control study. Int J Epidemiol 20: 1037–42

Crapper RM, Bhathaland PS, Mackay IR (1983) Chronic active hepatitis in alcoholic patients. Liver 3: 327–37

Cross CE, Halliwell B, Borish ET, et al. (1987) Oxygen radicals and human disease. Ann Int Med 107: 526–45

Daft FS, Sebrell WH, Lillie RD (1941) Production and apparent prevention of a dietary liver cirrhosis in rats. Proc Soc Exp Biol Med 48: 228–29

D'Amico G, Morabito VS, Pagliaro L, et al. (1986) Survival and prognostic indicators in compensated and decompensated cirrhosis. Dig Dis Sci 5: 468–75

Derr RF, Porta EA, Larkin CA, et al. (1990) Is ethanol per se hepatotoxic? J Hepatol 10: 381–86

Devor EJ, Reich T, Cloninger CR (1988) Genetics of alcoholism and related end-organ damage. Semin Liver Dis 8: 1–11

Diehl AM (1989) Alcoholic liver disease. Med Clin North Am 73: 815–30

DiLuzio NR, Hartman AD (1967) Role of lipid peroxidation on the pathogenesis of the ethanol-induced fatty liver. Fed Proc 26: 1436–42

DiPadova C, Worner TM, Julkunen RJK, Lieber CS (1987) Effects of fasting and chronic alcohol consumption on the first-pass metabolism of ethanol. Gastroenterology 92: 1169–73

DiPadova C, Frezza M, Lieber CS (1988) Gastric metabolism of ethanol; implications for its bioavailability in men and women. In: Kuriyama K, Takada A, Ishii H (eds), Biomedical and social aspects of alcohol and alcoholism. Elsevier, Barking, pp. 81–84

Duffy JC, Latcham RW (1986) Liver cirrhosis mortality in England and Wales compared to Scotland: an age-period-cohort analysis 1941–81. J R Stat Soc A 149: 45–49

Durbec JP, Bidart JM, Sarles H (1979) Etude des variations du risque de cirrhose du foie en function de la consommation d'alcool. Gastroenterol Clin Biol 3: 725–34

Edmondson HA, Peters RL, Reynolds TB (1963) Sclerosing hyaline necrosis of the liver in the chronic alcoholic. Ann Intern Med 59: 646–53

Edmondson HA, Peters RL, Frankel HH (1967) The early stage of liver injury in the alcoholic. Medicine 46: 119–20

Eghöje KN, Juhl E (1973) Factors determining liver damage in chronic alcoholics. Scand J Gastroenterol 8: 505–12

Farchi G, Fidanza F, Mariotti S, et al. (1992) Alcohol and mortality in the Italian rural cohorts of the Seven Countries Study. Int J Epidemiol 21: 74–82

Fernandez-Checa JC, Ookhtens M, Kaplowitz N (1987) Effect of chronic ethanol feeding on rat hepatocyte glutathione. Compartmentation, afflux and response to incubation with ethanol. J Clin Invest 80: 57–62

Fiessinger N, Bernard H, Courtial J, et al. (1936) Combustion de l'alcool éthylique au cours de la perfusion du foie. C R Soc Biol 122: 1255–58

Fisher MM, Rankin JG, eds (1977) Alcohol and the liver. Plenum Press, New York, vol 3

Fong TL, Govindarajan S, Valinluck B, et al. (1988) Status of hepatitis B virus DNA in alcoholic liver disease: a study of a large urban population in the United States. Hepatology 8: 1602–04

Forsander OA, Räihä N, Salaspuro M, et al. (1985) Influence of ethanol on the liver metabolism of fed and starved rats. Biochemical J 94: 259–65

French SW (1981) The Mallory body: structure composition and pathogenesis. Hepatology 1: 76–83

French SW (1989) Biochemical basis for alcohol-induced liver injury. Clin Biochem 22: 41–49

French SW, Benson NC, Sun PS (1984) Centrilobular liver necrosis induced by hypoxia in chronic ethanol-fed rats. Hepatology 4: 912–17

French SW, Miyamoto K, Tsukamoto H (1986) Ethanol-induced hepatic fibrosis in the rat: role of the amount of dietary fat. Alcohol Clin Exp Res 10: 13S–19S

Frezza M, DiPadova C, Pozzata G, et al. (1990) High blood alcohol levels in women: role of decreased gastric alcohol dehydrogenase activity and first pass metabolism. New Engl J Med 322: 95–99

Furst CJ, Beckman LJ (1981) Alcohol-related mortality and alcohol consumption statistics. Stability of estimates for small areas. J Stud Alcohol 42: 57–63

Gaines KC, Sakhany JM, Tuma DJ, et al. (1977) Reaction of acetaldehyde with human erythrocyte membrane proteins. FEBS Lett 74: 115–19

Galambos JT (1987) Natural history of cirrhosis due to alcohol. In: Tygstrup N, Orlandi F (eds), Cirrhosis of the liver: methods and fields of research. Elsevier, Amsterdam, pp. 307–22

Gallagher RP, Elwood JM (1980) Increase in alcohol related mortality in Canada, 1965–77 (letter). Lancet ii: 775–76

Garagliano CF, Lilienfeld AM, Mendeloff AI (1979) Incidence rates of liver cirrhosis and related diseases in Baltimore and selected areas of the United States. J Chron Dis 32: 543–53

Ginés P, Quintero E, Arroyo V, et al. (1987) Compensated cirrhosis: natural history and prognostic factors. Hepatology 7: 122–28

Goedde HW, Harada S, Agarwal DP (1979) Racial differences in alcohol sensitivity: a new hypothesis. Hum Genet 51: 331–34

Goedde HW, Agarwal DP (1989) Acetaldehyde metabolism: genetic variation and physiological implications. In: Goedde HW, Agarwal DP (eds.), Alcoholism: biomedical and genetic aspects. Pergamon Press, New York, pp. 21–56

Goldberg SJ, Mendenhall CL, Connell AM, et al. (1977) "Non-alcoholic" chronic hepatitis in the alcoholic. Gastroenterology 72: 598–604

Goldschmith RH, Iber FL, Miller BA (1983) Nutritional status of alcoholics of different socioeconomic class. J Am Coll Nutr 2: 215–20

Grant BF, Dufour MC, Harford TC (1988) Epidemiology of alcoholic liver disease. Semin Liver Dis 1: 12–25

Graudal N, Leth P, Marbjerg L, et al. (1991) Characteristics of cirrhosis undiagnosed during life: a comparative analysis of 73 undiagnosed cases and 149 diagnosed cases of cirrhosis, detected in 4929 consecutive autopsies. J Intern Med 230: 165–71

Haberman PW, Weinbaum DF (1990) Liver cirrhosis with and without mention of alcohol as cause of death. Br J Addict 85: 217–22

Hall P, ed. (1985a) Alcoholic Liver Disease. Edward Arnold, London

Hall PM (1985b) Pathological spectrum of alcoholic liver disease. Pathology 17: 209–18

Halliday ML, Coates RA, Rankin JG (1991) Changing trends of cirrhosis mortality in Ontario, Canada, 1911–1986. Int J Epidemiol 20: 199–208

Handler JA, Bradford BU, Glassman EB, et al. (1987) Inhibition of catalase-dependent ethanol metabolism in alcohol dehydrogenase-deficient deermice by fructose. Biochem J 248: 415–21

Handler JA, Forman DT, Glassman EB, et al. (1988a) Hepatic catalase-dependent ethanol oxidation. In: Kuriyama K, Takada A, Ishii H (eds), Biomedical and social aspects of alcohol and alcoholism. Elsevier/Excerpta Medica, Amsterdam/New York, pp. 71–75

Handler JA, Koop DR, Coon MJ, et al. (1988b) Identification of P-450ALC in microsomes from alcohol dehydrogenase-deficient deermice: contribution to ethanol elimination in vivo. Arch Biochem Biophys 264: 114–24

Hasumura Y, Teschke R, Lieber CS (1974) Increased carbon tetrachloride hepatotoxicity, and its mechanism, after chronic ethanol consumption. Gastroenterology 66: 415–22

Hasumura Y, Teschke R, Lieber CS (1975) Acetaldehyde oxidation by hepatic mitochondria. Decrease after chronic ethanol consumption. Science 189: 727–29

Hawkins RD, Kalant H, Khanna JM (1966) Effects of chronic intake of ethanol on rate of ethanol metabolism. Can J Physiol Pharmacol 44: 241–57

Hempel J, Bühler R, Kaiser R, et al. (1984) Human liver alcohol dehydrogenase. 1. The primary structure of the B1B1 isoenzyme. Eur J Biochem 145: 437–45

Hempel JD, Pietruszko R (1979) Human stomach alcohol dehydrogenase: isoenzyme composition and catalytic properties. Alcohol Clin Exp Res 3: 95–98

Hernandez-Munoz R, Caballeria J, Baraona E, et al. (1990) Human gastric alcohol dehydrogenase: its inhibition by H2-receptor antagonists, and its effect on the bioavailability of ethanol. Alcohol Clin Exp Res 14: 946–50

Hillers VN, Massey LK (1985) Interrelationships of moderate and high alcohol consumption with diet and health status. Am J Clin Nutr 41: 356–62

Hislop WS, Bouchier IA, Allan JG, et al. (1983) Alcoholic liver disease in Scotland and Northeastern England: presenting features in 510 patients. Q J Med 206: 232–43

Hodges JR, Millward GH, Wright R (1982) Chronic active hepatitis: the spectrum of disease. Lancet i: 550–55

Hrubec Z, Omenn GS (1981) Evidence of genetic predisposition to alcoholic cirrhosis and psychosis: twin concordances for alcoholism and its biological end points by zygosity among male veterans. Alcohol Clin Exp Res 5: 207–15

Hsu LC, Tani K, Fujiyoshi T, et al. (1985) Cloning of cDNAs for human aldehyde dehydrogenases 1 and 2. Proc Natl Acad Sci USA 82: 3771–75

Hunter DJW, Halliday ML, Coates RA, et al. (1988) Hospital morobidity from cirrhosis of the liver and per capita consumption of absolute alcohol in Ontario, 1978 to 1982: a descriptive analysis. Can J Public Health 79: 243–48

Hunter DJW, Halliday ML, Coates RA, et al. (1989) Mortality and hospital morbidity from cirrhosis of the liver in relation to per capita consumption of absolute alcohol, education and native status, Ontario; 1978 to 1982. Clin Invest Med 12: 230–34

Hurt RD, Higgins JA, Nelson RA, et al. (1981) Nutritional status of a group of alcoholics before and after admission to an alcoholism treatment unit. Am J Clin Nutr 34: 386–92

Hyman MM (1981) "Alcoholic", "unspecified" and "other specified" cirrhosis mortality: a study in validity. J Stud Alcohol 42: 336–43

Ijiri I (1974) Studies on the relationship between the concentrations of blood acetaldehyde and urinary catecholamine and the symptoms after drinking alcohol. Jpn J Stud Alcohol 9: 35–39

Inoue K, Fukunaga M, Yamasawa K (1980) Correlation between human erythrocyte aldehyde dehydrogenase activity and sensitivity to alcohol. Pharmacol Biochem Behav 13: 295–97

IARC (1988) Alcohol drinking. IARC Monograph on the Evaluation of Carcinogenic Risks in Humans vol 44. International Agency for Research on Cancer

International Group (1981) Alcoholic liver disease: morphological manifestations. Lancet ii: 707–11

Ishak KG, Zimmerman HJ, Ray MB (1991) Alcoholic liver disease: patho-logic, pathogenetic and clinical aspects. Alcohol Clin Exp Res 15: 45–66

Israel Y, Oporto B, Macdonald AD (1984) Simultaneous pair-feeding system for the administration of alcohol-containing liquid diets. Alcohol Clin Exp Res 8: 505–08

Israel Y, Orrego H (1981) Hepatocyte demand and substrate supply as factors in susceptibility to alcoholic liver injury. Clin Gastroenterol 10: 355–73

Israel Y, Orrego H, Schmidt W, et al. (1991) Trauma in cirrhosis: an indicator of the pattern of alcohol abuse in different societies. Alcohol Clin Exp Res 15: 433–37

Israel Y, Videla L, Bernstein J (1975) Liver hypermetabolic state after chronic ethanol consumption: hormonal interrelationships and patho-genic implications. Fed Proc 34: 2052–59

Iturriaga H, Bunout D, Hirsch S, et al. (1988) Overweight as a risk factor or a predictive sign of histologic liver damage in alcoholics. Am J Clin Nutr 47: 235–38

Jauhonen P, Baraona E, Miyakawa H, et al. (1982) Mechanism of selective perivenular hepatotoxicity of ethanol. Alcohol Clin Exp Res 6: 350–57

Jauhonen P, Baraona E, Lieber CS, et al. (1985) Dependence of ethanol-induced redox shift on hepatic oxygen tensions prevailing in vivo. Alcohol 2: 163–67

Jennett RB, Sorrell MF, Saffar-Fard A, et al. (1989) Preferential covalent binding of acetaldehyde to the alpha-chain of purified rat liver tubulin. Hepatology 1: 57–62

Johnson RD, Williams R (1985) Genetic and environmental factors in the individual susceptibility to the development of alcoholic liver disease. Alcohol Alcoholism 20: 137–60

Joliffe N, Jellinek EM (1941) Vitamin deficiencies and liver cirrhosis in alcoholics. Part VII. Cirrhosis of the liver. J Stud Alcohol 2: 544–83

Jones BR, Barrett-Connor E, Criqui MH, et al. (1982) A community study of calorie and nutrient intake in drinkers and nondrinkers of alcohol. Am J Clin Nutr 35: 135–39

Julkunen RJK, DiPadova C, Lieber CS (1985a) First pass metabolism of ethanol: a gastrointestinal barrier against the systemic toxicity of ethanol. Life Sci 37: 567–73

Julkunen RJK, Tannenbaum L, Baraona E, et al. (1985b) First pass metabolism of ethanol: an important determinant of blood levels after alcohol consumption. Alcohol 2: 437–41

Junge J, Bentsen KD, Christoffersen P, et al. (1988) Fibronectin as predictor of development of cirrhosis in alcohol abusing men. Br Med J 296: 1629–30

Kaklamani E, Thrichopoulus D, Tzonou A, et al. (1991) Hepatitis B and C viruses and their interaction in the origin of hepatocellular carcinoma. JAMA 256: 1974–76

Kalish GH, Di Luzio NR (1966) Peroxidation of liver lipids in the pathogenesis of the ethanol-induced fatty liver. Science 152: 1390–92

Kawase T, Kato S, Lieber CS (1989) Lipid peroxidation and antioxidant defence system in rat liver after chronic ethanol feeding. Hepatology 10: 815–21

Kenney WC (1982) Acetaldehyde adducts of phospholipids. Alcohol 6: 412–16

Kessler BJ, Liebler JB, Bronfin GJ, et al. (1954) The hepatic blood flow and splanchnic oxygen consumption in alcoholic fatty liver. J Clin Invest 33: 1338–45

Kim C-I, Leo MA, Lowe N, et al. (1988) Effects of vitamin A and ethanol on liver plasma membrane fluidity. Hepatology 4: 735–41

Klatskin G (1961) Alcohol and its relation to liver damage. Gastroenterology 41: 443–51

Klatsky AL, Friedman GD, Siegelaub AB (1981) Alcohol and mortality. A ten-year Kaiser-Permanente experience. Ann Intern Med 95: 139–45

Klatsky AL, Friedman GD, Siegelaub AB (1992) Alcohol and mortality. Ann Intern Med 117: 646–54

Kono S, Ikeda M, Ogata M, et al. (1989) The relationship between alcohol and mortality among Japanese physicians. Int J Epidemiol 12: 437–41

Kono S, Ikeda M, Tokudome S, et al. (1989) Alcohol and mortality: a cohort study of male Japanese physicians. Int J Epidemiol 15: 527–32

Kreitman N, Duffy J (1989) Alcoholic and non-alcoholic liver disease in relation to alcohol consumption in Scotland, 1978–84. Part I: epidemiology of liver diseases. Br J Addict 84: 607–18

Lamboeuf Y, de Saint Blanquat G, Derache R (1981) Mucosal alcohol dehydrogenase- and aldehyde dehydrogenase-mediated ethanol oxidation in the digestive tract of the rat. Biochem Pharmacol 30: 542–45

Lambouef Y, la Droitte P, De Saint DP (1983) The gastrointestinal metabolism of ethanol in the rat. Effect of chronic alcoholic intoxication. Arch Int Pharmacodynam Ther 261: 157–69

Laskus T, Slusarczyk J, Lupa E, et al. (1990) Liver disease among Polish alcoholics. Contribution of chronic active hepatitis to liver pathology. Liver 10: 221–28

Lauterburg BH, Bilzer M (1988) Mechanism of acetaldehyde hepatotoxicity. J Hepatol 7: 384–90

La Vecchia CL, DeCarli A, Mezzanotte G, et al. (1986) Mortality from alcohol related disease in Italy. J Epidemiol Commun Health 40: 257–61

Lee FI (1966) Cirrhosis and hepatoma in alcoholics. Gut 7: 77–85

Leevy CM (1968) Fatty liver: a study of 270 patients with biopsy proven fatty liver and a review of the literature. Medicine 41: 1445–51

Lelbach WK (1967) Leberschäden bei chronischem Alkoholismus. Teil III: Bioptisch-Histologische Ergebnisse. Teil IV: Diskussion und Schluss-folgerungen. Acta Hepatosplenol 14: 9–39

Lelbach WK (1975) Cirrhosis in the alcoholic and its relation to the volume of alcohol abuse. Ann NY Acad Sci 252: 85–105

Lelbach WK (1976) Epidemiology of alcoholic liver disease. In: Popper H, Schaffner F (eds.), Progress in liver diseases. Grune & Stratton, New York, pp. 494–515

Leloir LF, Munoz JM (1938) Ethyl alcohol metabolism in animal tissues. Biochem J 31: 299–307

Leo MA, Lieber CS (1982) Hepatic vitamin A depletion in alcoholic liver injury in men. N Engl J Med 37: 597–601

Leo MA, Sato M, Lieber CS (1983) Effect of hepatic vitamin A depletion on the liver in humans and rats. Gastroenterology 84: 562–72

Leo MA, Lieber CS (1985) New pathway for retinol metabolism in liver microsomes. J Biol Chem 260: 5228–31

Lewis KO, Paton A (1982) Could superoxide cause cirrhosis? Lancet ii: 188–89

Lieber CS (1975) Liver disease and alcohol: fatty liver, alcoholic hepatitis, cirrhosis, and their interrelationships. Ann NY Acad Sci 252: 63–84

Lieber CS (1977a) Metabolism of ethanol. In: Lieber CS (ed.), Metabolic aspects of alcoholism. University Park Press, Baltimore, MD, pp. 1–29

Lieber CS (1977b) Pathogenesis of alcoholic liver disease: an overview. In: Fisger MM, Rankin JG (eds.), Alcohol and the liver. Plenum Press, New York, pp. 197–225

Lieber CS (1982) Medical disorders of alcoholism: pathogenesis and treatment. W.B. Saunders, Philadelphia

Lieber CS (1983) Precursor lesions of cirrhosis. Alcohol Alcoholism 18: 5–20

Lieber CS (1984) Alcohol and the liver: 1984 update. Hepatology 6: 1243–60

Lieber CS (1988a) Metabolic effects of ethanol and its interaction with other drugs, hepatotoxic agents, vitamins, and carcinogens: a 1988 update. Semin Liver Dis 8: 47–68

Lieber CS (1988b) Biochemical and molecular basis of alcohol-induced injury to liver and other tissues. New Engl J Med 319: 1639–50

Lieber CS (1991a) Perspectives: do alcohol calories count? Am J Clin Nutr 54: 976–82

Lieber CS (1991b) Hepatic, metabolic and toxic effects of ethanol: 1991 update. Alcohol Clin Exp Res 15: 573–92

Lieber CS (1991c) Alcohol, liver and nutrition. J Am Coll Nutr 10: 602–32

Lieber CS (1992) Alcoholic liver injury. Curr Opin Gastroenterol 8: 449–57

Lieber CS, Schmid R (1961) The effect of ethanol on fatty acid metabolism: stimulation of hepatic fatty acid synthesis *in vitro.* J Clin Invest 40: 394–99

Lieber CS, Jones DP, DeCarli LM (1965) Effects of prolonged ethanol intake: production of fatty liver despite adequate diets. J Clin Invest 44: 1009–21

Lieber CS, Lefevre A, Spritz N, et al. (1967) Difference in hepatic metabolism of long- and medium-chain fatty acids: the role of fatty acid chain length in the production of the alcoholic fatty liver. J Clin Invest 46: 1451–60

Lieber CS, DeCarli LM (1968) Ethanol oxidation by hepatic microsomes: adaptive increase after ethanol feeding. Science 162: 917–18

Lieber CS, DeCarli LM (1970a) Hepatic microsomal ethanol-oxidizing system: *in vitro* characteristics and adaptive properties *in vivo.* J Biol Chem 245: 2505–12

Lieber CS, DeCarli LM (1970b) Quantitative relationship between amount of dietary fat and severity of alcoholic fatty liver. Am J Clin Nutr 23: 474–78

Lieber CS, DeCarli LM (1974) An experimental model of alcohol feeding and liver injury in the baboon. J Med Primatol 3: 153–63

Lieber CS, Savolainen M (1984) Ethanol and lipids. Alcohol Clin Exp Res 8: 409–23

Lieber CS, Leo MA, Mak K, et al. (1985) Choline fails to prevent liver fibrosis in alcohol-fed baboons but causes toxicity. Hepatology 5: 561–72

Lieber CS, DeCarli LM (1986) The feeding of ethanol in liquid diets: 1986 update. Alcohol Clin Exp Res 10: 550–53

Lieber CS, Lasker JM, DeCarli LM, et al. (1988) Role of acetone, dietary fat and total energy intake in the induction of the hepatic microsomal ethanol oxidizing system. J Pharm Exp Ther 247: 792–95

Lieber CS, Baraona E, Hernandez-Munoz R, et al. (1989) Impaired oxygen utilization: a new mechanism for the hepatotoxicity of ethanol in subhuman primates. J Clin Invest 83: 1682–90

Lieber CS, Pignon J-P (1989) Ethanol and lipids. In: Fruchart JC, Shepherd J (eds.), Human plasma lipoproteins: chemistry, physiology and pathology. Walter de Gruyter, New York, pp. 245–80

Lieber CS, Casini A, DeCarli LM, et al. (1990) *S*-adenosyl-L-methionine attenuates alcohol-induced liver injury in the baboon. Hepatology 11: 165–72

Lieber CS, DeCarli LM, Mak KM, et al. (1990a) Attenuation of alcohol-induced hepatic fibrosis by polyunsaturated lecithin. Hepatology 12: 1390–98

Lieber CS, DeCarli LM (1991) Hepatotoxicity of ethanol. J Hepatol 12: 394–401

Lieber CS, Salaspuro M (1992) Alcoholic liver disease. In: Millward-Sadler GH, Wright R, Arthur MJP (eds.), Wright's liver and biliary disease. Saunders, London, pp. 900–64

Lin GWJ, Lester D (1980) Significance of the gastrointestinal tract in the in vivo metabolism of ethanol in the rat. Adv Exp Med Biol 131: 281–86

Lin RC, Smith RS, Lumeng L (1988) Detection of a protein-acetaldehyde adduct in the liver of rat fed alcohol chronically. J Clin Invest 81: 615–19

Lindros KO, Stowell A, Pikkarainen P, et al. (1980) Elevated blood acetaldehyde in alcoholics with accelerated ethanol elimination. Pharmacol Biochem Behav 13 (suppl 1): 119–24

Lindros KO, Stowell A, Väänänen H, et al. (1983) Uninterrupted prolonged ethanol oxidation as a main pathogenetic factor of alcoholic liver damage: evidence from a new liquid diet animal model. Liver 3: 79–91

Lint JD (1981a) Alcohol consumption and liver cirrhosis mortality. The Netherlands, 1950–78. J Stud Alcohol 42: 48–56

Lint JD (1981b) The influences of much increased alcohol consumption on mortality rates: The Netherlands between 1950 and 1975. Br J Addict 76: 77–83

Lischner MW, Alexander JF, Galambos JT (1971) Natural history of alcoholic hepatitis. 1. The acute disease. Dig Dis Sci 16: 481–94

Lumeng L (1978) The role of acetaldehyde in mediating the deleterious effect of ethanol on pyridoxal 5-phosphate metabolism. J Clin Invest 62: 286–93

Lundsgaard E (1938) Alcohol oxidation as a function of the liver. Compt Rend Trav Lab Carlsberg (København) 22: 333–37

Maddrey WC (1988) Alcoholic hepatitis: clinicopathologic features and therapy. Semin Liver Dis 8: 91–102

Maier KP, Seitzer D, Haag G, et al. (1979) Verlaufsformen alkoholischer Lebererkrankungen. Klin Wochenschr 57: 311–17

Mann RE, Smart RG, Anglin L, et al. (1988) Are decreases in liver cirrhosis rates a result of increased treatment for alcoholism? Br J Addict 83: 683–88

Mann RE, Smart RG, Anglin L, et al. (1991) Reductions in cirrhosis deaths in the United States: associations with per capita consumption and AA membership. J Stud Alcohol 52: 361–65

Marbet UA, Bianchi L, Meury U, et al. (1987) Long-term histological evaluation of the natural history and prognostic factors of alcoholic liver disease. J Hepatol 4: 364–72

Martin NG, Perl J, Oakshott JG, et al. (1985) A twin study of ethanol metabolism. Behav Genet 15: 93–109

Matsuda Y, Baraona E, Salaspuro M, et al. (1979) Effects of ethanol on liver microtubules and Golgi apparatus. Possible role in altered hepatic secretion of plasma proteins. Lab Invest 41: 455–63

Matsuda Y, Takada A, Sato H, et al. (1985) Comparison between ballooned hepatocytes occurring in human alcoholic and nonalcoholic liver diseases. Alcohol Clin Exp Res 9: 366–70

Mauch TJ, Donuhue TM, Zetterman RK, et al. (1984) Covalent binding of acetaldehyde to purified enzymes. Fed Proc 43: 960–64

Maxwell JD (1985) Effect of coroner's rules on death certification for alcoholic liver disease. Br Med J 291: 708

McGlashan ND (1980) The social correlates of alcohol-related mortality in Tasmania, 1971–1978. Soc Sci Med 14D: 191–203

McSween RNM, Burt AD (1986) Histological spectrum of alcoholic liver disease. Semin Liver Dis 6: 221–32

Medina VA, Donohue Jr TM, Sorrell MF, et al. (1985) Covalent binding of acetaldehyde to hepatic proteins during ethanol oxidation. J Lab Clin Med 105: 5–10

Mendenhall CL (1985) VA Cooperative Study Group on Alcoholic Hepatitis: clinical and therapeutic aspects of alcoholic liver disease. In: Seitz HK, Kommerell B (eds.), Alcohol related diseases in gastroenterology. Springer-Verlag, Berlin, pp. 304–23

Mendenhall CL, Anderson S, Weesner RE, et al. (1984) Protein-calorie malnutrition associated with alcoholic hepatitis. Veterans Administration Cooperative Study Group on Alcoholic Hepatitis. Am J Med 76: 211–22

Metcalf JP, Casey CAS, Sorrell MF, et al. (1987) Chronic ethanol administration alters hepatic surface membranes as evidenced by decreased concavalin A binding. Proc Soc Exp Biol Med 185: 1–5

Mezey E (1989) Animal models for alcoholic liver disease. Hepatology 9: 904–05

Mezey E (1991) Interaction between alcohol and nutrition in the pathogenesis of alcoholic liver disease. Semin Liver Dis 11: 340–48

Mezey E, Potter JJ, Slusser RJ, et al. (1980) Effect of ethanol feeding on hepatic lysosomes in the monkey. Lab Invest 43: 88–93

Mezey E, Potter JJ, French SW, et al. (1983) Effect of chronic ethanol feeding on hepatic collagen in monkeys. Hepatology 3: 41–44

Mirsky IA, Nelson N (1939) The role of the liver in ethyl alcohol oxidation. Am J Physiol 126: P587–P588

Mizoi Y, Ijiri I, Tatsuno Y, et al. (1979) Relationship between facial flushing and blood acetaldehyde levels after alcohol intake. Pharmacol Biochem Behav 10: 303–11

Montull S, Parés A, Bruguera M, et al. (1989) Alcoholic foamy degeneration in Spain. Prevalence and clinico-pathological features. Liver 9: 79–85

Morgan MY (1981) Alcoholic liver disease: its clinical diagnosis, evaluation and treatment. Br J Alcohol Alcoholism 16: 62–76

Morgan MY (1991) Alcoholic liver disease: natural history, diagnosis, clinical features, evaluation, management, prognosis, and prevention. In: McIntyre N, Benhamou J-P, Bircher J, et al. (eds.), Oxford Textbook of Clinical Hepatology. Oxford University Press, Oxford, pp. 815–55

Morgan MY, Sherlock S (1977) Sex-related differences among 100 patients with alcoholic liver disease. Br Med J 1: 939–41

Morgan MY, Sherlock S, Scheuer PJ (1978) Acute cholestasis, hepatic failure and fatty liver in the alcoholic. Scand J Gastroenterol 13: 299–303

Morgan M, Camilo ME, Luck W (1981) Macrocytosis in alcohol related liver disease. Its value for screening. Clin Lab Haematol 3: 35–44

Morton S, Mitchell MC (1985) Effects of chronic ethanol feeding on glutathione turnover in the rat. Biochem Pharmacol 34: 1559–63

Nakano M, Worner TM, Lieber CS (1982) Perivenular fibrosis in alcoholic liver injury: ultrastructure and histologic progression. Gastroenterology 83: 777–85

Nanji AA, French SW (1984) Increased susceptibility of women to alcohol: is beer the reason? (letter). N Engl J Med 311: 1075–80

Nanji AA, French SW (1985) Relationship between pork consumption and cirrhosis. Lancet i: 681–83

Nanji AA, French SW (1986a) Correlations between deviations from expected cirrhosis mortality and serum uric acid and dietary protein intake. J Stud Alcohol 47: 253–55

Nanji AA, French SW (1986b) Dietary factors and alcoholic cirrhosis. Alcohol Clin Exp Res 10: 271–73

Nanji AA, Mendenhall CL, French AW (1989) Beef fat prevents alcoholic liver disease in the rat. Alcohol Clin Exp Res 13: 15–19

Nasralah SM, Nassar VH, Galambos JT (1980) Importance of terminal hepatic venule thickening. Arch Pathol Lab Med 104: 84–86

Natta PV, Malin H, Bertolucci D, et al. (1985) The influence of alcohol abuse as a hidden contributor to mortality. Alcohol 2: 535–39

Nebert DW, Adesnik M, Coon MJ, et al. (1987) The P450 gene superfamily: recommended nomenclature. DNA 6: 1–11

Neville JN, Eagles JA, Samson G, et al. (1986) Nutritional status of alcoholics. Am J Clin Nutr 21: 1329–40

Niemelä O, Juvonen T, Parkkila S (1990) Immunohistochemical demonstration of acetaldehyde-modified epitopes in human liver after alcohol consumption. J Clin Invest 87: 1367–74

Nikkilä EA, Ojala K (1963) Role of hepatic l-glycerophosphate and triglyceride synthesis in the production of fatty liver by ethanol. Proc Soc Exp Biol Med 113: 814–17

Nomura F, Lieber CS (1981) Binding of acetaldehyde to rat liver microsomes: enhancement after chronic alcohol consumption. Biochem Biophys Res Commun 100: 131–37

Norstrom T (1987) The impact of per capita consumption on Swedish cirrhosis mortality. Br J Addict 82: 67–75

Norton R, Batey R, Dwyer T, et al. (1987) Alcohol consumption and the risk of alcohol related cirrhosis in women. Br Med J 295: 80–82

Nuutinen H, Lindros KO, Salaspuro M (1983) Determinants of blood acetaldehyde level during ethanol oxidation in chronic alcoholics. Alcohol Clin Exp Res 7: 163–68

Ohnishi K, Lieber CS (1977) Reconstitution of the microsomal ethanol oxidizing system: qualitative and quantitative changes of cytochrome P-450 after chronic ethanol consumption. J Biol Chem 252: 7124–31

Ontko JA (1973) Effects of ethanol on the metabolism of free fatty acids in isolated liver cells. J Lipid Res 14: 78–85

Orholm M, Sorensen TIA, Bentsen KD, et al. (1985) Mortality of alcohol abusing men prospectively assessed in relation to history of abuse and degree of liver injury. Liver 5: 253–60

Orrego H, Blake JE, Blendis LM, et al. (1987) Long-term treatment of alco-holic liver disease with propylthiouracil. N Engl J Med 312: 1921–27

Orrego H, Carmichael FJ (1989) Alcohol, liver hypoxia and treatment of alcoholic liver disease with propylthiouracil. Alcohologia 1: 15–30

Pagliaro L, Saracci R, Bardelli D, et al. (1982) Chronic liver disease, alcohol consumption and HBsAg antigen in Italy: a multiregional case-control study. Ital J Gastroenterol 14: 90–95

Pagliaro L, Simonetti RG, Craxi A (1983) Alcohol and HBV infection as risk factors for hepatocellular carcinoma In Italy: a multicentric, controlled study. Hepatogastroenterology 30: 48–50

Parés A, Bosch J, Bruguera M, et al. (1978) Características clínicas y criterios pronósticos en la hepatitis alcohólica. Gastroenterol Hepatol 1: 118–23

Parés A, Caballería J, Bruguera M, et al. (1986) Histological course of alcoholic hepatitis: influence of abstinence, sex and extent of hepatic damage. J Hepatol 2: 33–42

Parés A, Prats E, Bruguera M, et al. (1987) Predictive value of histological features in the progression of alcoholic fatty liver. J Hepatol 5: S177

Parés A, Barrera JM, Caballería J, et al. (1990) Hepatitis C virus antibodies in chronic alcoholic patients: association with severity of liver injury. Hepatology 12: 1295–99

Parrish KM, Higuchi S, Muramatsu T, et al. (1991) A method for estimating alcohol-related liver cirrhosis mortality in Japan. Int J Epidemiol 20: 921–26

Patek Jr AJ, Toth IG, Saunders MG, et al. (1975) Alcohol and dietary factors in cirrhosis. An epidemiological study of 304 alcoholic patients. Arch Intern Med 135: 1053–57

Patek AJ, Bowry SC, Sabesin SM (1976) Minimal hepatic changes in rats fed alcohol and high casein diet. Arch Pathol Lab Med 100: 19–24

Paton A (1988) Alcohol: lessons from epidemiology. Proc Nutr Soc 47: 79–83

Pequignot G (1961) Die Tolle des Alkohols bei der Ätiologie von Leberzirrhosen in Frankreich. Münch Med Wochenschr 31: 1464–68

Pequignot G, Tuyns AJ, Berta JL (1978) Ascitic cirrhosis in relation to alcohol consumption. Int J Epidemiol 7: 113–20

Pestalozzi DM, Bühler R, von Wartburg JP, et al. (1983) Immuno-histochemical localization of alcohol dehydrogenase in the human gastrointestinal tract. Gastroenterology 85: 1011–16

Peters RL (1977) Patterns of hepatic morphology in jejunoileal bypass patients. Am J Clin Nutr 30: 53–57

Polokoff MA, Simon TJ, Harris A, et al. (1985) Chronic ethanol increases liver plasma membrane fluidity. Biochem 24: 3114–20

Popper H, Lieber CS (1980) Histogenesis of alcoholic fibrosis and cirrhosis in the baboon. Am J Pathol 98: 695–716

Porta EA, Hartroft WS, De la Iglesia FA (1965) Hepatic changes associated with chronic alcoholism in rats. Lab Invest 14: 1437–55

Porta EA, Hartroft WS, Comez-Dunn CLA, et al. (1967) Dietary factors in the progression and regression of hepatic alterations associated with experimental chronic alcoholism. Fed Proc 26: 1449–57

Prytz H, Skinhoj P (1980) Morbidity, mortality and incidence of cirrhosis in Denmark, 1976–1978. Scand J Gastroenterol 16: 839–44

Prytz H, Anderson H (1988) Underreporting of alcohol-related mortality from cirrhosis is declining in Sweden and Denmark. Scand J Gastroenterol 23: 1035–43

Qiao ZK, Halliday ML, Coates RA, et al. (1988) Relationship between liver cirrhosis death rate and nutritional factors in 38 countries. Int J Epidemiol 17: 414–18

Rao GA, Larkin EC, Porta EA (1986) Two decades of chronic alcoholism research with the misconception that liver damage occurred despite adequate nutrition. Biochem Arch 2: 223–27

Rao GA, Larkin EC, Porta EA (1989) Is alcohol itself hepatotoxic independent of nutritional factors in nonalcoholic humans? Biochem Arch 5: 1–9

Ray MB, Mendenhall CL, French SW, et al. (1988) Serum vitamin A deficiency and increased intrahepatic expression of cytokeratin antigen in alcoholic liver disease. Hepatology 8: 1019–26

Raymond L, Infante F, Voirol M, et al. (1985) Interaction des facteurs alcool et nutrition dans l'étiologie de la cirrhose hépatique, chez les hommes. Schweiz Med Wochenschr 115: 998–1000

Rissanen A, Sarlio-Lähteenkorva S, Alfthan G, et al. (1987) Employed problem drinkers: a nutritional risk group? Am J Clin Nutr 45: 456–61

Rogers AE, Fox JG, Gottlieb LS (1981) Effect of ethanol and malnutrition on nonhuman primate liver. In: Berk PD, Chalmers TCh (eds.), Frontiers in liver disease. Georg Thieme Verlag, New York, pp. 167–75

Roine RP, Salmela KS, Höök-Nikanne J, et al. (1992a) Alcohol dehydrogenase mediated acetaldehyde production by *Helicobacter pylori*: a possible mechanism behind gastric injury. Life Sci 51: 1333–37

Roine RP, Salmela KS, Höök-Nikanne J, et al. (1992b) Colloidal bismuth subcitrate and omeprazole inhibit alcohol dehydrogenase mediated acetaldehyde production by *Helicobacter pylori*. Life Sci 51: 195–200

Romelsjo A, Agren G (1985) Has mortality related to alcohol decreased in Sweden? Br Med J 291: 167–70

Rotily M, Durbec JP, Berthezene P, et al. (1990) Diet and alcohol in liver cirrhosis: a case-control study. Eur J Clin Nutr 44: 595–603

Rubin E, Lieber CS (1968) Alcohol induced hepatic injury in non-alcoholic volunteers. N Engl J Med 278: 869–76

Salaspuro M (1989) The organ pathogenesis of alcoholism: liver and gastrointestinal tract. In: Goedde HW, Agarwal DP (eds.), Alcoholism: biomedical and genetic aspects. Pergamon Press, New York, pp. 133–66

Salaspuro M (1991) Epidemiological aspects of alcohol and alcoholic liver disease, ethanol metabolism, and pathogenesis of alcoholic liver injury. In: McIntyre N, Benhamou J-P, Bircher J, et al. (eds.), Oxford textbook of clinical hepatology. Oxford University Press, Oxford, pp. 791–810

Salaspuro MP, Lieber CS (1980) Comparison of the detrimental effects of chronic alcohol intake in humans and animals. In: Eriksson K, Sinclair JD, Kiianmaa K (eds.), Animal models in alcohol research. Academic Press, London/New York, pp. 359–76

Salaspuro MP, Shaw S, Jayatilleke E, et al. (1981) Attenuation of the ethanol induced hepatic redox change after chronic alcohol consumption in baboons: metabolic consequences *in vivo* and *in vitro*. Hepatology 1: 33–38

Salaspuro M, Lindros K (1985) Metabolism and toxicity of acetaldehyde. In: Seitz HK, Kommerell B (eds.), Alcohol related diseases in gastro-enterology. Springer-Verlag, Berlin/Heidelberg/New York/Tokyo, pp. 106–23

Sales J, Duffy J, Peck D (1989) Alcohol consumption, cigarette sales and mortality in the United Kingdom: an analysis of the period 1970–1985. Drug Alcohol Depend 24: 155–60

Salmela KS, Roine RP, Koivisto T, et al. (1993) Characteristics of *Helicobacter pylori* alcohol dehydrogenase. Gastroenterology 105: 325-30

Sato M, Lieber CS (1981) Hepatic vitamin A depletion after chronic ethanol consumption in baboons and rats. J Nutr 111: 2015–23

Sato N, Kamada T, Kawano S, et al. (1983) Effect of acute and chronic ethanol consumption on hepatic tissue oxygen tension in rats. Pharmacol Biochem Behav 18: 443–47

Saunders JB (1989) Treatment of alcoholic liver disease. Baillieres Clin Gastroenterol 3: 39–65

Saunders JB, Davis M, Williams R (1981a) Do women develop alcoholic liver disease more readily than men? Br Med J 282: 1140–43

Saunders JB, Walters JRF, Davies P, et al. (1981b) A 20 year prospective study of cirrhosis. Br Med J 282: 263–66

Saunders JB, Wodak AD, Morgan-Capner P, et al. (1983) Importance of markers of hepatitis B virus in alcoholic liver disease. Br Med J 286: 1851–54

Saunders JB, Wodak AD, Williams R (1984) What determines susceptibility to liver damage from alcohol? (discussion paper). J R Soc Med 77: 204–16

Schmidt, W (1977) The epidemiology of cirrhosis of the liver: a statistical analysis of mortality data with special reference to Canada. In: Fisher MM, Rankin JG (eds.), Alcohol and the liver. Plenum Press, New York, pp. 1–26

Seeff LB, Cuccherini BA, Zimmerman HJ, et al. (1986) Acetaminophen hepatotoxicity in alcoholics (clinical review). Ann Intern Med 106: 399–404

Seitz HK, Kommerell B, eds. (1985) Alcohol related diseases in gastroenterology. Springer-Verlag, Berlin

Shaw S, Jayatilleke E, Ross WA, et al. (1981) Ethanol induced lipid peroxidation: potentiation by long-term alcohol feeding and attenuation by methionine. J Lab Clin Med 98: 417–24

Shaw S, Rubin K, Lieber CS (1983) Decreased hepatic glutathione and increased diene conjugates in alcoholic liver disease: evidence of lipid peroxidation. Dig Dis Sci 28: 585–89

Shaw S, Jayatilleke E, Lieber CS (1988) Lipid peroxidation as a mechanism of alcoholic liver injury: role of iron mobilization and microsomal induction. Alcohol 5: 135–40

Shibuya A, Yoshida A (1988) Genotypes of alcohol-metabolizing enzymes in Japanese with alcohol liver diseases: a strong association of the usual Caucasian-type aldehyde dehydrogenase gene (ALDH) with the disease. Am J Hum Gen 43: 744–48

Skinhoj P, Prytz H (1981) Changing mortality from cirrhosis in Denmark 1965–1978. Scand J Gastroenterol 16: 833–37

Skog OJ (1980) Liver cirrhosis epidemiology: some methodological problems. Br J Addict 75: 227–43

Skog OJ (1984) The risk function for liver cirrhosis from lifetime alcohol consumption. J Stud Alcohol 45: 199–208

Skog OJ (1985) The wetness of drinking cultures: a key variable in epidemiology of alcoholic liver cirrhosis. Acta Med Scand 703(suppl): 157–84

Smart RG (1988) Recent international reductions and increases in liver cirrhosis deaths. Alcohol Clin Exp Res 12: 239–42

Smart RG, Mann RE (1987) Large decreases in alcohol-related problems following a slight reduction of alcohol consumption in Ontario 1975–83. Br J Addict 82: 285–91

Smart RG, Mann RE (1991) Factors in recent reductions in liver cirrhosis deaths. J Stud Alcohol 52: 232–40

Smith DI, Burwell PW (1985) Epidemiology of liver cirrhosis morbidity and mortality in Western Australia, 1971–82: some preliminary findings. Drug Alcohol Depend 15: 35–45

Smith T, DeMaster EG, Furne JK, et al. (1992) First-pass gastric mucosal metabolism of ethanol is negligible in the rat. J Clin Invest 89: 1801–06

Sorensen TIA (1989) Alcohol and liver injury: dose-related or permissive effect. Br J Addict 84: 581–89

Sorensen TIA, Bentsen KD, Eghoje K, et al. (1984) Prospective evaluation of alcohol abuse and alcoholic liver injury in men as predictors of development of cirrhosis. Lancet ii: 241–44

Sorrell MF, Tuma DJ (1985) Hypothesis: alcoholic liver injury and the covalent binding of acetaldehyde. Alcohol Clin Exp Res 9: 306–09

Suematsu T, Matsumura T, Sato N, et al. (1981) Lipid peroxidation in alcoholic liver disease in humans. Alcohol Clin Exp Res 5: 427–36

Svendsen HO, Mosbech J (1977) Alcoholic cirrhosis of the liver in the Scandinavian countries 1961–1974. Int J Epidemiol 6: 345–47

Takada A, Nei J, Matsuda Y (1982) Clinicopathological study of alcoholic fibrosis. Am J Gastroenterol 77: 660–66

Takahashi H, Wong K, Jui L, et al. (1991) Effect of dietary fat on Ito cell activation by chronic ethanol intake: a long-term serial morphometric study on alcohol-fed and control rats. Alcohol Clin Exp Res 15: 1060–66

Takase S, Takada N, Enomoto N, et al. (1991) Different types of chronic hepatitis in alcoholic patients: does chronic hepatitis induced by alcohol exist? Hepatology 13: 876–81

Taraschi TF, Rubin E (1985) Biology of disease. Effects of ethanol on the chemical and structural properties of biologic membranes. Lab Invest 52: 120–31

Teschke R, Stutz G, Strohmeyer G (1979) Increased paracetamol-induced hepatoxicity after chronic alcohol consumption. Biochem Biophys Res Commun 91: 368–74

Tsukamoto H, Towner SJ, Ciofalo LM, et al. (1986) Ethanol-induced hepatic fibrosis in the rat: role of the amount of dietary fat. Hepatology 6: 814–22

Tsutsumi M, Lasker JM, Shimizu M, et al. (1989) The intralobular distribu-tion of ethanol-inducible P450IIE1 in rat and human liver. Hepatology 10: 437–46

Tuma DJ, Smith SL, Sorrell MF (1991) Acetaldehyde and microtubules. Ann NY Acad Sci 625: 786–92

Tuyns AJ, Esteve J, Pequignot G (1984) Ethanol is cirrhogenic, whatever the beverage. Br J Addict 79: 389–93

Tuyns AJ, Pequignot G (1984) Greater risk of ascitic cirrhosis in females in relation to alcohol consumption. Int J Epidemiol 13: 53–57

Tygstrup N, Juhl E (1971) The treatment of alcoholic cirrhosis. The effect of continued drinking and prednisone on survival. In: Gerok W, Sickinger K, Hennekeuser HH (eds.), Alcohol and the liver. F.K. Schattauer Verlag, Stuttgart/New York, pp. 519–36

Uchida T, Kao H, Quispe-Sjogren M (1983) Alcoholic foamy degeneration. A pattern of acute alcoholic injury of the liver. Gastroenterology 84: 683–92

Valentine GD, Ogden KA, Kortje DK, et al. (1987) Role of acetaldehyde in the ethanol-induced impairment of hepatic glycoprotein secretion in the rat in vitro. Hepatology 7: 490–95

Välimäki M, Alfthan G, Pikkarainen J, et al. (1987) Blood and liver selenium concentrations in patients with liver diseases. Clin Chim Acta 166: 171–76

Van Waes LV, Lieber CS (1977) Early perivenular sclerosis in alcoholic fatty liver, an index of progressive liver injury. Gastroenterology 73: 646–50

Videla L, Israel Y (1970) Factors that modify the metabolism of ethanol in rat liver and adaptive changes produced by its chronic administration. Biochem J 118: 275–81

Videla LA, Iturriaga H, Pino ME, et al. (1984) Content of hepatic reduced glutathione in chronic alcoholic patients: influence of the length of abstinence and liver necrosis. Clin Sci 66: 283–90

von Wartburg JP, Bühler R (1984) Biology of disease. Alcoholism and aldehydism: new biomedical concepts. Lab Invest 50: 5–15

Wagner JG (1986) Lack of first-pass metabolism of ethanol at blood concentrations in the social drinking range. Life Sci 39: 407–14

Wallgren H, Barry III H (1970) Prolonged exposure to alcohol. In: Wallgren H, Barry H (eds.), Actions of alcohol. Elsevier, Amster-dam/London/New York, vol II, pp. 480–583

Wilkinson P, Santamaria JN, Rankin JG (1969) Epidemiology of alcoholic cirrhosis. Australas Ann Med 18: 222–26

Williams GD, Grant BF, Stinson FS, et al. (1988) Trends in alcohol-related morbidity and mortality. Public Health Rep 103: 592–97

Wilson RA (1984) Changing validity of the cirrhosis mortality-alcoholic beverage sales construct: U.S. trends, 1970–1977. J Stud Alcohol 45: 53–58

Worner TM, Lieber CS (1985) Perivenular fibrosis as precursor lesion of cirrhosis. JAMA 253: 627–30

Yamada S, Mak KM, Lieber CS (1985) Chronic ethanol consumption alters rat liver plasma membranes and potentiates release of alkaline phosphatase. Gastroenterology 88: 1799–1806

Yoshida A, Hsu LC, Yasunami M (1991) Genetics of human alcohol-metabolizing enzymes. Prog Nucl Acid Res Mol Biol 40: 255–87

Zeisel SH, Da Costa K-A, Franklin PD, et al. (1991) Choline, an essential nutrient for humans. FASEB J 5: 2093–98

Zysset T, Polokof MA, Simon FR (1985) Effect of chronic ethanol administration on enzyme and lipid properties of liver plasma membranes in long and short sleep mice. Hepatology 5: 531–37

Abbreviations

AANB .... α-amino-N-butyric acid
ADH .... alcohol dehydrogenase
ALAT .... alanine aminotransferase (transaminase)
ALD .... alcoholic liver disease
ALDH .... aldehyde dehydrogenase
ALP .... alkaline phosphatase
ARBD .... alcohol-related birth defects
ASAT .... aspartate aminotransferase (transaminase)
BAC .... blood alcohol concentration
BMC .... bone mineral content
BMD .... bone mineral density
BMI .... body mass index
BW .... body weight
CAD .... coronary artery disease
CDT .... carbohydrate-deficient transferrin
CHD .... coronary heart disease
CI .... confidence interval
CNS .... central nervous system
CVD .... cardiovascular disease
CYP2E1 .... cytochrome P450 2E1
DRD2 .... dopamine D2 receptor
DSM .... Diagnostic and Statistical Manual of Mental
                          Disorders (with suffix in Roman numerals for edition
                          and R for revision)
EEG .... electroencephalogram
EIT .... ethanol-induced thermogenesis
ERP .... event-related potential
FAAS .... foetal alcohol abuse syndrome
FAE .... foetal alcohol effects
FAEE .... fatty acid ethyl esters
FAS .... foetal alcohol syndrome
FFF .... free fatty acids
GABA .... γ-aminobutyric acid
GGT .... γ-glutamyltransferase
GST .... glutathione transferase
HDL .... high-density lipoprotein
5-HT .... 5-hydroxytryptamine (serotonin)
LDL .... low-density lipoprotein
MAO .... monoamine oxidase
MCV .... mean corpuscular volume
MEOS .... microsomal ethanol oxidation system

MI .... myocardial infarction
NAD .... nicotinamide adenine dinucleotide
NADH .... the reduced form of NAD
NMDA .... *N*-methyl-D-aspartate
OR .... odds ratio
PTH .... parathyroid hormone
QTL .... quantitative trait loci
RR .... relative risk
SES .... socioeconomic status
TNF .... tumour necrosis factor
TRH .... thyrotropin-releasing hormone

Subject Index